Essentials of Correctional Nursing

Lorry Schoenly, PhD, RN, CCHP-RN, has over 25 years of experience in nursing and health care education and management, with current specialization in corrections. She was a leading member of the taskforce that launched the new CCHP-RN certification, the primary nursing specialty certification for correctional nurses, and a frequent contributing writer to the National Commission on Correctional Health Care (NCCHC). Her blog (CorrectionalNurse.net) represents the current state of correctional nursing. Previous experience in correctional nursing includes Clinical Education Manager, Correctional Medical Services (CMS), now Corizon, a company providing ambulatory, chronic, and emergency health care to 250,000 individuals incarcerated in 280 jails and prisons in 24 states, and Director, Staff Development CMS, NJ Region, with responsibility for creating and implementing in-service and continuing education for physicians, nurses, dentists, and ancillary health care staff for a 14-unit state prison system. Currently, she is a visiting professor at Chamberlain College of Nursing while managing a private consulting business in correctional health care risk management and professional development. She has published 14 peer-reviewed articles and several chapters in nursing books.

Catherine M. Knox, MN, RN, CCHP-RN, has over two decades of experience in correctional health care. She is an independent consultant with nursing and leadership experience in the Oregon Department of Corrections and as Statewide Director of Nursing for the Washington Department of Corrections, and Assistant Statewide Chief Nurse Executive for the California Prison Health Care Services. Catherine has a master's degree in psychiatric mental health nursing and has both administrative and clinical experience in this field. She is a recipient of the "Distinguished Service Award" from the American Correctional Health Services Association (ACHSA) and the "Bernard Harrison Award of Merit" from the NCCHC. She has published several articles in peer-reviewed journals and presents frequently in the United States.

Essentials of Correctional Nursing

Lorry Schoenly, PhD, RN, CCHP-RN
Catherine M. Knox, MN, RN, CCHP-RN

Editors

SPRINGER PUBLISHING COMPANY

NEW YORK

Springer Publishing Company, LLC
11 West 42nd Street
New York, NY 10036
www.springerpub.com

Acquisitions Editor: Allan Graubard
Composition: Techset

ISBN: 978-0-8261-0951-4
E-book ISBN: 978-0-8261-0952-1

12 13 14 15/ 5 4 3 2 1

The author and the publisher of this Work have made every effort to use sources believed to be reliable to provide information that is accurate and compatible with the standards generally accepted at the time of publication. Because medical science is continually advancing, our knowledge base continues to expand. Therefore, as new information becomes available, changes in procedures become necessary. We recommend that the reader always consult current research, specific institutional policies, and current drug references before performing any clinical procedure or administering any drug. The author and publisher shall not be liable for any special, consequential, or exemplary damages resulting, in whole or in part, from the readers' use of, or reliance on, the information contained in this book. The publisher has no responsibility for the persistence or accuracy of URLs for external or third-party Internet websites referred to in this publication and does not guarantee that any content on such websites is, or will remain, accurate or appropriate.

CIP data is available from the Library of Congress.

Printed in the United States of America by Gasch Printing.

Contents

III: NURSING CARE PROCESSES

IV: PROFESSIONAL ROLE AND RESPONSIBILITIES

Contributors

Margaret M. Collatt, BSN, RN, CCHP-RN, CCHP-A, Training and Development Specialist II, Oregon Department of Corrections, Health Services, Salem, Oregon

Rosanne E. Harmon, MN, RN, Psychiatric Mental Health Nurse Practitioner, Oregon Department of Corrections, Health Services, Oregon City, Oregon

Susan Laffan, RN, CCHP-RN, CCHP-A, Consultant in Correctional Health Care, Toms River, New Jersey

Jacqueline Moore, PhD, RN, CCHP-A, CCHP-RN, Correctional Health Care Consultant, Jacqueline Moore & Associates, Greenwood, Colorado

Mary Muse, MS, RN, CCHP-A, CCHP-RN, Chief Nursing Officer, Wisconsin Department of Corrections, Correctional Health Care Consultant, Madison, Wisconsin

Ellyn Presley, RN, CCHP-RN, Nursing Supervisor, Prince William County Juvenile Detention Center, Manassas, Virginia

Sue Smith, MSN, RN, CCHP-RN, Clinical Nursing Instructor/Academic Coach, Chamberlain College of Nursing/Instructional Connections, Columbus, Ohio

Patricia Voermans, MS, RN, APN, CCHP-RN, Nursing Coordinator and Medical Consultant, Wisconsin Department of Corrections, Madison, Wisconsin

Reviewers

Patricia Blair, PhD, LLM, JD, MSN, CCHP, Nurse Attorney, Patricia Blair Law Firm, Adjunct Associate Professor, University of Texas, Tyler School of Nursing, Tyler, Texas

Madeleine LaMarre, MN, FNP-BC, Correctional Health Care Consultant, Madeleine LaMarre PC, Atlanta, Georgia

Linda Lawrence, RN, CCHP-RN, Regional Clinical Coordinator for Alabama, Corizon, Calera, Alabama

Susan J. Loeb, PhD, RN, Associate Professor, School of Nursing, Department of Medicine, The Pennsylvania State University, University Park, Pennsylvania

Peggy Minyard, BSN, MSHCA, CCHP-RN, Regional Director of Nursing for Alabama, Corizon, Calera, Alabama

Denise M. Panosky, DNP, RN, CCHP, FCNS, Assistant Clinical Professor, University of Connecticut, Storrs, Connecticut

Becky Pinney, MSN, RN, CCHP-RN, Chief Nursing Officer, Senior Vice President, Corizon, Nashville, Tennessee

Deborah Shelton, PhD, RN, NE-BC, CCHP, FAAN, E. Jane Martin Professor & Associate Dean of Research, West Virginia University, School of Nursing, Morgantown, West Virginia

Sue Smith, MSN, RN, CCHP-RN, Clinical Nursing Instructor/Academic Coach, Chamberlain College of Nursing/Instructional Connections, Columbus, Ohio

Kathleen Tauer, MSN, RN, PNP, Pediatric Nurse Practitioner, Department of Juvenile Justice, Commonwealth of Virginia, Richmond, Virginia

Preface

Essentials of Correctional Nursing reviews the body of knowledge and practice standards that define the specialty of correctional nursing. The text also describes the health care needs of the youth, men, and women who are incarcerated in jails, prisons, and detention centers across the country. This is a population that is disenfranchised from society, often stigmatized, and invisible to the general community.

The intent of this book is to support correctional nurses by providing guidance and resources about the best practices to deliver nursing care that reduces suffering and improves the quality of life for incarcerated individuals, their families, and the community at large. Nurses who work in other settings also encounter patients who are incarcerated or who have been incarcerated. These settings include emergency departments, specialty clinics, hospitals, psychiatric treatment units, community health clinics, substance abuse treatment programs, and long-term care settings. Explanations and resources are provided in the book so that nurses in other settings are comfortable assessing and responding to the health needs of these patients. Students in graduate and undergraduate nursing programs may use the text to prepare for a learning experience in the correctional setting or to understand health care needs of this population in relation to community health.

Correctional nursing practice is complex. Nearly 1 of every 100 people in the United States is incarcerated in a jail, prison, or juvenile detention facility. Health needs of this population are characterized by disproportionate rates of mental illness, alcohol and drug dependence, victimization, traumatic injury, and both chronic and infectious disease. Minorities are overrepresented among the incarcerated, so correctional nurses are vigilant in the identification and treatment of conditions that represent greater morbidity and mortality for these groups and deliver care with cultural competence. Chapters are devoted to the nursing care provided to patients who have chronic disease, infectious disease, mental illness, or pain, or who are in withdrawal. Other chapters describe the unique health needs and resulting nursing care for specific populations, including women, juveniles, or individuals at the end of life.

The setting for delivery of nursing care is challenging. Correctional facilities operate to carry out criminal sanctions imposed by the court, not to deliver health care. Yet correctional facilities are obligated by state and federal law to provide health care to prisoners and other detainees. The operation of correctional settings and the legal obligation for care can create ethical challenges for nurses dealing with such issues as patient privacy and self-determination. The setting also challenges a central tenet of nursing, the concept of caring. *Essentials of Correctional Nursing* describes how nurses safely navigate the correctional environment to create a therapeutic alliance to center their nursing care on the patient.

Nurses have been described as the backbone of correctional health care. They are the eyes, ears, hands, heads, and hearts that respond to medical and mental health emergencies. During daily sick call and other routine health care encounters, correctional nurses listen to patients' health concerns and watchfully encourage other individuals who are unable or unwilling to raise a health concern. Nurses must apply their knowledge, skill, and ability to the assessment and diagnosis of the full range of health conditions presented by this population and determine both the urgency and priority of subsequent care. Nurses are often the primary gatekeeper to other health care professionals in the correctional setting. Chapters devoted to health screening, medical emergencies, sick call, and dental care describe how nurses identify, respond to, and manage these health concerns in the correctional setting.

The American Nurses Association (ANA) recognized correctional nursing as a specialty within professional nursing in 1985 with the publication of *Corrections Nursing: Scope and Standards of Practice*. The ANA standards are interwoven into each chapter of *Essentials of Correctional Nursing* and are used by correctional nurses to guide nursing practice with resulting improvements in patient care.

Improvements in the delivery of care have been achieved by the establishment of standards and accreditation offered by the American Correctional Association (ACA) and the National Commission on Correctional Health Care (NCCHC). Both the ACA and NCCHC offer certification exams for nurses to demonstrate their expertise in correctional health care. *Essentials of Correctional Nursing* was written to provide the content and structure to support nurses in studying for these certification examinations.

Correctional nurses participate in all of the interdisciplinary organizations, including the American Correctional Health Services Association, the NCCHC, the ACA, and the Academy of Correctional Health Professionals, often serving in leadership positions on boards and committees. *Essentials of Correctional Nursing* was written and reviewed by experienced correctional nurses who have devoted thousands of hours to the work of these organizations.

There is much to be done in correctional nursing to develop the evidence on which best practice is based. Correctional nurses need to further define and develop this area of professional practice, to transform health care delivery to improve patient outcomes in correctional settings, and to advocate on behalf of individual patients as well as the population for adequate health care. *Essentials of Correctional Nursing* provides a framework for review and application of research to promote quality patient care. Finally, nurses are invited to reflect on their own practice and challenged to consider the future of correctional nursing, setting the stage for growth of the specialty.

Readers are invited to visit Dr. Lorry Schoenly's blog that explores essential skills and competencies in correctional nursing at http://essentialsofcorrectionalnursing.com.

ONE

Context of Correctional Nursing

Lorry Schoenly

C orrectional nursing is "... the practice of nursing and the delivery of patient care within the unique and distinctive environment of the criminal justice system ..." (ANA, 2007, p. 1). This criminal justice system includes county jails, state and federal prisons, juvenile detention centers, and substance-abuse treatment centers.

Correctional nurses practice in a specialized environment, one that does not embrace health care as its primary mission. The patient population, inmates and detainees, is unique as well. Although professional nursing practice is based on universal concepts, the application of these care concepts in this specialized environment to this unique patient population provides the primary components of the nursing specialty. An understanding of the care environment, patient population demographics, and the culture of correctional professionals helps to frame the practice of a correctional nurse and informs the care provided.

There are both rewards and challenges to the practice of correctional nursing. Initial investigation of the correctional nursing role indicates that nurse responsibilities can vary greatly depending on the size and type of facility. The role can provide increased autonomy of practice and potential for reduced conflict with other health care professionals (Flanigan & Flanigan, 2001; Shelton, 2009; Smith, 2005). The majority of jail nurses responding to a survey described the reaction of their peers when the nurse said that they provided health care to offenders as most often consisting of respect, interest, and fascination (Hardesty, Champion, & Champion, 2007). These researchers also found that socialization to the role of correctional nurses (such as a rotation during school or having a member of the family who works in a correctional facility) and prior work experience in emergency or mental health environments contributed to jail nurse job satisfaction. The variety of daily activities

TABLE 1.1   Daily Functions of Correctional Health Care Nurses

FUNCTION	PERFORMED DAILY
Patient education	70%
Physical exams	55%
Medication distribution	52%
First aid	49%
Counseling	41%
Health screening	38%
Staff education	22%
Postoperative care	4%
Drawing blood	3%
Detoxification	1%

Source: Adapted from Flanigan and Flanigan (2001).

and potential for novel situations can also be attractive. Table 1.1 describes the types of activities in which the nurses responding to this survey were engaged and how often they performed each activity.

Correctional nursing practice is a challenging nursing specialty for several reasons. Health care units in jails and prisons are often underequipped and do not have appropriate space for delivery of health care. The location of the health care unit may have been an afterthought in facilities that were built before the advent of organized onsite health care. Some correctional facilities were built in isolated, rural locations, making it difficult to recruit health care professionals. Professional isolation can be a problem in retaining nurses once recruited. Many correctional facilities are overcrowded, leaving little room for privacy in dealing with health care concerns. Privacy issues are also increased by the need for correctional officer oversight of the health care delivery areas in order to maintain safety of staff and other inmates. Some inmates must be isolated in higher security units with restricted movement, making it necessary to deliver health care in the housing area.

The implications of a caring relationship between the correctional nurse and the inmate-patient also create a challenge to practice. Correctional nurses must establish a therapeutic relationship with individuals convicted of crimes, some of a violent nature. Reconciling the humanity of the patient in need of health care with the criminal behavior of the inmate is an important aspect of providing care. Correctional patients have been described as "difficult, manipulative, aggressive, and demanding" (Flanigan & Flanigan, 2001, p. 75). A significant number of inmate-patients seek health care services for secondary gain such as additional privileges, reduced work assignments, or special clothing (Paris, 2006). This can cloud the nurse's evaluation and treatment decisions. The increased autonomy of the correctional nurse and the need to sort out desire for secondary gain from true medical need requires solid assessment and critical thinking skills. Finally, creative patient education plans are required due to limited healthy living options such as fresh fruits and vegetables or adequate exercise.

Negotiating with other entities in the care environment also brings challenge. Strict boundaries set by the corrections system can prove frustrating to nurses desiring to show compassion for patients (Weiskopf, 2005). In the custody environment, nurses may feel that they are forbidden from entering into a caring relationship with an inmate-patient (Maeve, 1997; Maroney, 2005). The noncaring attitudes of others in the work environment such as security officers, other staff members, and the inmate population can influence nursing attitudes over time (Weiskopf, 2005). Some correctional nurses must balance the conflicting roles of being employed by an organization with a mission of public safety and security while upholding a professional mission of health and well-being for the inmate population (ANA, 2007).

Finally, the need to be ever-vigilant about personal security in a potentially unsafe environment can erode the caring relationship with patients. Unlike many other care environments, nurses must await an evaluation of the safety of an environment before entering to assist in emergency treatment. The continual concern for personal safety while delivering care can challenge basic principles of caring. Therefore, it has been said that correctional nurses "walk a tightrope between providing therapeutic treatment and maintaining a secure environment" (Weiskopf, 2005, p. 341).

EXHIBIT 1.1
Principles of Correctional Nursing

- A registered nurse's primary duty in the corrections setting is to restore and maintain the health of patients in a spirit of compassion, concern, and professionalism.
- Each patient, regardless of circumstances, possesses intrinsic value and should be treated with dignity and respect. Each encounter with patients and families should portray professionalism, compassion, and concern. Each patient should receive quality care that is cost effective and consistent with the latest treatment parameters and clinical guidelines.
- Patient confidentiality and privacy should be preserved. Nurses should collaborate with other health care team members, correctional staff, and community colleagues to meet the holistic needs of patients, which include physical, psychosocial, and spiritual aspects of care.
- Nurses should encourage each individual through patient and family education to take responsibility for disease prevention and health promotion. Each nurse maintains responsibility for monitoring and evaluating nursing practice necessary for continuous quality improvement.
- Nursing leadership should promote the highest quality of patient care through application of fair and equitable policies and procedures in collaboration with other health care services team members and corrections staff.
- Nursing services should be guided by nurse administrators who foster professional and personal development. These responsible leaders are sensitive to employee needs; give support, praise, and recognition; and encourage continuing education, participation in professional organizations, and generation of knowledge through research.

Correctional nurses maintain the professional nature of their practice through a principled approach to patient care. These ANA-affirmed principles focus correctional nursing practice on the health and safety needs of the patient population while providing a compass to navigate the correctional system for themselves as well as their patients. The essence of correctional nursing is caring for and respecting the human dignity of the incarcerated (ANA, 2007). Limited resources, challenging patients, competing security priorities, and ongoing concern for personal safety can mitigate against principled nursing practice. A frequent return to the core values and goals undergirding correctional nursing practice helps re-center nurses on the meaning and importance of their role (Exhibit 1.1).

HISTORY OF CORRECTIONAL NURSING

Although health care has been delivered in the U.S. correctional environment as early as 1797 with the opening of Newgate Prison in New York City (ANA, 2007), the establishment of the correctional nursing specialty came much later. The correctional setting for nursing practice began to emerge in the professional literature in the 1970s as nurses became involved in developing working systems of health care in this setting (Murtha, 1975). Prison riots, the civil rights movement, and civil litigation shed light on the invisible prison health care setting. In addition, health care for the incarcerated received a legal mandate with the 1976 Supreme Court decision of *Estelle v Gamble*. This case established the constitutional obligation to provide health care to any citizen in the custody of the government.

While still in its infancy in comparison to more mature nursing specialties, correctional nursing has been recognized by the American Nurses Association (ANA) since 1985, when the Task Force on Standards of Nursing Practice in Correctional Facilities under the direction of the Executive Committee of the Council of Community Health Nurses published *Standards of Nursing Practice in Correctional Facilities* (C. Bickford, personal communication, July 1, 2011). Professional development of the specialty has included certification through at least two multidisciplinary groups (American Corrections Association, National Commission on Correctional Health Care). Most nurses who have worked in traditional settings such as a hospital or clinic before entering corrections find the specialty to be unique. Others have described it as similar to nursing care delivered in a psychiatric, military, or public health clinic setting (Flanigan & Flanigan, 2001).

Nurses are the predominant health care providers in the correctional setting. They are often the first to see a patient in need of service as well as the ones to assure that appropriate treatment is received. The limited and fragmented nature of health services in corrections requires solid care delivery processes and reliable follow-through. Nurses are often the managers of care delivery processes in this setting. Establishing efficient and effective care delivery in the midst of the conditions cited makes this specialty both challenging and rewarding.

CARE DELIVERY ENVIRONMENT

Over 7.2 million people are under some form of correctional supervision in the United States (Glaze, 2010). The size and type of correctional facility and the level of security can affect the types of health care services delivered and therefore the provision of nursing care. Generally, nursing care is not delivered in parole and probation settings. Individuals complete these supervised experiences in the community and have access to community or public health service resources. Correctional nursing takes place in jails, prisons, and juvenile detention settings.

Correctional Nursing in Jails

Local jails are managed by counties or cities and hold individuals awaiting court hearings, trials, or sentencing. In addition, individuals may remain in the jail setting to serve out sentences of 12 months or less rather than be processed and classified into a state or federal prison system (Minton, 2011). The temporary and transient nature of a jail stay lends an emergent nature to the health care delivered; however, chronic conditions must still be considered and treated. Drug and alcohol withdrawal is a frequent issue and patients with mental health conditions may not be currently taking their medications. Stabilizing the health condition of newly entering inmates is a priority.

Rapid turnover can result in incomplete treatments, missed diagnoses, and uncontained communicable diseases. It is important for nurses working in a jail setting to have strong links with local community and public health services to extend treatment past the facility walls.

Correctional Nursing in Prisons

Prisons house individuals who have been convicted of a crime with sentences generally longer than 12 months. The extended nature of the stay leads to health management of a more long-standing nature that can include managing chronic conditions and surgical procedures. There are two systems managing prisons based on sentencing. The Federal Bureau of Prisons (FBOP) manages a prison system of 102 facilities housing inmates serving sentences related to a federal crime (Bureau of Justice, 2008). These facilities are spread throughout the United States but have centralized management and similar standards of practice.

By contrast, state prison systems are under the jurisdiction of the state's government and practice standards are consistent throughout the network of state facilities but may differ among the states. Several states (Delaware, Rhode Island, Massachusetts) have combined jail and prison facilities, where both detainees and sentenced inmates reside.

Correctional Security Levels

Inmates are brought into a prison system from jail custody after sentencing. State and federal prison systems designate intake facilities where incoming inmates are evaluated and classified on a number of factors that lead to a facility assignment. Intake facilities are arranged to rapidly evaluate an individual's psychological, criminological, and medical status for placement. Nurses working in a prison intake facility develop excellent assessment skills.

Although terminology can vary from state to state, prisons are categorized by the degree of security needed to maintain the safety of inmates, staff, and the public. Security level designates the degree of external and internal environmental controls in place, as well as the security staff to inmate ratio. Higher levels of security require lower ratios and greater environmental controls.

The security level of a prison will determine the degree of restriction, particularly on the movement of inmates to and from the medical area and the level of custody involvement in the medical unit. Some large prison complexes may have a mix of security levels among buildings within a common external perimeter. It is important to know the security level of a facility, as this indicates characteristics of the patient and the nursing care environment.

Minimum Security

Minimum or low security facilities house inmates designated as low risk for violence or elopement (FBOP, n.d). Minimum security facilities focus on personal responsibility and inmates may be involved in community work assignments. Minimum security facilities may also include working farms, machine shops, and military-style boot camps (North Carolina Department of Corrections, n.d.).

Health care may only be available part of the time. Nurses working in these facilities are involved in medical clearance for work programs. In addition, care activities can include evaluation and treatment of work-related injuries.

Medium Security

Inmates designated for a medium security setting have been determined to be an escape risk and pose a threat to others (Executive Office of Public Safety and Security, n.d.). Inmates in these facilities have more direct supervision and more restricted movement. Medium security settings have more work and self-improvement projects within the external security perimeter and fewer patient transports or contact with the public.

Health Units in medium security prisons are usually staffed 24 hours a day and involve a full array of ambulatory services. They are more likely to include infirmary care and initiate treatments such as IV therapy and tube feedings as needed. Health care is delivered primarily in the health care unit, although nursing staff must be able to deal with emergencies (man-down) in the housing and exercise areas. Permanent security staffs are often assigned to the health care units in medium security settings and inmate-patients are observed at all times.

High Security (Maximum)

Inmates designated for high security settings have been determined to be a serious escape or violence risk. High security prisons have a variety of descriptors including penitentiary, maximum, super max, and close security. Death row inmates and those convicted of particularly violent or heinous crimes will be assigned to high security prisons. The internal environment of high security settings includes a greater degree of physical barriers and checkpoints.

Nurses working in maximum security prisons must deliver a greater percentage of care cell-side due to the security nature of the setting. Inmate movement is limited and security staff escorts are required for movement to the health care unit. Sentences are typically long in maximum security prisons and so the health care trajectory can also be longer than in other settings. A full array of health care services is provided including ambulatory care, infirmary care, and chronic disease management.

Special Housing

Correctional facilities also have special housing areas for increased security purposes or for vulnerable inmate populations. Correctional nurses may have responsibilities for providing nursing care in these specialized environments. Terminology may differ across systems and within various regions of the country. It is important, therefore, to understand the meaning of the various special housing situations within the system or facility of employment.

Segregation

This specialized unit, also called Seg, Administrative Seg, Protective Housing, or Secure Housing Unit (SHU), is a restricted security area within a jail or prison for inmates who continue to violate security rules, threaten, or otherwise place other inmates and staff members in danger. Inmates placed in segregation have their movement severely restricted. Health care must be provided in the housing area with an escort by correction officers. Delivery of medication and treatments can be challenging and if appropriate facilities and equipment are not available, nurses may be expected to deliver such care cell-side. Nurses must be prepared for the possibility of verbal abuse or attempts at physical disruption such as spitting or throwing of bodily excrement. Patient privacy during examination and history-taking can be difficult. Special arrangements and additional security are required when segregated inmates are transported to the medical unit for evaluation or treatment.

Medical, Sheltered, or Protective Housing

Medical, sheltered, and protective housing units are created in large correctional institutions or systems to provide added safety for inmates with physical or mental impairment that could lead to victimization in the general inmate population. The older inmate, adolescents sentenced as adults, and those with significant disability require extra protection, as do those with severe mental health issues such as schizophrenia or psychoses. Medical, sheltered, and protective housing units are often located near the health care unit.

Prerelease

Prerelease facilities and half-way houses are used to prepare inmates nearing the end of incarceration by developing independent skills for community living. Prerelease facilities generally have minimal health care staff and frequently refer inmates with chronic or serious acute conditions to a nearby higher-level prison medical unit for treatment.

CORRECTIONAL MANAGEMENT STRUCTURE AND HEALTH CARE DELIVERY

Correctional health care units can be managed in several ways. Unlike hospitals or clinics in the community, the health care staff in a correctional setting may not report directly to the same leadership as other staff in the facility (Table 1.2). Having an understanding of lines of authority within the facility can improve effectiveness and decrease message confusion.

Governmental Agencies (Self-Operated)

The majority of nurses working in corrections are employed by the same governing body as their custody peers. Also called self-operated or self-op, health care managers in this management structure are a part of the organizational hierarchy and reporting framework. This organizational framework has advantages in allowing for parity

TABLE 1.2   Management Systems for Correctional Health Care Units

MANAGEMENT TYPE	PORTION OF THE U.S. CORRECTIONAL SYSTEM
Government agencies (self-operated)	58%
Independent health care service companies	30%
State university medical systems	12%

Source: Adapted from Corizon (2011).

among the services and can foster support for inmate medical needs. Although the wellbeing of the inmate population is a common goal for both custody and nursing staff, professional frameworks and guiding principles can differ. Nurses in these organizations must be vigilant to maintain professional nursing judgment in all matters of care delivery.

Independent Health Care Service Companies

Another way correctional health care is provided through contracts with independent health care service companies. These companies contract with county or state governments to deliver needed health care services within correctional facilities. Nurses are most often employees of the health care service company and report to managers within the company. When working for a company independent of the correctional authority, nurses must understand the contractual relationship with the Department of Corrections and the communication and reporting structure. Health care staff in this situation are guests in the facility and must strive to develop collaborative working relationships with custody staff.

State University Medical Systems

Several state prison systems provide health care to inmates through the state university system. For example, in Connecticut, inmates receive care through the University of Connecticut medical system, and in New Jersey, health care services are provided through the state's University of Medicine and Dentistry. Nurses working in these systems have the advantage of access to academic resources while nursing, medical, and dentistry students have an opportunity to experience the correctional environment. The corollary in jails is for the county health department to provide the health care at the jail. In this circumstance, nurses have the advantage of access to resources of the county health department. Although health care staff are not employees of the same entity as corrections staff, a common relationship exists among the government bodies.

CORRECTIONAL OFFICER DEMOGRAPHICS

The environment in which correctional nurses provide patient care is shaped by the professionals managing the primary service of security within the facility. Correctional officers, also called CO's, custody officers, or security officers, are professionals with their own perspective and worldview gained during training for their role and assimilation into their work environment. Primary concerns of correctional officers are order, control, and discipline (Maroney, 2005). These themes provide a framework for the systems and processes that help manage the corrections environment.

The work environment shapes the actions and reactions of correctional officers. High levels of work stress, ongoing potential for workplace violence, and a perceived lack of public support can create bonds of solidarity among the custody staff (Garcia, 2008). Correctional nurses must somehow bridge this solidarity without compromising nursing professional principles when collaborating with custody staff to accomplish care goals.

From the Experts ...

"Mutual respect will go a long way to facilitate collaboration with security staff. Correctional officers and administrators have a hard job. Correctional nurses need to recognize this and refrain from being overly critical or judgmental about security perspectives about prisoners—without sacrificing their nursing perspective. Simply put—the words "please" and "thank you," professional courtesy, and consideration will help nurses collaborate with their security colleagues."

Sue Smith, MSN, RN, CCHP-RN
Columbus, OH

PATIENT POPULATION DEMOGRAPHICS

Individuals detained or in the custody of the corrections system have several terms used as identifiers. Individuals held in pretrial settings such as county jails can be called detainees or arrestees. Once sentenced, the most common terminology is offender or inmate. For the purposes of this discussion, the terms inmate or patient will be used to designate the patient population receiving correctional nursing care.

The U.S. inmate population has grown considerably over the last three decades for a variety of reasons. In fact, the United States has the largest incarcerated population in the world, at 2.3 million inmates. The second largest inmate population, China, is far behind with 1.5 million. Russia is a distant third with less than a million behind bars. Reasons given for the higher incarceration rate include tougher sentencing rules, three-strikes measures, and reduction of mental health hospitalization options (The PEW Center on the States, 2008; Torrey, Kennard, Eslinger, Lamb, & Pavle, 2010).

Slightly more than one in every 100 Americans is behind bars (Pew, 2008). The incarcerated population does not mirror general population statistics as to gender, race, education, or age. The contrast helps to frame the type of necessary health care services provided by correctional nurses.

Gender

The majority of incarcerated Americans are male adults. The Bureau of Justice Statistics for 2009 indicates male individuals are imprisoned at a rate 14 times the rate for female individuals. Local jail detainee populations are, on average, almost 88%

male (Glaze, 2010). Male inmates are more likely than female to be alcohol dependent (Binswanger et al., 2010). Although women make up only 10% of those incarcerated, their numbers are increasing nearly twice as fast as men (Pew, 2008). Stricter sentencing laws bring in a greater number of female individuals who were part of a domestic violence disturbance or an accomplice to a male-directed criminal activity such as driving a boyfriend or spouse to a theft or drug deal (Kelly, Parlaz-Dieckmann, Chang, & Collins, 2010).

Female inmates are more likely than their male counterparts to have custody of their children and to have been a victim of sexual abuse or domestic violence (Belknap, 2006; Kelly et al., 2010). The health issues of incarcerated women expand to also include reproductive health issues. In addition, women have a disproportionately higher rate of treated mental illness (Binswanger et al., 2010) with increased prescription of psychotropics and tranquilizers (Belknap, 2006). Those providing health care in female institutions find a higher use of medical and psychiatric services than similarly sized male institutions (Binswanger et al., 2010; Drapalski, Youman, Stuewig, & Tangney, 2009).

Race

African Americans and Hispanics are disproportionately represented in the U.S. inmate population. Although Black Americans make up 12.6% of the general population, they make up 39.3% of the incarcerated population (West, Sabol, & Greenman, 2010). While one in 106 White men over age 18 are imprisoned in America, one in 15 Black men in this age group are behind bars (Pew, 2008). Likewise, one in 36 Hispanic men aged 18 or older are incarcerated. Hispanic/Latinos make up 15.8% of the jail population (Minton, 2011) and 21% of the prison population (West et al., 2010).

Disproportionately higher numbers of minority inmates will impact the frequency of certain medical conditions treated in correctional settings. Not only are Black Americans three times more likely to have diabetes and stroke, but they are 11 times more likely to die of HIV disease. Black men have higher rates of prostate, lung, stomach, and colorectal cancers. Black women are more prone to prenatal diseases and cancers of the colon, pancreas, and stomach (CDC, 2005).

Health disparities in the Latino community also impact the inmate population. Hispanics have a disproportionately higher disease profile with increased death from stroke, chronic liver disease, diabetes, and HIV disease. Also, this population segment has a much higher rate of cancers of the stomach and cervix than the general population (CDC, 2004).

Education

Education levels of the U.S. inmate population are lower than the general population. Harlow (2003) reports less than 50% of the total incarcerated population have a high school diploma. This figure is under 20% for the general U.S. population. Inmates are more than twice as likely as other citizens to have learning disabilities (Greenberg, Dunleavy, & Kutner, 2007a).

Literacy, a component of education level, that is of particular importance for health education, is also below normal levels in the inmate population. Using a three-factor scale of literacy evaluation (prose, document, quantitative), researchers found inmates, on average, were more likely to have only basic levels of literacy and below compared to the general population. In addition, very few prisoners were able to read and comprehend at the highest level (Greenberg, Dunleavy, Kutner, & White, 2007b).

Basic literacy allows interpretation of simple instruction and graphic material. Special consideration should be given to the reading level of printed health information provided to the inmate population. In addition, correctional nurses need to evaluate the patient's understanding of health information provided. Case Example 1.1 provides an opportunity to apply this information.

CASE EXAMPLE 1.1

Nurses at a large maximum security prison are teaching patients about sexually transmitted diseases. While the inmates await their chronic care appointment in the clinic holding area, they are given written material from the Centers for Disease Control website. During the nurse portion of the chronic care visit, each inmate is asked if they received the material and if they have any questions. If they have no questions, the nurse documents successful patient teaching on the topic in the medical record. Describe flaws in this process and suggest improvements in the teaching method.

Age

Generally speaking, the majority of inmates in adult facilities are young male individuals. For example, the average inmate age in the federal prison system is 39 years (Bureau of Prisons, 2011). Inmates aged 20 to 39 make up 64% of the 1.45 million sentenced prisoners at the end of 2009 (Bureau of Justice, 2011a). The growing edges of the age continuum, youth and elderly, have specific health needs to consider.

Elderly

By all accounts, the U.S. inmate population is aging along with the general population as baby boomers move into retirement and geriatric care. However, due to many factors, inmates age earlier in life and elder inmates are growing in number behind bars due to maximum sentencing formulas developed in prior decades (Aday, 2003). Although the definition of elderly differs across systems, there is general agreement that inmates in their 50s are considered to be in this category (Anno, Graham, Lawrence, & Shansky, 2004; Loeb & AbuDagga, 2006). Elderly inmates use more medical and mental health resources. They require additional protection from abuse and predation. They often need protective housing and assistive devices. Both correctional officers and nurses must be vigilant to identify decreasing functionality and increasing disease burden in this segment of the inmate population (Anno et al., 2004).

Youth

The youth or juvenile designation is generally given to those under 18 years of age in the U.S. prison system. The majority of youth are detained and serve sentences in residential-styled facilities with an environment created to meet the needs of adolescents. Correctional nurses working in juvenile facilities deal with growth and development issues, psychosocial concerns, and parental custody matters.

A growing number of youth are given adult sentences and sent to adult facilities to serve out their time. Upwards of 25% of juvenile offenders are in adult prisons. Young inmates in adult prisons have increased rates of suicide and prison rape (Campaign for Youth Justice, 2007). Young offenders are a vulnerable population that should have additional protections from the general prison population. It is important for correctional nurses in adult facilities to know about and monitor the youth segment of the inmate population. Youth nutritional needs and medical conditions are unique to their season of life and should be considered at every health care encounter.

PHYSICAL HEALTH
Chronic Illness

When age is standardized with the U.S. general population, inmates in jails and prisons were found to have higher rates of diabetes, hypertension, prior myocardial infarction, and persistent asthma (Wilper et al., 2009). Details of this difference are found in Table 1.3. Correctional nurses have an opportunity to improve inmate health and thereby public health through the evaluation and treatment of these chronic conditions during incarceration.

Infectious Diseases

Poor nutrition, substance abuse, homelessness, lack of medical care, and risky sexual behaviors lead to a disproportionately higher rates of HIV, Hepatitis C (HCV), sexually transmitted infections (STIs), and tuberculosis (TB; Hammett, 2006). Rates of HIV in federal and state prisons are nearly four times the general population, while up to 35% of inmates have chronic HCV infection (Gough et al., 2010). Tuberculosis in the corrections population is a growing concern, with reported rates at least 3 times that of the general population (MacNeil, Lobato, & Moore, 2005). STIs are also common in this patient group. Syphilis, chlamydia, and gonorrhea rates among jail and prison inmates are surprisingly high compared to the general population (Table 1.4).

Awareness of the increased likelihood of any particular patient to have one or more of these conditions can lead to early identification and treatment. Correctional nurses can help limit the spread of these diseases through patient education and encouragement of risk-reduction practices.

MENTAL HEALTH

Mental illness among the inmate population is also more frequent than in the general population (Table 1.5). While 11% of Americans meet criteria for a mental health disorder, more than half of the jail and prison population have recent history or

TABLE 1.3 Age-Standardized Prevalence of Selected Chronic Conditions Among Adult Federal and State Prisoners, Jail Inmates, and the Noninstitutionalized U.S. Population

CONDITION	FEDERAL (%)	STATE (%)	JAIL (%)	GENERAL POPULATION (%)
Diabetes	11.1	10.1	8.1	6.5
Hypertension	29.5	30.8	27.9	25.6
Prior myocardial infarction	4.5	5.7	2.1	3.0
Persistent asthma	7.7	9.8	8.6	7.5

Source: Adapted from Wilper et al. (2009).

TABLE 1.4   Comparison of Sexually Transmitted Infections Among U.S. General and Inmate Populations

SEXUALLY TRANSMITTED INFECTIONS	GENERAL POPULATION (%)[a]	INMATE POPULATION (%)[b]
Chlamydia	0.4	2.4
Gonorrhea	0.1	1.0
Syphilis	0.005	2.6–4.3

[a]Centers for Disease Control (2009). [b]National Commission on Correctional Health Care (2002).

symptoms of a mental health problem (James & Glaze, 2006). This almost fivefold difference includes symptoms of mania, major depression, and psychotic disorders.

Borderline Personality Disorder (BPD) is also overrepresented in the inmate population. This mental health condition is characterized by poor impulse control, self-injury, and substance abuse with increased rates of diagnosis in the female population (National Institutes of Mental Health, n.d.). Studies vary widely; however, BPD rates in the general U.S. population are well below 5%, while estimates in the jail and prison population vary from 25% to 50% (Sansome & Sansome, 2009).

Correctional nurses need to understand mental illnesses to identify, refer, and support the patient's treatment. Nurses must also understand the implications of mental illness co-morbidity in managing other medical conditions. Vigilant monitoring for drug–drug interactions, preventing adverse reactions, and helping patients to tolerate and manage side effects are key aspects in nursing care of this population.

Traumatic Brain Injury

Traumatic brain injury (TBI) and its effects are common in the inmate population. Although an estimated 2% of the general population has sustained a TBI with continuing disability (Langlois, Rutland-Brown, & Wald, 2006) a meta analysis of studies in the inmate population indicates a prevalence of over 60% (Shiroma, Ferguson, & Pickelsimer, 2010). This condition can be caused by a variety of brain traumas such as assault, falls, motor vehicle crashes, and military duty blasts (Centers for Disease Control, n.d.). TBI can lead to depression, anxiety, failed anger

TABLE 1.5   Diagnosed Mental Conditions Among Inmates of State and Federal Prisons and Local Jails

CONDITION	FEDERAL (%)	STATE (%)	JAIL (%)
Any diagnosed mental condition	14.8	25.5	25.0
History of medication for emotional or mental problems (among those diagnosed with a mental condition)	71.6	74.6	73.7
History of counseling for mental or emotional problems (among those diagnosed with a mental condition)	63.6	62.9	63.4

Source: Adapted from Wilper et al. (2009).

management control, and substance abuse. It can also predispose to seizure disorders, Alzheimer's, and Parkinson's diseases (Centers for Disease Control, n.d.). Correctional nurses must consider the impact of TBI aftermath on the functioning of the patient population. Case Example 1.2 provides opportunity to apply this information.

CASE EXAMPLE 1.2

A 23-year-old male is being medically evaluated in a large urban jail, detained for disorderly conduct at a local bar. The inmate is belligerent and argumentative during the assessment. He is a large man, was a linebacker for his high school football team, and has a military history with deployment in Afghanistan. Based on his history, what primary and secondary conditions might the nurse assess for in this patient?

Posttraumatic Stress Disorder

Another condition common in the inmate-patient population is posttraumatic stress disorder (PTSD). PTSD is an anxiety disorder that develops following a terrifying event or when an individual is frequently placed in dangerous or deadly situations (NIMH, 2011). Inmates enter the system with a variety of backgrounds leading to this condition, such as high levels of physical or sexual abuse and involvement in violent crime (Haugebrook, Zgoba, Maschi, Morgen, & Brown, 2010). Added to this is the trauma of incarceration with concerns over victimization, coercion, and assault. Military veterans make up 13% of state and 15% of federal prison populations and have high rates of PTSD from combat duty (Bureau of Justice, 2000). This condition is also common among female inmates due, in part, to the high level of child, domestic, and sexual abuse in their history (Binswanger et al., 2010). PTSD symptoms can affect the nurse–patient relationship. Triggers such as confinement, perceived coercion, and loud aggressive voice tones can cause PTSD victims to experience flashbacks and respond to perceived threat in nontypical fashion. An understanding of this condition and its prevalence in the patient population can aid the delivery of nursing care in the corrections setting.

Drug and Alcohol Involvement

A staggering 84.8% of all U.S. inmates are substance involved, whether alcohol or illegal drug use (National Center on Addiction and Substance Abuse, 2010). Even those serving time for nonsubstance-related offenses have extremely high rates of dependence. More than half of those convicted of violent or property crime were alcohol involved at the time of the crime. In addition, substance involvement is frequently found to co-occur with mental health problems. Nearly one in four inmates have both a substance use disorder and a diagnosis of mental illness (National Center on Addiction and Substance Abuse, 2010).

Alcohol and drug withdrawal, therefore, is a major concern for correctional nurses working in corrections, particularly jails. Regardless of the setting for incarceration, inmates should be supported in the development of alternative coping mechanisms because the evidence is clear that treating substance abuse reduces criminal recidivism.

From the Experts ...

"In the jail environment, nurses are challenged to treat individuals who are coming straight from the street and in many cases have had no health care prior to incarceration. They may have drug or alcohol addictions in addition to other chronic illnesses. In the prison population, the patients have had their chronic care needs identified and a treatment plan has already been established by the transferring jail. Jails would therefore be compared to an acute care setting and prisons would be considered more of a long-term care facility in regards to health care."

Dyni Brookshire, RN, MSN, CCHP-RN
Lumberton, TX

Tobacco Use

Those entering the correction system are more likely to smoke tobacco. At least one-third of the prison population was smoking at the time of arrest, compared with one-quarter of the general population (The National Center on Addiction and Substance Abuse at Columbia University, 2010). Of particular note is the high rate of smoking among inmates with other substance issues. With the current trend for correctional facilities to become smoke-free, correctional nurses must look for ways to assist inmate-patients to cope with nicotine withdrawal.

Suicidality

The inmate population, especially in jails, has greater potential for attempted and completed suicide than any other population (Hayes, 2010). Although the rate has dropped significantly since first tracked in 1980 (see Table 1.6), it is still a major concern that should be attended to by all correctional staff. Correctional nurses must consider suicide potential in all inmate contacts, but especially on intake, after sentencing or when at-risk for in threats while in custody such as rape, gang activity, or personal violence (Hanson, 2010).

TABLE 1.6   Progress in U.S. Prison and Jail Suicide Rates 1983–2006 (per 100,000)

YEAR	U.S. POPULATION	JAIL	PRISON
1983	12.4	129	27
2006	11.3	36	17

Source: Condensed from Bureau of Justice Statistics (2011b), Centers for Disease Control, National Center for Health Statistics, National Vital Statistics System (2002).

SUMMARY

Correctional nurses work in the challenging environment of jails, prisons, and juvenile detention facilities, sometimes with little resources, respect, or recognition. The correctional environment including the level of facility security, correctional officer, and administrative staff, and the inmate-patients, create a framework for the provision of nursing care. An understanding of the unique needs of the patient population and the specific restraints of the corrections environment allow nurses to be effective in maximizing health, decreasing illness, and reducing infection. Correctional nurses choose to use their knowledge and skills to care for a marginalized community of vulnerable patients who are often difficult to care for and care about. Many nurses find this a rich and fulfilling career choice.

DISCUSSION QUESTIONS

1. What are some differences in jail and prison nursing based on information in this chapter?
2. Based on the context of correctional nursing, what would be key skills and characteristics for nurses in this environment?
3. What challenges to care delivery are found in the information in this chapter?
4. What are the similarities and differences between the population at your facility and the statistics describing the inmate population in this chapter?

REFERENCES

Aday, R. H. (2003). *Aging prisoners: Crisis in American corrections.* Westport, CT: Praeger.

American Nurses Association (ANA). (2007). *Corrections nursing: Scope & standards of practice.* Silver Spring, MD: Author.

Anno, B. J., Graham, C., Lawrence, J. E., & Shansky, R. (2004). *Addressing the needs of elderly, chronically ill, and terminally ill inmates.* Retrieved from nicic.gov/Library/Files/018735.pdf

Belknap, J. (2006). *The invisible woman: Gender, crime, and justice.* Belmont, CA: Wadsworth/Thompson Learning.

Binswanger, I. A., Merrill, J. O., Krueger, P. M., White, M. C., Booth, R. E., & Elmore, J. G. (2010). Gender differences in chronic medical, psychiatric, and substance-dependence disorders among jail inmates. *American Journal of Public Health, 100*(3), 476–482.

Bureau of Justice. (2000). *Special report: Veterans in prison or jail.* NCJ 178888. Retrieved from http://bjs.ojp.usdoj.gov/content/pub/pdf/vpj.pdf

Bureau of Justice. (2008). *Census of state and federal correctional facilities, 2005.* Retrieved from http://bjs.ojp.usdoj.gov/content/pub/pdf/csfcf05.pdf

Bureau of Justice. (2011a). *Bureau of justice statistics: Key facts at a glance.* Retrieved from http://bjs.ojp.usdoj.gov/content/glance/corr2.cfm

Bureau of Justice. (2011b). *Deaths in custody statistical tables.* Retrieved from http://bjs.ojp.usdoj.gov/content/dcrp/dcst.pdf

Bureau of Prisons. (2011). *Quick facts about the bureau of prisons.* Retrieved from http://www.bop.gov/news/quick.jsp

Campaign for Youth Justice. (2007). *Jailing juveniles: The dangers of incarcerating youth in adult jails in America.* Retrieved from http://www.campaignforyouthjustice.org/Downloads/NationalReportsArticles/CFYJ-Jailing_Juveniles_Report_2007-11-15.pdf

Centers for Disease Control. (n.d.). *Traumatic brain injury: A guide for criminal justice professionals.* Retrieved from http://www.tbiwashington.org/professionals/documents/Prisoner_Crim_Justice_Prof.pdf

Centers for Disease Control. (2004). *Morbidity & mortality weekly report: Health disparities experienced by Hispanics — United States.* Retrieved from http://www.cdc.gov/mmwr/preview/mmwrhtml/mm5340a1.htm

Centers for Disease Control. (2005). *Morbidity & mortality weekly report: Health disparities experienced by Black or African Americans—United States.* Retrieved from http://www.cdc.gov/mmwr/preview/mmwrhtml/mm5401a1.htm

Centers for Disease Control. (2009). *Trends in sexually transmitted diseases in the United States: 2009 National data for gonorrhea, chlamydia and syphilis.* Retrieved from http://www.cdc.gov/std/stats09/tables/trends-table.htm

Centers for Disease Control, National Center for Health Statistics, National Vital Statistics System. (2002). *Age-adjusted death rates for 72 selected causes by race and sex using year 2000 standard population: United States, 1979–1998.* Unpublished table NEWSTAN 79-98S. Retrieved June 30, 2011, from http://www.cdc.gov/nchs/data/mortab/aadr7998s.pdf

Corizon. (2011). *U.S. correctional healthcare spending: Market share analysis.* Unpublished internal document used with permission.

Drapalski, A. L., Youman, K., Stuewig, J., & Tangney, J. (2009). Gender differences in jail inmates' symptoms of mental illness, treatment history and treatment seeking. *Criminal Behavior and Mental Health, 19,* 193–206. doi:10.1002/cbn.733

Executive Office of Public Safety and Security. (n.d.). *Security levels.* Retrieved June 20, from http://www.doc.state.nc.us/dop/custody.htm

FBOP. (n.d.). *Federal bureau of prisons: Prison types and general information.* Retrieved June 20, 2011, from http://www.bop.gov/locations/institutions/index.jsp

Flanagan, N. A., & Flanagan, T. J. (2001). Correctional nurses' perceptions of their role, training requirements, and prisoner health care needs. *Journal of Correctional Health Care, 8*(1), 67–85.

Garcia, R. M. (2008). *Individual and institutional demographic and organizational climate correlates of perceived danger among federal correctional officers.* Unpublished dissertation. Retrieved from http://www.ncjrs.gov/pdffiles1/nij/grants/222678.pdf

Glaze, L. (2010). *Bureau of justice statistics bulletin: Correctional populations in the United States, 2009.* Retrieved from http://bjs.ojp.usdoj.gov/content/pub/pdf/cpus09.pdf

Gough, E., Kempf, M., Graham, L., Manzanero, M., Hook, E., Bartolucci, A. et al. (2010). HIV and hepatitis B and C incidence rates in US correctional populations and high risk groups: A systematic review and meta-analysis. *BMC Public Health,* http://www.biomedcentral.com/1471-2458/10/777

Greenberg, E., Dunleavy, E., & Kutner, M. (2007a). *Literacy behind bars: Results from the 2003 National Assessment of Adult Literacy Prison Survey (NCES 2007-473).* U.S. Department of Education. Washington, DC: National Center for Education Statistics.

Greenberg, E., Dunleavey, E., Kutner, M., & White, S. (2007b). *Literacy prison survey (NCES 2007-473).* U.S. Department of Education. Washington, DC: National Center for Education Statistics. Retrieved from http://nces.ed.gov/pubs2007/2007473.pdf

Hammett, T. M. (2006). Epidemiology of HIV/AIDS and other infectious diseases in correctional facilities. In M. Puesis (Ed.), *Clinical practice in correctional medicine* (2nd ed.). Chicago: Mosby/Elsivier.

Hanson, A. (2010). Correctional suicide: Has progress ended? *Journal of the American Academy of Psychiatry Law, 38,* 6–10.

Hardesty, K. N., Champion, D. R., & Champion, J. E. (2007). Jail nurses: Perceptions, stigmatization, and working styles in correctional health care. *Journal of Correctional Health Care, 13,* 196–205.

Harlow, C. W. (2003). *Education and correctional populations.* Bureau of Justice Statistics Special Report NCJ 195670. Retrieved from http://www.policyalmanac.org/crime/archive/education_prisons.pdf

Haugebrook, S., Zgoba, K. M., Maschi, T., Morgen, K., & Brown, D. (2010). Trauma, stress, health, and mental health issues among ethnically diverse older adult prisoners. *Journal of Correctional Health Care, 16*(3), 220–229.

Hayes, L. (2010). *National study of jail suicide: 20 years later.* Retrieved from http://www.ncianet.org/suicideprevention/documents/SuicideStudy-20YearsLater.pdf

James, D. J., & Glaze, L. E. (2006). *Bureau of justice statistics special report: Mental health problems of prison and jail inmates.* Retrieved from http://www.nami.org/Content/ContentGroups/Press_Room1/2006/Press_September_2006/DOJ_reportmental_illness_in_prison.pdf

Kelly, P. J., Parlaz-Dieckmann, E., Chang, A. L., & Collins, C. (2010). Profile of women in a county jail. *Journal of Psychosocial Nursing, 48*(4), 38–45.

Langlois, J. A., Rutland-Brown, W., & Wald, M. M. (2006). The epidemiology and impact of traumatic brain injury: A brief overview. *Journal of Head Trauma Rehabilitation, 21,* 375–378.

Loeb, S. J., & AbuDagga, A. (2006). Health-related research on older inmates: An integrative literature review. *Research in Nursing and Health, 29,* 556–565.

MacNeil, J., Lobato, M., & Moore, M. (2005). An unanswered health disparity: Tuberculosis among correctional inmates, 1993 through 2003. *American Journal of Public Health, 95*(10), 1800–1805.

Maeve, M. K. (1997). Nursing practice with incarcerated women; Caring within mandated alienation. *Issues in Mental Health Nursing, 18,* 495–510.

Maroney, M. K. (2005). Caring and custody: Two faces of the same reality. *Journal of Correctional Health Care, 11*(1), 157–169.

Minton, T. D. (2011). *Jail inmates at mid-year 2010—Statistical tables.* Retrieved from http://bjs.ojp. usdoj.gov/content/pub/pdf/cpus09.pdf

Murtha, R. (1975). Change in One City's System: It started with a director of nursing. *American Journal of Nursing, 75*(3), 421–422.

National Commission on Correctional Health Care. (2002). *The health status of soon-to-be-released inmates: A report to Congress.* Retrieved from http://www.ncchc.org/stbr/Volume1/Preface. pdf

National Institutes of Mental Health. (n.d.) *Borderline personality disorder: Symptoms.* Retrieved from http://www.nimh.nih.gov/health/publications/borderline-personality-disorder-fact-sheet/ index.shtml

NIMH. (2011). *National Institute of Mental Health: Post traumatic stress disorder (PTSD).* Retrieved from http://www.nimh.nih.gov/health/topics/post-traumatic-stress-disorder-ptsd/index. shtml

North Carolina Department of Corrections. (n.d.). *Assigning inmates to prison.* Retrieved from http://www.doc.state.nc.us/dop/custody.htm

Paris, J. E. (2006). Interaction between correctional staff and health care providers in the delivery of medical care. In M. Puisis (Ed.), *Clinical practice in correctional medicine* (2nd ed.). Philadelphia: Mosby Elsevier.

Pew Center on the States. (2008). *One in 100: Behind bars in America 2008.* Retrieved from http:// www.pewcenteronthestates.org/uploadedFiles/One%20in%20100.pdf

Sansome, R. A., & Sansome, L. A. (2009). Borderline personality and criminality. *Psychiatry, 6*(10), 16–20.

Shelton, D. (2009). Forensic nursing in secure environments. *Journal of Forensic Nursing, 5,* 131–142.

Shiroma, E. J., Ferguson, P. L., & Pickelsimer, E. E. (2010). Prevalence of traumatic brain injury in an offender population: A meta-analysis. *Journal of Correctional Health Care, 16*(2), 147–159.

Smith, S. (2005). Stepping through the looking glass: Professional autonomy in correctional nursing. *Corrections Today, 67,* 54–70.

The National Center on Addiction and Substance Abuse at Columbia University. (2010). *Behind bars II: Substance abuse and America's prison population.* New York, NY: The National Center on Addiction and Substance Abuse at Columbia University. Retrieved from http://www. casacolumbia.org/articlefiles/575-report2010behindbars2.pdf

Torrey, E. F., Kennard, A. D., Eslinger, D., Lamb, R., & Pavle, J. (2010). *More mentally ill persons are in jails and prisons than hospitals: A survey of the states.* Treatment Advocacy Center: National Sheriffs' Association. Retrieved from http://www.treatmentadvocacycenter.org/storage/ documents/final_jails_v_hospitals_study.pdf

Weiskopf, C. S. (2005). Nurses experience of caring for inmate-patients. *Journal of Advanced Nursing, 49,* 336–343.

West, H. C., Sabol, W. J., & Greenman, S. J. (2010). *Bureau of justice statistics: Prisoners in 2009.* Retrieved from http://bjs.ojp.usdoj.gov/content/pub/pdf/p09.pdf

Wilper, A. P. O., Woolhandler, S., Boyd, J. W., Lasser, K. E, McCormick, D., Bor, D. H., et al. (2009). The health and health care of US prisoners: Results of a nationwide survey. *American Journal of Public Health 99*(4), 666–672.

TWO

Ethical Principles for Correctional Nursing

Lorry Schoenly

E thical issues abound in any nursing practice and may be acute in correctional nursing. Correctional nurses can use professional codes and values to guide their actions in an ethically challenging environment. By understanding the ethical foundations of professional practice, nurses working in corrections can make thoughtful patient-centered decisions about their responsibilities in any particular situation.

The Corrections Nursing Scope and Standards of Practice (ANA, 2007) provides a framework for making appropriate decisions in the face of ethical dilemmas in practice. Ethics is a standard of professional correctional nursing practice and is multidimensional (Exhibit 2.1). This standard will guide a discussion of professional nursing ethics in the correctional setting.

CODES OF ETHICS FOR NURSES

Foremost in the practice of ethical nursing is the use of a professional code. A professional code distinguishes professional practice from mere occupational pursuit. It establishes the responsibilities and obligations a professional has toward those they serve (Davis, 2008). Codes of ethics professionalize moral values and make explicit the "ethical virtues, values, ideals, and norms of a profession" (Fowler, 2008a, p. xvii). The nine provisions of the Code of Ethics for Nurses can be categorized into three themes: fundamental values, duty and loyalty, and expanded duties beyond patient care (Table 2.1).

Although the ANA Code of Ethics is explicitly cited in the Corrections Nurse Scope and Standards as the basis for ethical practice, two other codes are available for consultation and can provide additional support for practice decisions. The International Council of Nurses (ICN) Code of Ethics for Nurses (2006) guides

EXHIBIT 2.1
Corrections Nursing Scope and Standards of Practice Standard 12: Ethics

The corrections nurse integrates ethical provisions in all areas of practice

- Uses Code of Ethics for Nurses with Interpretive Statements to guide practice
- Delivers care in a manner that preserves and protects patient autonomy, dignity, and rights
- Maintains patient confidentiality within legal and regulatory parameters, considering the unique corrections environment
- Serves as a patient advocate and assists patients in developing skills for self-advocacy
- Maintains a therapeutic and professional patient–nurse relationship with appropriate professional role boundaries
- Demonstrates a commitment to practicing self-care, managing stress, and connecting with self and others
- Contributes to resolving ethical issues of patients, colleagues, or systems as evidenced in such activities as participating in ethical committees
- Reports illegal, incompetent, or impaired practices

Source: Copyright 2007 by American Nurses Association, p. 40. Reprinted with permission. All rights reserved.

international nursing practice. Ethical principles are categorized according to the nurse relationship to patients, coworkers, the profession, and the practice. A common theme in the ANA and ICN ethical codes is the prime importance of compassionate nursing care and the alleviation of suffering (Butts, 2008).

The Code of Ethics for Correctional Health Care (ACHSA, n.d.) provides ethical guidelines for nurses and others working in correctional health care (Table 2.2). Many of the basic principles and values found in the ANA and ICN codes are translated for the unique corrections environment. Key elements of these two additional codes will be mentioned in the continuing discussion of core themes of the ANA Code of Ethics for Nurses.

FUNDAMENTAL VALUES OF THE PROFESSIONAL NURSE

The first three provisions of the ANA Code of Ethics speak to fundamental values of the profession. These values are further developed by the American Association of Colleges of Nursing (2008) to include five essential values for nursing practice (Table 2.3). These values are applied to correctional practice as nurses use the Code of Ethics for Nurses with Interpretive Statements to guide practice and deliver care in a manner that preserves and protects patient autonomy, dignity, and rights (ANA, 2007).

Altruism

Altruism is an outward-facing value speaking to the direction of interests held by the nurse. Altruism is described as seeking the welfare and well-being of others (AACN, 2008). Professional nursing practice is altruistic in maintaining a primary

TABLE 2.1   Provisions of the Code of Ethics for Nurses

Fundamental Values of the Professional Nurse	
Provision 1	The nurse, in all professional relationships, practices with compassion and respect for the inherent dignity, worth, and uniqueness of every individual, unrestricted by consideration of social or economic status, personal attributes, or the nature of health problems.
Provision 2	The nurse's primary commitment is to the patient, whether an individual, family, group, or community.
Provision 3	The nurse promotes, advocates for, and strives to protect the health, safety, and rights of the patient.
Duty and Loyalty	
Provision 4	The nurse is responsible and accountable for individual nursing practice and determines the appropriate delegation of tasks consistent with the nurse's obligation to provide optimum patient care.
Provision 5	The nurse owes the same duties to self as to others, including the responsibility to preserve integrity and safety, to maintain competence, and to continue personal and professional growth.
Provision 6	The nurse participates in establishing, maintaining, and improving health care environments and conditions of employment conducive to the provision of quality health care and consistent with the values of the profession through individual and collective action.
Expanded Duties Beyond Direct Patient Care	
Provision 7	The nurse participates in the advancement of the profession through contributions to practice, education administration, and knowledge development.
Provision 8	The nurse collaborates with other health professionals and the public in promoting community, national, and international efforts to meet health needs.
Provision 9	The profession of nursing, as represented by associations and other members, is responsible for articulating nursing values, for maintaining the integrity of the profession and its practice, and for shaping social policy.

Source: Adapted from ANA (2001) and Hook and White (2009).

commitment to the patient (Provision 2) rather than to other possible competing concerns. Altruism as a professional value leads to seeing patients as ends in themselves rather than means to ends. Correctional nurses reflect the value of altruism when seeking the well-being of the inmate community from both a health improvement and disease treatment perspective. When confronted by a dilemma of competing priorities, evaluating the situation from the perspective of the patient's welfare can often lead to an appropriate nursing action.

Autonomy

The value of autonomy as it relates to the patient is also affirmed in the ANA Code of Ethics. Autonomy is described as a right of self-determination (ANA, 2001). Much of an inmate's autonomy has been abrogated by the incarceration experience. However, autonomy as it regards health care decisions and actions can still often be maintained.

TABLE 2.2   ACHSA Code of Ethics

Preamble	Correctional health professionals are obligated to respect human dignity and act in ways that merit trust and prevent harm. They must ensure autonomy in decisions about their inmate patients and promote a safe environment
Principles	The correctional health professional should: • Evaluate the inmate as a patient or client in each and every health care encounter. • Render medical treatment only when it is justified by an accepted medical diagnosis. Treatment and invasive procedures shall be rendered after informed consent. • Afford inmates the right to refuse care and treatment. Involuntary treatment shall be reserved for emergency situations in which there is grave disability and immediate threat of danger to the inmate or others. • Provide sound privacy during health services in all cases and sight privacy whenever possible. • Provide health care to all inmates regardless of custody status. • Identify themselves to their patients and not represent themselves as other than their professional license or certification permits. • Collect and analyze specimens only for diagnostic testing based on sound medical principles. • Perform body cavity searches only after training in proper techniques and when they are not in a patient–provider relationship with the inmate. • Not be involved in any aspect of execution of the death penalty. • Ensure that all medical information is confidential and health care records are maintained and transported in a confidential manner. • Honor custody functions but not participate in such activities as escorting inmates, forced transfers, security supervision, strip searches, or witnessing use of force. • Undertake biomedical research on prisoners only when the research methods meet all requirements for experimentation on human subjects and individual prisoners or prison populations are expected to derive benefits from the results of the research.

Source: ACHSA, n.d. Used with permission.

Limits to autonomy can happen in some situations where the welfare of the larger community is jeopardized by the decision of an individual. An example of this is the need to treat a contagious disease such as tuberculosis so that spread to other inmates and staff is reduced.

TABLE 2.3   Five Essential Values of Nursing Practice

VALUE	DEFINITION
Altruism	Concern for the welfare and well-being of others
Autonomy	Right to self-determination
Human Dignity	Respect for the inherent worth and uniqueness of individuals and populations
Integrity	Acting in accordance with an appropriate code of ethics and accepted standards of practice
Social Justice	Acting in accordance with fair treatment regardless of economic status, race, ethnicity, age, citizenship, disability, or sexual orientation

Source: Adapted from American Association of Colleges of Nursing (2008).

Informed consent is fundamental to ethical care delivery and supports patient autonomy (Hook & White, 2009). Correctional nurses, in particular, have a need to assure the patient has full understanding of the patient decision in question and consequences of various options when determining informed consent. The literacy level of the inmate population can affect comprehension in the health care decision-making process. Attendance to the nursing value of autonomy will lead nurses in this situation to seek additional means for obtaining patient understanding so that an informed decision can be made.

The ACHSA Code of Ethics applies the value of autonomy in asserting that inmates have a right to refuse care and treatment. This right is overshadowed in occasions where there is "immediate threat of danger to the inmate or others" (ACHSA, n.d. p. 1).

Human Dignity

Professional nurses value the human dignity of every individual in their care, no matter the socioeconomic status, personal characteristics, or life choices they have made. Human dignity is described as "respect for the inherent worth and uniqueness of individuals and populations. In professional practice, concern for human dignity is reflected when the nurse values and respects all patients and colleagues" (AACN, 2008, p. 26). Honoring the inherent worth of every person undergirds the entire nursing profession and is of particular importance as a basis for correctional nursing practice. Correctional nurses are often challenged by the need to care and respond to individuals who may have committed heinous crimes, who show disregard themselves for basic human worth, or are guided by a destructive personal code. It is through a continual reaffirmation of this basic nursing value that correctional nurses can honestly care for and about the patients they serve. Provision 1 of the ANA Code makes clear the significant importance of human dignity as a nursing value.

Valuing human dignity also concerns interactions with others in the care community, whether other health care staff, support, or custody staff. Respectful communication and actions among staff members indicate a value-based perspective.

Integrity

As a professional nursing value, integrity refers to consistent honesty of action. This term also emphasizes acting on the basis of a professional code of conduct (AACN, 2008). Nurses act with integrity when actions are regularly based on an ethical code such as the ANA Code advocated by the Corrections Nursing Scope and Standards of Practice (2007). Incremental deviations from professional ethical principles can be deemed acceptable in challenging situations, leading to a slow loss of integrity over time. Correctional nurses must be especially vigilant about professional practice in a prison or jail setting. For example, it may be difficult to maintain a primary commitment to patient autonomy when pressured by unruly patient behavior and the need by custody to maintain control. Correctional nurses in every setting must consider their professional duty when confronted with ethical conflict encouraging an easy answer that may breach integrity of practice.

Acting with integrity, as with all other professional nursing values, is important for the nurse–patient relationship, but also relationships with others on the health care team. Patient outcomes are enhanced when team members are trustworthy and share the patient's welfare as a common goal.

Integrity can be breached when nurses are asked to act inconsistently with professional beliefs and values. Pressure to treat inmates inhumanely or provide substandard care can cause moral distress and threaten wholeness of character. Correctional nurses placed in a situation of this nature can use moral reasoning to guide actions that maintain integrity and professional nursing values (Butts, 2008).

From the Experts ...

"Trustworthiness is the foundation for working in a correctional setting. Never have the words *firm, fair,* and *constant* been as important to achieve our goals and set the guidelines for our success with those around us. Patients, staff, and the community see that what we do for one, we do for all, and this builds respect others can depend on. Inmates are our patients and we serve them as well as our staff members and the community by being the best nurse we can be—to do otherwise is a travesty and disservice to our profession."

Royanne Schissel, RN, CCHP
Santa Fe, NM

Social Justice

The professional value of social justice is of significant importance in correctional nursing practice, where there is increased contact with vulnerable and marginalized people and population groups in a dehumanizing environment devoid of many comforts. The value of social justice guides correctional nursing practice as the basis for fair treatment that looks beyond the outward characteristics or "labels" of an individual to the core human who deserves the best treatment that can be offered them. Nurses may be called upon to advocate for basic rights and needs for patients in the correctional setting. A balance must often be struck between nursing care delivery and criminal justice requirements. When faced with an ethical dilemma among conflicting goals, correctional nurses can be guided by the value of social justice, along with other professional nursing values, in determining appropriate action.

Provision 3 of the ANA Code of Ethics (2001) gives voice to the need for all nurses to promote, advocate for, and strive to protect the patient's health, safety, and rights. In addition, the ICN Code (2006) encourages nurses to promote an "environment in which the human rights, values, customs, and spiritual beliefs of the individual, family and community are respected" (p. 2). These concepts are applied to the correctional setting through the ACHSA Code in Element 5—provide health care to all inmates regardless of custody status. Correctional nurses have a significant opportunity to improve the welfare of the inmate population through a value-based approach to nursing practice.

DUTY AND LOYALTY

Provisions 4 through 6 of the ANA Code of Ethics consider the duties and loyalties of the nurse. Duties and loyalties identify the individuals and groups a nurse is responsible for and accountable to. These provisions emphasize respect for persons, including self-respect, in the application of values expressed in prior provisions (Hook & White, 2009). This section closely aligns with the Nurses and Practice segment of the ICN Code of Ethics (2006), where accountability, responsibility, competence, and personal health are addressed.

Accountability and Responsibility

Differentiating these terms can be helpful in understanding the moral power of a professional nurse. Accountability is the overarching term in a professional practice. Nurses are accountable to themselves and others for judgments and actions taken as a nurse. Nurses are bound by a moral standard of practice that transcends any specific responsibilities conferred by a particular role or job description. Professional codes, scopes of practice, and licensure standards provide the framework for professional accountability and are a higher authority than any employer requirement (Badzak, 2008).

Responsibility, on the other hand, refers to the requirements of a specific nursing role or position (Hook & White, 2009). Correctional nurses may be responsible for providing nursing care according to health care unit policies and procedures but accountable to perform them ethically according to professional nursing practice standards. When organizational requirements are less than professional ethics demand, nurses are accountable to go beyond role responsibilities.

A professional code of ethics provides the moral authority to question potentially unethical requirements or conditions of employment. Correctional nurses may be placed in situations where professional nursing values are thwarted by competing organizational values such as financial constraint or punitive action. Nurses must understand their moral autonomy in these situations and consider appropriate action based on accountability to self and patient.

Delegation of nursing functions can be a concern when considering professional responsibility and accountability. Nurses must understand the scope of practice of licensed individuals on the care team as well as the job responsibilities of unlicensed staff. Professional nurses are responsible for delegating to individuals competent to perform the requested tasks and remain accountable for the care provided under their direction. Therefore, nurses must assess their own competency as well as the competency of others they direct to perform components of patient care (Hook & White, 2009).

Duty to Self

Nurses are called to consider their professional duty to self, as well as others. Provision 5 identifies duty to self and others as preserving integrity and safety, maintaining competence, and continuing personal and professional growth. Practically speaking, the nurse has always owed the same duty to self as to individuals in their care or on their care team. However, this duty has not always been explicitly stated (Fowler, 2008b). Work–life balance assists nurses to maintain perspective and motivation to deliver meaningful patient care. Duty to self includes attending to personal safety and well-being.

In addition, duty to self includes a need to maintain competence and continuous personal and professional growth. Ongoing self-evaluation and peer review are practices that assist in motivating professional growth (Fowler, 2008b). Competence and continuous learning benefit the patient and health care team, in addition to the individual nurse. However, the enhancement of personal self-esteem and the satisfaction of ethical good that come from professional growth are of great benefit to the individual nurse (ANA, 2001).

Finally, nurses have a duty to self in maintaining professional integrity and wholeness of character in the midst of ethical decision-making. The ANA Code of Ethics identifies the need for integrity-preserving compromise and conscientious objection as actions open to nurses in dealing with an ethical situation that challenges personal and professional moral standards. Correctional nurses can easily find themselves in situations where nursing values are jeopardized. Professional ethics requires that nurses preserve their moral integrity while determining a satisfying compromise among competing principles. Agreeing upon an integrity-preserving compromise is the most satisfying conclusion to an ethical dilemma. When this is not possible, conscientious objection is an avenue open to professional nurses. This stance is not taken lightly but is necessary in situations where the requested action is a violation of a "deeply held moral value, personal, or professional" (Fowler, 2008b, p. 68). Instances in correctional nursing are described later in the chapter and can include involvement in deceiving a patient with placebo treatment or allowing suffering when treatment is available. The ACHSA Code of Ethics applies this principle in prohibiting correctional health care staff from performing body cavity searches or participating in execution of the death penalty.

Conscientious objection is an action reserved for serious moral objection and allows for the preservation of a nurse's moral integrity. Correctional nurses have a responsibility to alert employers to clinical activities that cause severe moral distress and proactively seek satisfying solutions to the situation.

Environments and Conditions

Accountability for professional nursing practice also includes a nurse's participation in the improvement of the care environment and conditions of employment to advance quality health care (Provision 6). These factors provide a context for ethical nursing care by providing the necessary resources. Poorly staffed and equipped care environments risk patient safety and health. This also jeopardizes the quality of health care delivered. Nurses are charged to work individually and in groups to improve the environment and conditions of care. This may be accomplished through professional association work or collective bargaining activity.

Expanded Duties Beyond Direct Patient Care

The final three provisions of the ANA Code of Ethics involve the expanded duties of professional nursing beyond direct patient care activities. Nurses have an ethical responsibility to advance the profession through contributions that will increase knowledge development and shape public policy. Nurses advance global health goals through community, national, and international efforts to meet health needs (ANA, 2001).

For correctional nurses, this involves advancing the specialty practice and professional stature of those nurses working in the specialty. Correctional nurses have opportunity to advance the specialty even if not involved in professional speaking or writing. Curiosity from family, friends, and other nurses provide opportunity to present a positive image of correctional nursing practice which can enhance the professional status of nurses working in jails and prisons. In addition, correctional nurses represent the profession to other correctional professionals in their interactions and demeanor while on the job. This includes both interactions among the care team and with custody staff.

ETHICS OF THE NURSE–PATIENT RELATIONSHIP

Nursing is a relationship-based practice. Values inherent in ethical relationships are addressed throughout the ANA Code of Ethics. Indeed, relationship is the context in which ethics is practiced in the profession. Relationship-based care, a model of nursing practice, provides a framework for considering ethical relationships in nursing (Koloroutis, 2004). This model suggests that a caring, therapeutic nurse–patient relationship is central to professional nursing practice. Exhibit 2.2 provides selected elements of the relationship-based care model.

EXHIBIT 2.2
Selected Elements of Relationship-Based Care

- Patients desire an individual relationship with care providers
- The nurse–patient relationship is the foundation of excellent care delivery
- Nurses are accountable for a therapeutic patient relationship
- Interdisciplinary communication and teamwork are vital as they promote mutual respect and role clarity
- Patient involvement in their care is increased by positive relationships with their care providers

Source: Adapted from Koloroutis (2004).

Nurse relationships with patients are therapeutic in nature and always patient focused. Although nurses often gain personal satisfaction from a patient relationship, the goal is always patient benefit. The nurse–patient relationship, as well as the nurse colleague relationship, is for the purpose of preventing illness, alleviating suffering, promoting health, and preventing illness (Hall, 2011). These goals provide boundaries and direction to the nurse–patient relationship. Several types of patient relationship situations are of particular ethical concern in the correctional setting.

Informed Consent

The ethical concern in informed consent comprises two parts. First, has the patient received and fully understood all the information needed to make a decision? Second, does the patient agree, or consent, to have the treatment? Informed consent is more than just obtaining the patient signature on a legal form (Dempski, 2009). Key components of informed consent are found in Table 2.4.

TABLE 2.4   Informed Consent Components

CATEGORY	COMPONENTS
Information	• Description of procedure • Risks and benefits of procedure • Reasonable alternatives and their risks and benefits
How much information	• Material risks and benefits reasonable person would want to know before undergoing or refusing procedure
Assessment of patient competence	• Communicates understanding of procedures and information given

Source: From Dempski (2009, p. 77). Used with permission.

The nurse's ethical responsibility is to confirm both the understanding and agreement that constitute informed consent. This can be challenging in the corrections environment where patients can feel coerced by the imbalance of power in operation during incarceration. In addition, low literacy levels and miscommunication can lead to a misunderstanding of information. Some inmates can be suspicious of the underlying factors of a particular medical procedure or have motivations other than health in making treatment decisions. Correctional nurses can assist in the informed consent process through a therapeutic nurse–patient relationship and established trustworthiness.

Supporting Decision Making

Nurses must also support patient decision making in other health care situations. As patient advocates, correctional nurses are often in a position to support the patient decision-making process. Elements of decision-making support include interpretation and explanation of complex medical information, suggesting benefits and detrimental outcomes that require consideration, and protecting the patient from coercion. In addition, nurses can facilitate decision analysis by guiding the patient toward concrete actions, such as listing pros and cons of a particular course of action.

Confidentiality

An important component of any nurse–patient relationship is confidentiality. The ethical nurse "holds in confidence personal information and uses judgment in sharing information" (ICN, 2006, p. 2). Health care providers obtain a variety of confidential information from patients that could be used to their detriment if revealed in other situations. This can be acutely significant in a correctional environment, where health information shared inappropriately could render the person vulnerable to physical, emotional, or psychological harm. Heightened awareness is necessary for particularly sensitive health information, such as HIV status.

Some information about a patient's condition must necessarily be shared with custody so that appropriate health measures can be taken. The extent of information given is determined by patient need rather than the needs of any other entity. For example, significant health needs may determine inmate classification and need for protective housing, limited work assignments, or disciplinary management (NCCHC, 2008). In cases of disclosure of personal health information, correctional nurses must limit information to what is necessary for the health and safety of the patient and confidentiality of the information maintained among those privy to the information. Accreditation standards suggest that communication about health needs be guided by written policy and documents. Exhibit 2.3 lists health needs that may require communication among health care and custody staff.

EXHIBIT 2.3
Health Needs That May Require Disclosure to Custody Staff

- Chronic illness
- Dialysis
- Adolescents in adult facilities
- Communicable diseases
- Physical disability
- Pregnancy
- Frail or elderly
- Terminal illness
- Mental illness or suicidal
- Developmental disability

Source: Adapted from NCCHC (2008).

Information provided to the nurse in the context of the nurse–patient relationship has always been considered confidential from an ethical perspective. Full disclosure from a patient is necessary to adequately treat health conditions. Sensitive information is less likely to be revealed without assumed confidentiality based on privacy rights. The right of privacy can be traced to the U.S. Constitution (Westrick, 2009).

There are several situations where it is appropriate and acceptable for health care information to be shared with a party other than the patient or care provider. Foremost is when the patient agrees to the disclosure. This permission should be in writing. Information can also be shared with other caregivers or agencies if they need to know based on the patient's health and safety needs. In addition, disclosure may be required if there is a legal duty to report, such as public health requirements for tracking communicable diseases, or statutory requirements to report child or domestic abuse situations (Westrick, 2009).

The 45 C.F.R. 164.512 (k) (5) (i) section of the HIPAA act allows for the sharing of health information with correctional institutions by health entities covered by the regulation. Once again, information disclosure is based on necessity for the individual's health and safety (Gostin, 2002). Exhibit 2.4 lists situations in which protected health information can be shared with correctional authorities.

THE CONCEPT OF CARING IN CORRECTIONAL NURSING

Caring is the essence of professional nursing practice (Koloroutis, 2004). Indeed, caring is described as a central concept to the ethical practice of nursing and primary to the nature of the nurse–patient relationship (Fyr & Johnstone, 2008). It is suggested that "the primary way of being in nursing is caring" (Bishop & Scudder, 2008, p. 216). Yet, caring in correctional nursing has sometimes been

EXHIBIT 2.4
HIPAA-Permitted Disclosure to Correctional Institutions

HIPAA permits disclosure if the correctional institution proves that such protected health information is necessary for:

- The provision of health care to such individuals
- The health and safety of such individuals or other inmates
- The health and safety of the officers or employees of or others at the correctional institution
- The health and safety of such individuals and officers or other persons responsible for the transporting of inmates or their transfer from one institution, facility, or setting to another
- Law enforcement on the premises of the correctional institution
- The administration and maintenance of the safety, security, and good order of the correctional institution

Source: Adapted from Gostin (2002).

discouraged and some have even questioned whether correctional nurses can care for their inmate patients (Brookshire, 2011). Ambivalence toward caring in the correctional setting may stem from the nature of the environment and the nature of the patient population. Weiskopf (2005) found caring in correctional nursing to be unique from all other settings.

Caring in correctional nursing practice may be moderated by several environmental factors. One factor is the incongruent missions of nursing and the prevailing security culture in which it is practiced (Brodie, 2001). Nurses must continually negotiate boundaries between the values of custody and the values of caring; continually guarding against co-opting security values in practice (Weiskopf, 2005). Caring can be difficult in an anti-therapeutic environment.

Unique boundaries also exist in the nurse–patient relationship. The real and potential danger to physical and psychological well-being when working closely with the inmate population threatens the ability to genuinely care for the patient over time. The manipulative nature of some patients in this setting encourages the development of cynicism and erodes the essential nurse–patient relationship (Brodie, 2001). Finally, the heinous crimes committed by some patients can make it difficult for nurses to overcome repugnance for what the patient has done to see the inherent humanity of who the patient is. Caring in nursing practice is challenging in the corrections environment.

Three nurse theorists have given voice to the concept of caring and therefore provide a language for interpretation and application to correctional nursing. Selected caring concepts from these theorists are of particular application to nursing in the correctional environment (Exhibit 2.5). Applying these caring principles to nursing in the correctional setting can enhance ethical practice and increase satisfaction. That being said, the boundaries of nursing practice and the constraints made necessary by the security environment limit the more intimate qualities of the care relationship envisioned by these theorists. More research is needed to better understand the nature of caring in correctional nursing practice.

> ## EXHIBIT 2.5
> ### Selected Caring Concepts From Nurse Theorists
>
> Benner's Primacy of Caring
>
> - Caring is necessary for the giving of help by the nurse and the receiving of help by the patient
> - A caring component of the nurse–patient relationship expressing connection and concern
> - The science of nursing is guided by an ethic of care and responsibility
>
> Leininger's Transcultural Caring
>
> - To care is to assist others with real or anticipated needs
> - Caring is an action or activity directed toward providing care
> - Care must be provided in the context of the patient culture—the learned, shared, and transmitted values, beliefs, norms, and lifeways of the patient
>
> Watson's Transpersonal Caring
>
> - Care is provided in a transpersonal relationship in which there is a moral commitment to protect and enhance human dignity
> - Caring is the intention of doing for another and being with another who is in need
> - Care is authentic presence where the nurse honors the patient's dignity and vulnerability
>
> *Source*: Adapted from Benner and Wrubrel (1989), Sitzman and Eichelberger (2004), and Watson (2012).

THE ETHICAL NURSE MAKING DECISIONS
Ethical Decision-Making Model

Correctional nurses confronted with an ethical dilemma must grapple with many variables in order to make a decision about necessary actions. Ethical decision making takes into account the personal beliefs and values of the nurse, ethical concepts for nursing, approaches to ethics, and standards for ethical behavior (Fry & Johnstone, 2008). Ethical debate in a practice setting is challenging but can be healthy; strengthening collaborative relationships around a common goal (Epstein & Delgado, 2010). Using a model for decision making can assist nurses in determining right actions in the face of ethical uncertainty.

Several ethical decision-making models are available to nurses (Fry & Johnstone, 2008). No one model is ideal for every situation. However, Johnstone's moral decision-making model provides a five-step format to help nurses sort out the issues involved in an ethical situation and provide clarity toward a satisfying solution (Johnstone, 2004). In addition, this ethical decision-making model follows the format of the nursing process, a natural way of thinking for the nurse. The five steps of the Johnstone Moral Decision Making Model are:

- Assess the situation
- Identify moral problems
- Set moral goals and plan moral actions

■ Implement moral plan of action
■ Evaluate moral outcomes

This model begins with a reflective assessment of the situation at hand. Reflection on the ethical situation allows the nurse to identify the conflicting values at play in a particular situation. Consideration should be given to identifying which professional values are at issue as well as determining any confounding personal and patient values. The nursing and health care Codes of Ethics reviewed earlier in this chapter provide a basis for reflection on professional values and duties.

Once a reflective assessment has been made, the nurse can move toward identifying and therefore diagnosing the moral problem. Giving language to an issue causing moral distress helps to clarify the concern and often makes visible the path to resolution. At this point, it can be helpful to dialog with other care providers concerned with the issue.

The next two steps of the process involve planning and implementing a course of action to address the ethical issue. These steps may involve collaboration with other disciplines, the involvement of organizational leadership, or negotiating with the patient. A thorough assessment and identification of the ethical concern gives moral strength and courage to mount an action plan toward resolution.

Finally, as with any implementation, an evaluation of the outcome is warranted. Resolution of ethical dilemmas is an opportunity for team development and personal growth. The time taken to debrief following action over an ethical dilemma is well spent and can speed resolution of future concerns.

Moral Distress and Moral Courage

Correctional nurses can suffer moral distress when they know the right action to take in an ethical situation but are constrained from acting (Epstein & Delgado, 2010). This constraint can come from the organization, the patient, or care providers with more authority than the nurse. Some ethical dilemmas have a clear, correct action based on professional values. In contrast, moral distress can be caused by ambiguous ethical situations where there are major concerns about any of the options for action. In addition, moral distress can be experienced when a nurse advocates unsuccessfully for a patient in a care situation (Gallagher, 2010). Schluter, Winch, Holshauser, and Henderson (2008) found three primary causes of moral distress for nurses working in an acute care setting: Poor quality and futility care, unsuccessful advocacy, and raising unrealistic hopes. This phenomenon has not yet been studied in the correctional setting.

Moral distress can build over time and cause physical, psychological, and emotional symptoms of severe stress. Nurses can experience anger, depression, frustration, and guilt. Physical symptoms can include headache, neck pain, and stomach upset (Gallagher, 2010). Further research is needed on strategies to prevent and respond to moral distress. Nurse awareness of the condition and education about coping mechanisms have been suggested, as has improving the organization's ethical climate (Schluter et al., 2008).

Moral courage is needed in the face of an ethically challenging work setting. Moral courage is a professional value that allows nurses to challenge unethical or illegal practices, behaviors, or attitudes (Gallagher, 2010). Many historic nursing figures have shown moral courage in creating positive change, including Florence Nightingale, Clara Barton, and Dorothea Dix. Overcoming fears in order to take action in a difficult situation is not easy. Nurses may also lack confidence in how to respond in a morally distressing situation. Lachman (2010) suggests a process for acting in response to fear that can be helpful in a situation needing moral courage. The four key elements of this response are: (1) Identify the risk you want to take; (2) Identify the situational fear you experience; (3) Determine the outcome you want and what you have to do to achieve this outcome; (4) Identify resources accessible to you; and (5) Take action (Lachman, 2010). Courage, practiced for the right reasons and in the appropriate context, can support the nursing ethical values of patient health and safety. Case Example 2.1 applies this information.

CASE EXAMPLE 2.1

Owing to financial cutbacks, jail administration has asked that intake medical screening be done by the officers who perform other screenings. The nursing staff are uncomfortable with this decision and are discussing options before requesting to speak to the sheriff about the change. What ethical considerations should be made in dealing with this issue? Suggest ways the nursing staff could summon the moral courage to address their concerns.

COMMON ETHICAL DILEMMAS IN CORRECTIONAL NURSING

Many ethical dilemmas confront nurses in the day-to-day activities of providing nursing care. Some specific to the corrections specialty are gathering forensic evidence, cavity searches, participating in executions, witnessing use of force, inmate discipline, and hunger strikes. The application of core professional values and a common professional code of ethics can assist in making satisfying decisions about actions to be taken. Care must be taken to frame the deliberation in the context of nursing values and ethical practice rather than the needs and values of the correctional or judicial interests in the situation.

From the Experts ...

"Nursing in correctional settings is fraught with ethical issues not seen in other health care settings. Nurses should be attentive to them through education and affirmative (positive) support groups."

Patricia Blair, PhD, LLM, JD, MSN
Lindale, TX

Body Cavity Search

Correctional nurses may be asked to participate in body cavity searches. In determining whether this activity is ethical, the context and goals of the search are of primary importance. A body cavity search for a medical reason is within the parameters of ethical practice, as the intent is for the health and safety of the patient. This search would not violate the nurse–patient relationship. Body cavity searches for punitive or judicial purposes are not a part of ethical nursing practices and violate the nurse–patient relationship. If a body cavity search of this type is needed and medical skill is needed for the safety of the patient, a health professional who does not have a provider–patient relationship should be sought. Options include a local emergency room or a provider from a nearby correctional setting who does not have or is unlikely to have a provider–patient relationship with the individual (Anno & Spencer, 2006).

Executions

Nursing values prohibit involvement in executions. Executions are purely procedures of criminal justice and serve no health care purpose. In addition, they are rarely performed with informed patient consent. The tenets of the nurse–patient relationship require that nurses always act in the best interest of the patient. Even if a nurse's personal values allow for capital punishment as a criminal sanction, involvement in the execution itself is prohibited by professional ethics (ANA, 2010). In support of the human dignity of a patient and as an offer of comfort, correctional nurses may, if requested, help inmate-patients prepare for execution. This preparation would not include taking part in the execution process. Suggested comfort care measures may include pain control, anxiety relief, or arranging chaplain services (ANA, 2010).

Hunger Strikes

Most hunger strikes in the correctional setting are self-limiting and do not become life threatening. In rare cases where a mentally competent inmate has chosen to refuse food for political or manipulative purposes, correctional nurses may be asked to assist in involuntary feeding to maintain the individual's life (Anno & Spencer, 2006). This ethical dilemma hinges on the nurse's professional obligation to save life and the patient's right of autonomy. Certainly, mental competence must be evaluated to determine if the patient has made a reasoned decision to forgo nourishment. In the face of a principled decision by an inmate to deny food, each correctional nurse must determine a course of action that is congruent with both personal and professional values in order to maintain professional integrity.

Inmate Discipline

Correctional nurses may be asked to participate in documenting institutional rule violation leading to inmate discipline. Whenever possible, health care staff should deal with rule infraction through other methods (Anno, 2001). Of particular importance is an understanding of how the institution views such medical-related issues as refusing treatment, not showing up for appointments, or "malingering." The involvement of nursing staff in punitive measures does not support a healthy nurse–patient relationship and can establish, instead, an adversarial relationship.

Treatment Refusal/Forced Medications

Patient autonomy supports the right to refuse treatment. Patient autonomy is a value expressed in all professional nursing codes of ethics. In the correction setting, however, the nature of the environment, the patient, and the treatment situation can make it difficult to determine the reason for refusal (Anno, 2001). Correctional nurses have a responsibility to assure that treatment refusal is based on independent patient judgment. Other reasons for refusal could include schedule conflicts such as visiting hours or work programs, or barriers to health care such as onerous scheduling requirements, custody regulation, or fee-for-service.

In the correctional setting, patient autonomy to refuse treatment may be limited by the need for health and safety of the greater patient community. For example, a patient refusing treatment for tuberculosis may jeopardize the health of those living in close proximity. Although it is always ideal to convince the patient to submit to treatment through information and collaboration, forced treatment may be necessary and accomplished through legal procedure (Anno & Spencer, 2006).

On rare occasions, patients may require involuntary medication. This situation most often involves a patient deemed mentally incompetent to make decisions about their health and who is jeopardizing the safety of themselves and others. Participation in forced medication administration should be guided by policy; of limited duration; and clearly for the patient's welfare and not for organizational, staff, or punitive purposes (NCCHC, 2008).

Witnessing Use of Force

The advent and wide use of video cameras has reduced the need for witnessing use of force in corrections and nurses are rarely asked to participate. Cell extractions and other operations deemed necessary for the control of inmates are clearly not health related and should not involve nurse participation. Correctional nurses may be requested to review the medical history of inmates prior to a planned use of force to determine any medical conditions that should be taken into consideration. This action is congruent with the professional values inherent in patient health and safety. In addition, health care staff should evaluate an inmate following a use of force procedure to determine and treat any injuries. Case Example 2.2 applies information from this section.

CASE EXAMPLE 2.2

A call is received in the medical unit from the 5-cell observation area of a county jail. The officers have determined a need for a cell extraction and are asking for medical assistance. Pepper spray will be used. They ask that the inmate's medical record be reviewed and a nurse report to the observation area to assist with the extraction. What ethical principles should guide the nurse's decision making about participation? What boundaries should be placed on nursing activities in a cell extraction?

SUMMARY

Correctional nurses have a professional obligation to practice ethically. Several codes of ethics are available to correctional nurses, including the ANA and ICN Code of Ethics for Nurses as well as the ACHSA Code of Ethics. These professional codes identify the foundational values, duties, and loyalties of the nurse to a patient. The nurse–patient relationship is primarily based on a caring ethic, even in the boundaries of a correctional environment. Correctional nurses face moral distress and have opportunities to practice moral courage in advocating for the health and safety of inmate patients. Correctional nurses can be faced with unique ethical dilemmas such as participation in body cavity searches, hunger strikes, and forced medication administration. The use of an ethical decision-making framework and application of professional codes of ethics can assist in determining appropriate action. Correctional nursing practice based on ethical principles can be satisfying as well as beneficial to the patient and colleagues.

DISCUSSION QUESTIONS

1. What are the ethical dilemmas recently encountered in your correctional nursing practice? How consistent were your responses with the principles from the ANA Code of Ethics for Nurses?
2. Describe examples of acceptable and unacceptable nurse–patient relationships from your own experiences. Consider ways to maintain appropriate relationship boundaries in these situations.
3. Discuss caring in the context of correctional nursing and the boundaries of the security environment. How would you describe the nurse–patient relationship to a new correctional nurse?

REFERENCES

American Association of Colleges of Nurses (AACN). (2008). *The essentials of baccalaureate education for professional nursing practice*. Retrieved from http://www.aacn.nche.edu/Education/pdf/BaccEssentials08.pdf

American Correctional Health Services Association (ACHSA). (n.d.) *Code of ethics*. Retrieved from http://www.achsa.org/displaycommon.cfm?an=9

American Nurses Association (ANA). (2001). *Code of ethics for nurses with interpretive statements*. Silver Spring, MD: Author. Retrieved from http://nursingworld.org/MainMenuCategories/Ethics-Standards/CodeofEthicsforNurses/Code-of-Ethics.aspx

American Nurses Association (ANA). (2007). *Corrections nursing: Scope & standards of practice*. Silver Spring, MD: Author.

American Nurses Association (ANA). (2010). *Position statement: Nurses' role in capital punishment*. Silver Spring, MD: Author. Retrieved from http://www.nursingworld.org/MainMenuCategories/EthicsStandards/Ethics-Position-Statements/prtetcptl14447.aspx

Anno, B. J. (2001). *Correctional health care: Guidelines for the management of an adequate delivery system*. Chicago, IL: National Commission on Correctional Health Care.

Anno, B. J., & Spencer, S. S. (2006). Medical ethics and correctional health care. In M. Puisis (Ed.), *Clinical practice in correctional medicine* (2nd ed.). St. Louis, MO: Mosby Elsevier.

Badzak, L. A. (2008). Provision four. In M. D. M. Fowler (Ed.), *Guide to the code for ethics for nurses: Interpretation and application*. Silver Spring, MD: American Nurses Association.

Benner, P., & Wrubel, J. (1989). *The primacy of caring: Stress and coping in health and illness*. Menlo Park, CA: Addison-Wesley.

Bishop, A. H., & Scudder, J. R. (2008). The primacy of caring practice in nursing ethics. In W. J. E. Pinch & A. M. Haddad (Ed.), *Nursing and health care ethics: A legacy and a vision*. Silver Spring, MD: American Nurses Association.

Brodie, J. S. (2001). Caring: The essence of correctional nursing. *Tennessee Nurse, 64*(2), 10–12.

Brookshire, D. (2011). *Can nurses provide a caring environment to patients in a correctional setting?* Unpublished thesis, Lamar University, Beaumont, TX.

Butts, J. B. (2008). Ethics in professional nursing practice. In J. B. Butts & K. L. Rich (Eds.), *Nursing ethics: Across the curriculum and into practice* (2nd ed.). Boston, MA: Jones & Bartlett.

Davis, A. J. (2008). Provision two. In M. D. M. Fowler (Ed.), *Guide to the code for ethics for nurses: Interpretation and application*. Silver Spring, MD: American Nurses Association.

Dempski, K. (2009). Informed consent. In S. J. Westrick & K. Dempski (Eds.), *Essentials of nursing law and ethics*. Boston: Jones & Bartlett.

Epstein, E. G. T., & Delgado, S. (2010). Understanding and addressing moral distress. *OJIN: The Online Journal of Issues in Nursing, 15*(3). DOI: 10.3912/OJIN.Vol15No03Man01

Fowler, M. D. M. (Ed.). (2008a). *Guide to the code for ethics for nurses: Interpretation and application*. Silver Spring, MD: American Nurses Association.

Fowler, M. D. M. (2008b). Provision five. In M. D. M. Fowler (Ed.), *Guide to the code for ethics for nurses: Interpretation and application*. Silver Spring, MD: American Nurses Association.

Fry, S. T., & Johnstone, M. J. (2008). *Ethics in nursing practice: A guide to ethical decision making* (3rd ed.). Oxford, UK: International Council of Nurses-Blackwell Publishing.

Gallagher, A. (2010). Moral distress and moral courage in everyday nursing practice. *OJIN: The Online Journal of Issues in Nursing, 16*(2). DOI: 10.3912/OJIN.Vol16No02PPT03

Gostin, L. L. (2002). *Public health law and ethics: A reader*. Retrieved from http://www.cmemsc.org/news/HIPAAregulations.pdf

Hall, K. (2011). Building a trusting relationship with patients. *Home Healthcare Nurse, 29*(4), 210–217.

Hook, K. D., & White, G. B. (2009). *Code of ethics for nursing with interpretive statements, 2001. Continuing education module*. Silver Spring, MD: American Nurses Association. Retrieved from http://www.nursingworld.org/mods/mod580/code.pdf

International Council of Nurses (ICN). (2006). *The ICN code of ethics for nurses*. Geneva: International Council of Nurses. Retrieved from http://www.icn.ch/images/stories/documents/about/icncode_english.pdf

Johnstone, M. (2004). *Bioethics: A nursing perspective* (3rd ed.). Sydney: Harcourt Saunders.

Koloroutis, M. (2004). *Relationship-based care: A model fortransforming practice*. Minneapolis, MN: Creative Health Care Management.

Lachman, V. D. (2010, September 30). Strategies necessary for moral courage. *OJIN: The Online Journal of Issues in Nursing, 15*(3), Manuscript 3. Retrieved from http://www.nursingworld.org/MainMenuCategories/ANAMarketplace/ANAPeriodicals/OJIN/TableofContents/Vol152010/No3-Sept-2010/Strategies-and-Moral-Courage.aspx

National Commission on Correctional Health Care (NCCHC). (2008). *Standards for health services in prisons*. Chicago, IL: Author.

Schluter, J., Winch, S., Holshauser, K., & Henderson, A. (2008). Nurses' moral sensitivity and hospital ethical climate: A literature review. *Nursing Ethics, 15*(3), 304–321.

Sitzman, K., & Eichelberger, L. W. (2004). *Understanding the work of nurse theorists: A creative beginning*. Boston, MA: Jones & Bartlett.

Watson, J. (2012). *Human caring science: A theory of nursing* (2nd ed.). Boston, MA: Jones & Bartlett.

Weiskopf, C. S. (2005). Nurses' experience of caring for inmate patients. *Journal of Advanced Nursing, 49*(4), 336–343.

Westrick, S. J. (2009). Confidential communication. In S. J. Westrick & K. Dempski (Eds.), *Essentials of nursing law and ethics*. Boston: Jones & Bartlett.

THREE

Legal Considerations in Correctional Nursing

Jacqueline Moore

*T*he legal basis of correctional nursing is governed by the current state nurse prac- tice acts and licensure standards. Because the body of federal and state case law related to the incarcerated also affects nursing practice in corrections, correctional nurses need an understanding of basic legal judgments, in particular the U.S. Supreme Court decision in *Estelle v. Gamble*. As in any movement for social change, litigation can be a major catalyst for reform. The issues of inadequate health care can ultimately be addressed by society through effective legislative changes and the resources necessary to sustain them.

EARLY LEGAL CONSIDERATIONS

Numerous conditions prevalent in the earlier portion of the past century contributed to the degeneration of inmates' health within jails and prisons. Barriers to quality health care for the incarcerated included overcrowding, insubstantial provision of food or food that consisted of insufficient nutrients, substandard heating/cooling and light- ing, unsanitary environment, and the presence of insects and vermin. As a result, inmates suffered from numerous diseases and maladies—not the least of which were born from resulting mental health issues physically manifested in stress, vio- lence, and suicide (Moore, 1986). These factors amplified the need to greatly improve medical attention and health care delivery in the correctional environment.

Courts and the "Hands-Off" Doctrine

In an archaic approach to incarceration, inmates were historically viewed as slaves to the county or state—an outlook reinforced by a societal view that Constitutional and often basic human rights were privileges rather than actual guaranteed rights for residents of the penal system because the incarcerated had transgressed upon societal standards (*Newman v Alabama*, 1972). Then, throughout much of the 20th century (until the 1960s–1970s), U.S. courts hid behind a "hands-off" doctrine, often dismissing inmate petitions for writs of habeas corpus, except for those that could prove that medical attention received or denied equated to cruel and unusual punishment to a degree that would "shock the conscience of the court" (Zalman, 1972, pp. 185–189). This doctrine was based on the belief that the courts lacked the necessary knowledge in penology to question the actions and protocols of correctional officials, exacerbated by a fear that interference with prison and jail officials' systems and actions could subvert disciplinary control within the penal system. In this "hands-off" doctrine, courts used the distinction between rights and privileges to defer power of judgment to correctional officials (Van Alstyne, 1968).

Reversal of the "Hands-Off" Doctrine

The courts have recognized in *Newman v. Alabama* that they have a duty to uphold the Constitutional rights of prisoners, as the incarcerated are unable to do so themselves. This case signaled the reversal of the "hands off" doctrine with respect to prisoners' rights. In this October 1972 decision, a U.S. District Court found the entire state of Alabama to be in violation of the 8th and 14th amendment rights by failing to provide inmates with adequate staff and medical care (Newman v. Alabama, 1972).

The legal vehicle of choice for inmate lawsuits against correctional agencies and staff is a civil rights suit filed under the provisions of Chapter 42 of the United States Code Section 1983 (hence the common phrase, "§1983 actions"). That statute, passed during the post-Civil War Construction, provides, in relevant part, that:

Every person under color of any statute, ordinance, regulation, custom or usage of any State or Territory of the District of Columbia, subjects or causes to be subjected, any citizen of the United States or any person within the jurisdiction thereof to the deprivation of any rights, privileges or immunities secured by the Constitution and laws, shall be liable to the party injured in an action at law, suit in equity of proper proceeding for redress (Chapter 42 of US Code Section [§] 1983). To understand the full implication of this statement, an understanding of the terminology used is necessary and is discussed below:

Person: A human being is obviously a person under the statute; however, "persons" can also include local government agencies such as counties. States and state agencies are not considered "persons" and cannot be sued in a "§1983 action." The State can, however, be sued for at least some purposes through suits against state officials in their "legal capacity" as opposed to their "individual capacity." When officials in their "official capacity" are found to have violated the rights of inmates, the court can issue an injunction against the named official and the official's successors—in essence, an order against the State.

Color of statute: The "color of any statute" paraphrased is acting under the "color of state law." In other words, the person is acting under some authority of state law. For example, a correctional officer may use excessive force, as allowed by the facility's policies, against an inmate in a cell extraction and would be considered as operating under the color of state law. That same officer who saw the released inmate in a local store in the community and got in a fight with him in the parking lot would, however, not be operating under the color of state law.

Causation: The "subjects" or "cause to be subjected" under the language of the §1983 is important. Someone suing under the law (the plaintiff) must show a causal link between what the defendant did (or failed to do) and the violation of the plaintiff's rights.

Liability: §1983 provides that a defendant found to have violated the rights of someone "... shall be liable in a suit of law or equity of other proper proceeding for redress." This portion of the statute describes the relief that can be awarded to the successful plaintiff. It means that a court can issue an injunction against a defendant, requiring some change in behavior, or it can award damages to the injured party.

In *Monroe v. Pape* (1961), the U.S. Supreme Court ruled that citizens could bring suits against state officials in federal courts without first exhausting all state judicial remedies. This section of the Civil Rights Act of 1871, which imposes civil liability on any person who deprives another of Constitutional rights, enabled inmates to more successfully challenge the constitutionality of prison life. In *Robinson v. California* (1962), the Court extended the Eighth Amendment's prohibition against cruel and unusual punishment to the states.

Although the pendulum has swung away from the former "hands-off" doctrine, the Supreme Court holds that the restriction and reduction of personal rights is in line with upholding the sentencing of the incarcerated, and should be maintained to such a degree as prison officials see fit for the maintenance of security.

Estelle v. Gamble

In 1977, Respondent J. W. Gamble, an inmate of the Texas Department of Corrections, filed a complaint initially in the District Court citing inadequate medical care received during his incarceration, following an injury to his back sustained in the course of prison work when a bale of cotton fell on him while unloading a truck. In the months that ensued, he received 17 examinations, multiple variations of pain relievers, and cell-pass to relieve him of prison work duty. He was taken before the prison disciplinary committee for his refusal to work, and though threatened to be placed on the "farm," Gamble maintained that his injury still caused him as much pain as the day it was received. A captain in the facility visited Gamble three times and then testified that Gamble was in "first class condition." With no further examination or testimony, Gamble was placed in solitary confinement. Four days later, he complained of chest pains and "black-outs," and was seen that evening by a medical assistant who ordered him to be hospitalized. Three days after hospitalization, completion of an electrocardiogram, and administration of medication for cardiac rhythm irregularity, he was returned to confinement. Gamble requested for two days to see the last doctor, but was refused. It was not until the third day that the inmate was seen and his medication was continued. Gamble filed a complaint two days later, citing cruel and unusual punishment in violation of the Eighth Amendment (*Estelle v. Gamble*, 1977).

After Gamble's complaint was reinstated by the Court of Appeals, the Supreme Court concluded that his pain and suffering resulting from a denial of medical care were found to have no legitimate penological purpose and were deemed "inconsistent with contemporary standards of decency" (*Estelle v. Gamble*, 1977, at 103). The court ruled that the complaint was predicated on a failure to provide additional diagnostic tests and alleged a claim of medical malpractice against the prison medical doctor.

In evaluation of *Estelle v. Gamble,* the Supreme Court considered the obligation of the government to provide care for an incarcerated individual who has no alternative source of treatment and is otherwise incapable of providing care himself. The court ruled that the proper standard to be applied in considering prisoner medical cases was "deliberate indifference" to the serious medical needs of prisoners: Deliberate indifference was defined as the "wanton infliction of unnecessary pain which can be manifested by doctors in their response to the prisoner's need or by the prison guards in intentionally interfering with the treatment once prescribed" (*Estelle v. Gamble,* 1977, at 104–105).

It was through this case that the Supreme Court ruled that proper standards be applied in the administration of medical care to inmates. Additionally, the term "deliberate indifference" was coined, which requires the court to consider the action or inaction of prison officials in regard to addressing "serious medical need." The uniform standard of "deliberate indifference" remains applicable to all courts in dealing with prison medical care claims today. Case Example 3.1 applies information from this section.

CASE EXAMPLE 3.1

A woman turned herself in on a failure-to-appear warrant. She charged that the health staff was deliberately indifferent to her serious medical need during the 12 hours she was held in custody before she could post bail. She had suffered from a spinal cord injury 3 years before the arrest, for which she still occasionally wore a neck brace and took medication for pain and muscle spasms. She claimed that the jail had confiscated her neck brace and her pain medication during booking and, despite alerting the nurse, did not get them back. The woman said she was in excruciating pain, suffering from muscle spasms and neck stiffness. Did the woman experience a serious medical need? What information is needed to determine if there was deliberate indifference?

CURRENT JUDICIAL CONSIDERATIONS

The judicial attitude has changed drastically from the de facto "hands-off" position of the past. Courts are now willing to intervene in correctional health care. Judicial definitions and decisions regarding rights of prisoners have evolved considerably over the past 35 years.

The "deliberate indifference" standard established by the Supreme Court in *Estelle v. Gamble* is cumbersome in redressing individual claims of inadequate medical treatment. The *Estelle* decision clearly established an inmate's right to medical treatment but left unanswered such questions as to what standard of care an inmate is entitled and whether every medical need must be met. Consequently, the application of the standard has been extended to include all claims pertaining to prisoners' medical needs. The standard is applied using various U. S. Constitutional Amendments that are discussed below.

Eighth Amendment

The Eighth Amendment to the U.S. Constitution succinctly states, "Excessive bail shall not be required, nor excessive fines imposed, nor cruel and unusual punishments inflicted." Its application in correctional health care correlates to the denial or delay of necessary medical treatment, with wanton intent to inflict pain upon an inmate (429 US at 104).

Courts use various phrases to define "serious medical need" as established by *Estelle v. Gamble.* Despite the various methods the courts have developed, the functional test is largely in the eye of the beholder. Some medical needs are universally accepted as "serious," while others are not so serious. If the failure to treat an injury results in further significant injury or the unnecessary and wanton inflection of pain, for example, the condition is serious. Epilepsy was found to be a serious medical condition (*Hattiwanger v. Mobley,* 2001). Acne, on the other hand, is not seen as a serious health concern (*Hudgins v. De Bruyn,* 1996; *Ware v. Fairman,* 1995).

Fourteenth Amendment

Section 1 of the Fourteenth Amendment to the U.S. Constitution states, "All persons born or naturalized in the United States, and subject to the jurisdiction thereof, are citizens of the United States and of the state wherein they reside. No state shall make or enforce any law which shall abridge the privileges or immunities of citizens of the United States; nor shall any state deprive any person of life, liberty, or property, without due process of law; nor deny to any person within its jurisdiction the equal protection of the laws."

For pretrial detainees, the phrase "... without due process of the law" specifically protects their rights, as they have not been convicted of any crime. At any given time a substantial portion of the jail population consists of pretrial detainees. The constitutional analysis of the Eighth Amendment (cruel and unusual punishment) applies only to convicted persons. It does not protect pretrial detainees. However, the Supreme Court long ago held that the due process clause of the Fourteenth Amendment prohibits detainees from being punished (*Bell v. Wolfish,* 441 US Constitution 320). Punishment was defined as exposing detainees to conditions including poor medical care that would violate the Eighth Amendment if applied to convicted persons.

"Due process" has two quite distinct meanings: substantive due process and procedural due process. *Substantive due process* is a concept that can limit or prohibit certain actions by a state. *Procedural due process* says that in order to lawfully deprive someone of life, liberty, or property, the decision must be made fairly. An example of both substantive and procedural due process arose in *Washington v. Harper,* 494 US 210 (1990). The issues in this case were under what circumstances, if any, the state could medicate a mentally ill inmate when the inmate did not consent to the medication (substantive due process) and, assuming the state could involuntarily medicate the inmate under some circumstances, what procedures the state must follow to assure fairness in determining that the circumstances did exist (procedural due process). In summary, the court found that there were circumstances where an inmate could be involuntarily medicated, and it approved a formal process for hearing and review.

Particular Issues Affecting §1983 Lawsuits

Cost of Care

Some medical procedures are very expensive. While inmates are not entitled to the most expensive medical treatment, the cost of treatment will not justify its denial if there are no other reasonable alternatives. An example of this would be releasing early those inmates diagnosed with serious medical needs that require costly treatments as a means to avoid the cost of the treatment. Courts have not addressed this practice uniformly; however, if an inmate were released and had no access to or funds for the necessary health care, the question arises whether early release could be seen as deliberate indifference.

Delayed Care

There may be circumstances, particularly in a jail setting, where there will be pressure to delay the provision of medical care. A typical example is when a medical procedure is expensive and the inmate in need may be either released or transferred in the near future. Can the jail simply not provide care because the inmate is leaving? The answer of whether this is acceptable under the Constitution depends on the effects of the delay. If the delayed care does not result in worsening condition or constant pain, it will be acceptable. If the inmate suffers as a result of delayed care, however, the delay becomes suspect.

Preexisting Conditions

Correctional officials cannot refuse to treat a preexisting condition. An example would be a new pretrial detainee seeking attention to dental concerns. It is obvious to the clinicians that the detainee has serious dental problems. The facility officials cannot refuse to treat the detainee's dental problems simply because he ignored the need for dental until he was detained.

LEGISLATION AFFECTING LITIGATION
Americans with Disabilities Act

The Americans with Disabilities Act (ADA) of 1990 protects Americans from discrimination on the basis of disability and requires special accommodations for these individuals, including modification of architectural surroundings, communication devices, and transportation availability. This further encompasses wheelchairs, prosthetic devices, and visual and hearing aids. This applies to the incarcerated handicapped and does not absolve correctional officials of their duty toward them (*Ruiz v. Estelle*, 1980). From local to federal detention facilities, these provisions must be afforded inmates or detainees, and failure to provide such aid can be construed as a violation of the Eighth Amendment. The ADA subjects all types of correctional facilities (local, county, state, and federal) to potential claims, damages, and suits for failure to comply (*Cummings v. Roberts*, 1980; *Johnson v. Hardin County, KY*, 1990).

Prison Litigation Reform Act

In 1996, the United States Congress passed the Prison Litigation Reform Act (PLRA) to minimize the number of nonmeritorious inmate civil rights lawsuits and limit the role of the federal courts in management of prison and jail operations. The law had two primary goals: "The first is to reduce what Congress felt was excessive, frivolous litigation by inmates by making it somewhat more difficult for inmates to pursue federal lawsuits against correctional officials. The most notable example of this goal is the new requirement that inmates pay a full $150 filing fee in order to file a §1983 case in federal court. The second goal was to reduce what Congress felt was excessive intervention by federal courts in jail and prison operations" (p. 14) (Collins, 2004). The constitutionality of the passage of this act is still the subject of great debate. If PLRA is sustained, it may have a tremendous impact on judicial enforcement of the Eighth Amendment protection against deliberate indifference to inmates' serious medical needs (Rold, 2006).

As tracked by *Prisoner Petitions Filed in U.S. District Courts, 2000, with Trends 1998–2000* (Scalia, 2002), the number of suits filed from 1970 to 1995 increased dramatically; however, the quantity of suits was found to be in line with the increased number of those incarcerated. It should be noted that, although the number of suits has reached administratively paralyzing proportions (40,000 in 1995), the PLRA grants the courts power to dismiss these cases before they reach an opportunity to settle or go to trial. Many cases are dismissed because most inmates file their claim *pro se*—without the assistance of a lawyer, who could help identify whether the case has merit or is, in fact, frivolous (Scalia, 2002).

The PLRA also diminishes the federal court's ability to impose imposing injunctions to provide relief where the courts find violation of inmate constitutional rights. Court ordered remedies to violations must be the "least intrusive means necessary to correct the violation of the federal right," and "extend no further than necessary to correct" (18 USC §3626[a][1]). Additionally, courts may not issue "prison release orders," which is defined to include both explicit release orders and population caps, until other less intrusive relief has been tried and found to be unsatisfactory (Collins, 2004).

Finally, the PLRA grants defendants the opportunity to move to terminate a lawsuit after 2 years. If Constitutional violations are still found, the remedial order must be reexamined to determine that it was drawn modestly enough, or rather, to "extend no further than necessary to correct" (*Laaman v. Warden*, New Hampshire State Prison, 283 F.3d 14 [1st Cir. 2001]. Should violations still exist, the order must be redrawn to correct them. Nonetheless, the burden of the initiation of termination rests upon the defendant.

MALPRACTICE AND THE CORRECTIONAL NURSE

Health professional liability is a type of negligence for which professionals can be sued. Because of their profession and the impact of their professional actions on others' lives, nurses are held to a higher standard of conduct than laypersons. Nurses are charged with utilizing the degree of skill and judgment commensurate with their experience and education. There are generally five elements required in a claim for negligence:

1. Duty was owed to the client (professional relationship);

2. Breach of Duty—the professional violated duty and failed to conform to the standard of care;
3. Causality—failure to act by the professional was the proximate cause of resulting injury;
4. Damages—actual damages resulted from the breach of duty (Catalano, 1996) and
5. Foreseeability—is the ability to see or know in advance; hence, the reasonable anticipation that harm or injury is a likely result of acts or omissions. (*Emery v. Thompson*, 347 Mo. 494, 148 S.W. 479, 480 [1941]).

The "'foreseeability' element of proximate cause is established by proof that actor, as person of ordinary intelligence and prudence, should reasonably have anticipated danger to others created by his negligent act, whether by event which occurred or some similar event, without regard to what actor believed would occur or anticipation as to just how injuries would grow out of dangerous situation created by him." (*Clark v. Waggoner*, Tex., 452 S.W. 2d 437 [1970]). Case Example 3.2 applies information from this section.

CASE EXAMPLE 3.2

An inmate with chest pain came to the infirmary. The nurse told the inmate to wait until she attended to several other inmates. The inmate left the infirmary and came back later. He was examined by another staff member, given an EKG, and taken to a hospital. Coronary artery blockages were discovered and an angioplasty was performed. Was the first nurse negligent?

Six major categories of negligence that prompt malpractice lawsuits have been identified:

1. Documentation describing negative behavior such as lack of, incomplete, ineffective, and/or improper charting;
2. Failure to follow the standards of care;
3. Failure to use equipment in a responsible manner;
4. Failure to communicate;
5. Failure to assess and monitor the patient; and
6. Failure to follow a physician's written or verbal order (Moore, 2003).

Standard of Care

Standard of care for most states can be summarized by three primary components:

1. An obligation to have accomplished the level of education and maintain a level of skill required within the position;
2. A responsibility to utilize the above-mentioned education and skill to provide care in the medical setting; and
3. "The duty to use reasonable diligence and best judgment in carrying out duties" (Hudgins, 2003, p. 3–3).

In legal cases, the standard of care is typically explained by expert witness(es) in detail as that standard relates to the case at hand. The expert witness then gives an opinion about whether or not that standard of care was met. Any alleged breach of standard of care must be proven to have caused injury for a plaintiff's case to prevail. This is causation. A plaintiff must, however, prove that the receipt of medical care, denial of treatment, and/or oversight of or ignorance to the existing health condition created injury, damage, loss, or harm—essentially creating or worsening a condition—to stand a chance of a favorable ruling in court.

Nursing licensure (including education, training, additional certification, and practice) is evidence of competence, capability, willingness, and earnestness to provide or exceed the standard of care in whatever state or facility the nurse is employed.

DELIBERATE INDIFFERENCE

Established in the 1976 U.S. Supreme Court case *Estelle v. Gamble*, the "deliberate indifference" standard governs inmates' right to medical care. Deliberate indifference can be interpreted as the denial, delay, or interference with providing care for an inmate's serious medical needs (Hudgins, 2003).

Distinction From Nursing Negligence

Distinguishing between deliberate indifference and negligence is inherently difficult insofar as "deliberate indifference" is, itself, an oxymoron: "deliberate" is defined as carefully considered or intentional, whereas "indifference" is defined by a lack of concern or interest. Deliberate indifference boils down to the ethics and morality of a choice or decision, whereas ignorance of practice and protocols, equates largely to negligence.

A serious medical need must either have been diagnosed by a physician as a condition requiring treatment, or is a need so blatantly obvious that a layperson could immediately recognize the inmate's need for medical attention. Components that could legally uphold the serious medical need of the case include:

1. The plaintiff had a serious medical need;
2. The defendant knew that the plaintiff had a serious medical need;
3. The effect of delayed medical care, either in assessment or treatment (or both), created harm to the plaintiff;
4. The plaintiff's harm was caused by the defendant's indifference; and
5. The failure to treat the need resulted in further damage to the patient's health or unnecessary infliction of additional pain (Hudgins, 2003).

Ignoring the existence of a serious medical need including any of the five subcategories or failing to investigate into any of these could be the basis for a court finding of deliberate indifference.

Right to Access Care

The right to receive care is a fundamental component of the deliberate indifference standard. When access to care is delayed or denied, patients are placed in jeopardy. Access to care includes both routine and emergency care, as well as specialist treatment and hospitalization when warranted (Anno, 2001). Access to care must be provided for any condition, whether it is medical, dental, or mental health. If care is denied or delayed, the result can be increased pain, suffering, or deterioration of the patient, and the court will be inclined to favor the plaintiff in a personal injury lawsuit. When adequate systems of care are not in place, the health care staff does not know which patients need emergency medical attention and which patients can afford to wait (Anno, 2001).

Right to Care That Is Ordered

Generally, courts assume that care would not have been ordered if it had not been needed. Thus, once a physician or mid-level provider orders care for a patient, the court, as a matter of constitutional law, protects the patient's right to receive that treatment without undue delay (Rold, 2006). To ensure that the care ordered is, in fact, delivered, the courts will require the treating provider to specify a time frame for the care to occur. As established in *Todaro v. Ward* (1977), failure to provide ordered care for a serious medical need violates the Eighth Amendment.

Right to a Professional Nursing Judgment

Generally, courts will not intervene and make a decision regarding treatments that are ordered or their efficacy. The courts will, however, review cases where the care (or lack of care) was so extreme or abusive as to be completely out of the range of professional judgment. Included in this category are issues related to equipment, staffing, and nature and timing of nursing decisions (Rold, 2006).

Serious Medical Need

The U.S. Constitution requires that correctional officials and health providers provide care for "serious medical needs." Generally, a medical need is deemed "serious" if:

- It has been diagnosed by a physician as needing treatment;
- The condition is so obvious that even a layperson would recognize the necessity for medical attention; and
- Failure to treat the medical condition could result in further significant injury and the subsequent unnecessary and wanton infliction of pain (Hudgins, 2003).

The U.S. Supreme Court has held that a guilty defendant must have had knowledge of a serious medical need and disregarded it, causing an excessive risk to the inmate's health or safety (*Farmer v. Brennan*, 1994). An example of a serious medical need can be found in *Lancaster v. Monroe County* (1997), where an action was brought by the estate of a detainee who allegedly died due to indifference of his medical needs. The court found that a jail official who is aware of but ignores the danger of alcohol withdrawal, and waits for it to manifest to an emergency before obtaining medical care, is deliberately indifferent to the inmate's Constitutional rights.

DEFENSES

There are a variety of defenses available to nurses that include causation, unforseeability, a Good Samaritan statute, and acting in good faith (Hudgins, 2003). The best defense to nursing negligence or deliberate indifference is an affirmation that the standard of care was met. This is most often accomplished through the testimony of an expert witness. The causation defense can also be successful because the plaintiff must show that the denial, delay, or interference with care caused the injury. The causation defense must prove that the alleged malpractice caused the injury. Most states have Good Samaritan statutes to insulate health care providers if they provide care in an emergency and act in their professional capacity. The defense that an outcome was unforeseeable can be used if a provider acted in good faith. Whether or not an action was performed in good faith is ultimately determined by a jury.

Summary Judgment

"A summary judgment allows the defendant to submit his version of the facts to the court through affidavits or sworn declarations. The plaintiff is allowed to submit counter affidavits" (Collins, 2004, p. 282). After examination of these written documents, if the court feels that material evidence is in order, a trial with live testimony will follow. Where the law is not clear, a summary judgment can be an effective defense, allowing the defendant (and plaintiff) to submit a series of detailed, written statements (and affidavits) explaining the situation—particularly where harsh allegations are asserted in the complaint.

Immunity

Government officials may be entitled to absolute immunity (unconditional immunity) from liability if their acts are based on carrying out a government function based on their job descriptions. It includes judicial, testimonial, and legislative immunities. In *Harlow v. Fitzgerald* (1982), the U.S. Supreme Court held that government officials performing discretionary functions are generally immune (absolutely immune) from civil liability unless their conduct violates an established Constitutional right that a reasonable person would have known about. Qualified immunity is a doctrine in U.S. federal law that arises in cases brought against state officials under 42 U.S.C Section 1983 and against federal officials under *Bivens v. Six Unknown Named Agents*, 403 U.S. 388 (1971). Qualified immunity shields government officials from liability for the violation of an individual's federal constitutional rights. This grant of immunity is available to state or federal employees performing discretionary functions where their actions, even if later found to be unlawful, did not violate "clearly established law." The defense of qualified immunity was created by the U.S. Supreme Court, replacing a court's inquiry into a defendant's subjective state of mind with an inquiry into the objective reasonableness of the contested action. A government agent's liability in a federal civil rights lawsuit no longer turns upon whether the defendant acted with "malice," but on whether a hypothetical reasonable person in the defendant's position would have known that his/her actions violated clearly established law. Qualified immunity has not been extended to private health care firms that contract with governmental entities (*Richardson v. McKnight*, 1997); however, it might apply to nurses who are employed by the state or county.

Nurse Practice Act

Nurses are subject to the laws and regulations established by the board of nursing and nurse practice act in the state or province in which they work. The regulations in each state, designed to ensure the public's safety, define the scope of practice for the various levels of licensed nurses. The practice of nursing requires rules and regulations to ensure patient safety and a competent level of behavior in the professional role of the nurse. Nurse practice acts, licensure, and standards of care are key elements in the regulation of nursing practice.

State nursing licensing laws define the scope of nursing practice and are used as evidence in determining whether nurses acted within the legal limits of the profession. Throughout their careers, nurses must maintain current knowledge of determinants of nursing practice. Lack of knowledge increases nurses' risk of an untoward event that could lead to disciplinary charges or malpractice litigation. Claiming ignorance of the nursing practice act is never a defense for a nurse (Catalano, 1996). When the state authorizes a nursing practice through licensure, the state licensing authority expects the nurse to assume responsibility for remaining current regarding the legal and acceptable standards of practice.

Nursing regulations are generally published in a compilation known as the administrative code. They can also be found online under the nurse practice act for a particular state. Inherent in the licensing is an obligation to abide by the state's laws and regulations as a condition of accepting licensure in the state. For nurses who wish to practice in multiple states, most states require licensure. The only exception are nurses who reside and are licensed in a compact state and may practice in the other states that are part of the compact. Travel nurses must abide by the laws of all states where they are practicing. Thus, complaints regarding a travel nurse would be processed in the state where the alleged violation occurred and would also be reported to the home state (Erickson, 2006).

Nurse–Patient Relationship

The nurse–patient relationship is imposed on both the inmate and the nurse by the governmental entity that is responsible for providing the medical service. The inmate cannot go elsewhere, and the nurse cannot refuse to treat. Studies of lawsuits arising in the community have shown that nurses who communicated well with their patients were at lower risk of being sued. Good communication includes explaining procedures, listening effectively, seeking the patient's opinion, conveying respect, and using humor. On the other hand, patients who sued nurses after a bad outcome complained that the nurses would not talk to them, performed cursory exams, rushed them, or ignored them. The crux of correctional nursing is to maintain open, honest, respectful relationships with the inmate-patient. Patients are less likely to sue if they feel that a nurse has been caring and professional (Ballard, 2011).

STANDARDS IN CORRECTIONAL HEALTH CARE

The American Nurses Association (ANA) defines nursing practice as protection, promotion, and optimization of health and abilities; prevention of illness and injury; alleviation of suffering through diagnosis and treatment of human responses; and advocacy in the care of individuals, families, communities, and the populations (2010). The basic philosophy, underscored by the ANA standards, is that health care in a correctional facility should be equivalent to that available in the community and subject to the same regulations. The Courts, in interpreting the U.S. Constitution, recognized that detainees and inmates in a correctional setting are totally dependent upon the facility's health professionals for their medical care. Thus, the responsibility of the nurses for assisting the incarcerated with their health care problems is increased.

Community Standard of Care

The community standard of care refers to the degree of attentiveness, caution, and prudence that a reasonable person would exercise in the circumstances. Should a person's conduct fall below such standard, one may be liable for injuries or damages resulting from one's conduct (Black's Law Dictionary, 2009). Failure to meet the community standard of care is negligence and holds the provider liable for any damages caused by such negligence (Black's Law Dictionary, 2009).

Accreditation for Correctional Health Facilities

The American Correctional Association (ACA) and the National Commission on Correctional Health Care (NCCHC) establish standards for correctional health care (ACA, 2011; NCCHC, 2011). The standards are broad in base and cover multiple topics such as facility governance and administration, health care services and support, inmate care and treatment, health promotion and disease prevention, special inmate needs and services, health records, medical legal issues, and environmental health and safety. Accreditation of correctional facilities is voluntary. Standards of care are the minimum criteria for a health care professional's proficiency on the job, enabling others to judge the quality of the health care they provide.

Correctional standards are guidelines for sound, safe nursing care in correctional institutions. Regardless of practice settings, nurses are expected to meet standards of care for every nursing task performed in correctional health care. One of the most important standards of nursing care is documentation in the health record of the nurse's interventions and response of the patient to the care provided. The court may interpret a lack of documentation as an absence of health care provided to inmates. Both the ACA and the NCCHC claim that accredited agencies have a stronger defense against litigation through good faith effort to improve the conditions of confinement. NCCHC argues that facilities that meet NCCHC accreditation are more favorably regarded by the courts (NCCHC, 2011). Voluntary compliance with NCCHC standards demonstrates to government officials, the public, and the courts that a facility understands the legal requirements of correctional health care. The ACA indicates that, as an incentive for agencies willing to participate in ACA's national accreditation program, insurance companies offer a reduction on liability premiums of 10% (ACA, 2011).

Certification and Correctional Nursing

The alleged absence of adequate health care has been cited as a factor in lawsuits that affect 35% of correctional facilities today. Court decisions regarding these lawsuits have declared unreasonable deprivation of medical, mental health, and dental care as unconstitutional; consequently, states and counties have been ordered to take remedial action. As a result of judicial decisions, governmental entities began to evaluate the level of care provided in their facility and have taken steps to enhance the delivery of medical services by hiring additional nursing staff.

As accreditation standards have emerged, so too have standards for professionals, aided by the development of certification programs by groups including the NCCHC and the ACA. Certification is the formal recognition of knowledge, skill, and experience that demonstrates competence and achievement of standards of a specialty that fosters and promotes optimal health outcomes (Muse, 2009).

The NCCHC offers certifications as Certified Correctional Health Professional (CCHP), Certified Correctional Health Professional Registered Nurse (CCHP-RN), and the ACA provides a certification as a Certified Correctional Nurses (CCN) and Certified Correctional Nurse Manager (CCN/M). The exams are developed by expert nurses with extensive experience in correctional nursing and are designed to improve the individual's practice in this field. The addition of a certification program will maintain the excellence of correctional nursing that is necessary in the practice of nursing and the development of patient care within the distinct environment of the criminal justice system. Because certification is still new to the field of correctional nursing, it is yet unknown whether certification will decrease liability.

MANAGING RISK

To establish an environment for patient safety, it is essential to undertake risk management evaluation with regard to nursing interventions in correctional clinical settings. Nurses are held accountable to the public for their professional judgment and the outcomes arising from that judgment. Malpractice litigation can be professionally and emotionally devastating, as well as financially disastrous. Table 3.1 provides some common-sense tips to reduce liability.

TABLE 3.1   Ways to Reduce Potential Liability

Communication
Never offer opinions when a patient asks you what you think is wrong—you may be rendering a medical diagnosis. Never criticize health care providers or their actions when with a patient. Never make a statement that a patient may interpret as an admission of fault or guilt.
Education
Regularly subscribe to and read professional journals (e.g., *Journal of Correctional Health Care, CorrectCare, Correctional Health Report, American Journal of Nursing*). Request a copy of your state's nurse practice act with initial licensure and all subsequent renewals. Maintain a personal library of the most recent publications in your field. Review the policies and procedures of your organization and place of employment. Attend relevant continuing education classes and in-service programs. Maintain copies of all certificates received indicating completion of a course.
Practice
Maintain competency in your area of specialty practice. Maintain membership in one or more professional associations (e.g., the Academy of Health Professionals, American Correctional Health Professionals, State Nurses Association, etc.) Seek appointment to a leadership position of various nursing committees both inside and outside of your workplace. Practice within the bounds of your professional licensure. Practice only the skills that are allowed by your professional license. Never accept a clinical assignment if you do not feel competent to perform it. Document all nursing care in an accurate and timely fashion. Care must be factual, accurate, complete, and timely. Remember the mnemonic: FACT.

Source: Adapted from Ballard (2011).

From the Experts . . .

"During the years of reviewing medical malpractice cases that took place in correctional settings, most of the litigation was due to nurses not advocating for the patient, resulting in delay of treatment. This includes nurses being judgmental in their charting (e.g. "malingering, drug seeking"), resulting in lack of access to care. Also, nurses' failure to follow the provider's orders for medications and treatments resulted in withholding or lack of care."

Kathleen E. Page MS, RN, CCHP
Aurora, OR

SUMMARY

The correctional health care model has greatly improved over the past century. Nonetheless, continued modification of prison health care systems across the nation—in an effort to achieve parity with health care systems within their communities, as well as attain accreditation and the standardization afforded by accreditation guidelines—seems to be the most effective path toward minimizing of inmate lawsuits. Additionally, this will protect inmates' human rights by affording correctional health care that is more available, more cost-effective, and does not jeopardize the security processes of the correctional environment.

Lawsuits are an unfortunate part of correctional health care. There is no way to guarantee a suit-free practice in this environment. The best approach to reduce the risk of legal action is for correctional nurses to have knowledge of the legal system, to practice within their licensure, have a strong code of ethics, and document well.

DISCUSSION QUESTIONS

1. How would you describe deliberate indifference to a colleague?
2. What are the key rights established by *Estelle v. Gamble*, 1977?
3. Which two constitutional amendments are cited in inmate legal cases?
4. List ways correctional nurses can reduce legal liability in their practice.

REFERENCES

American Correctional Association-Performance Based Standards for Correctional Health Care. Retrieved February 28, 2011, from http://www.aca.org/standards/healthcare/

American Nurses Association (ANA). (2010). *Scope and standards of practice* (2nd ed.). Washington, DC: Author.

Anno, B. J. (2001). *Correctional health care guidelines for the management of an adequate delivery system*. U.S. Department of Justice National Institute of Corrections.

Ballard, K. (2011). Beyond licensure: Determinants of nursing practice. *Nurse Service Organization*. Retrieved from http://www.nso.com/nursing-resources/article/45.jsp

Bivens v. Six Unknown Named Agents, 403 U.S. 388 (1971).

Catalano, J. (1996). *Nursing law and liability in nurses' legal handbook* (3rd ed., Chapter 8). North Wales, PA: Springhouse.

Clark v. Waggoner, Tex., 452 S.W. 2d 437 (1970).

Collins, W. C. (2004). *Jail and prison legal issues an administrators guide.* American Jail Association.

Cummings v. Roberts, 628 F.2d 1065 (1980).

Eighth Amendment, *U.S. Constitution.* Ratified 12/15/1791. *Emery v. Thompson*, 347 Mo. 494, 148 S.W. 479, 480 (1941).

Erickson, K. (2006). *The nurse practice act: A closer look.* Retrieved from www.BharatBhasha.com article URL:http://www.bharathhasa.com/legal.php/34665

Estelle v. Gamble, 429 U.S. 97, 102, 8th Am. (1976).

Farmer v. Brennan, 511 U.S. 825 (1994).

Fourteenth Amendment (Sec. 1), *U.S. Constitution.* Ratified 7/9/1868.

B. Garner (Ed.) (2009). *Black's law dictionary.* New York, NY: West Group Publisher.

Hattiwanger v. Mobley, 230 F 3d, 1363 (8th Circuit Court, 2001).

Harlow v. Fitzgerald, 457 U.S. 800, 818 (1982).

Hudgins, N. (2003). Correctional health care: The legal perspective. In J. Moore (Ed.), *Management and administration of correctional health care* (pp. 3–3). Kingston, NJ: Civic Research Institute.

Hudgins v. De Bruyn, 922 F Supp. 144 (S. D. OND, 1996).

Johnson v. Hardin County, KY 908 F2 1280 6th Circuit (1990).

Laaman v. Warden, New Hampshire State Prison, 283 F.3d 14 (1st Cir. 2001).

Lancaster v. Monroe County 116 F.3d 1419 (11th Circuit 1997).

Legal rights of prisoners — The beginnings of prisoners' rights law: The Civil Rights Era. (n.d.) Retrieved February 27, 2011, from http://law.jrank.org/pages/1762/Prisoners-Legal-Rights-beginnings-prisoners-rights-law-civil-rights-era.html

Moore, J. (1986). Prison health care: Problems and alternatives in the delivery of health care to the incarcerated, Part I. *Journal of Florida Medical Association, 73,* 531–534.

Monroe v. Pape, 365 U.S. 806, 81 S.Ct. 473 (1961).

Muse, M. (2009). Correctional nursing: The evolution of a specialty. *Correct Care, 23*(1), 3–4.

National Commission on Correctional Health Care. (2011). *NCCHC health services accreditation brochure.* Chicago, IL: Author.

Newman v Alabama, 503 F2d1320, 1324, 1330 5TH Cir. (1972).

Pierce v. LaVallee, 293 F.2d 223 (2d Cir. 1961).

Richardson v. McKnight, 521 U.S. 399 (1997).

Robinson v. California, 370 U.S. 660, 82 S.Ct. 1417 (1962).

Ruiz v. Estelle, 503 F. Supp. 1265, 1331 (S.D. Tex. 1980).

Rold, W. J. (2006). Legal consideration in the delivery of health care services in prisons and jails. In M. Puisis (Ed.), *Clinical practice in correctional health care.* St. Louis, MO: Mosby.

Scalia, J. (2002). *Prisoner petitions filed in U.S. District Court 1980–2000.* Bureau of Justice Statistics. NCJ 189430. Retrieved from http://bjs.ojp.usdoj.gov/content/pub/pdf/ppfusd00.pdf

Sewell v. Pegelow, 291 F.2d 196 (4th Cir. 1961).

Todaro v. Ward, 565 F.2d 48 (CA2 1977).

Van Alstyne, W. W. (1968). The demises of right-priviledge distinction in constitutional law. *Harvard Law Review, 81,* 1439–1464.

Ware v. Fairman, 884F. Supp. 1201 (N.D. III, 1995).

Washington v. Harper, 494 US 210 (1990).

Zalman, M. (1972). Prisoner's right to medical care. *Journal of Criminal Law, Criminology and Police Science, 2,* 185–189.

FOUR

Safety for the Nurse and the Patient

Lorry Schoenly

*U*nlike many other patient care environments, nursing in corrections requires that safety comes first, followed by therapy and treatment goals. The corrections environment necessitates the active establishment of personal and professional boundaries. Nurses must understand how to interact with custody and inmates to accomplish therapeutic goals while remaining ever vigilant for personal safety. Correctional nurses advocate for the vulnerable inmate-patient in the midst of an unforgiving and sometimes punitive environment. This requires developing a professional nursing practice that guards the safety of both the nurse and the patient.

Workplace violence is not new to nursing or particular to correctional nursing. It is, however, on the rise and of increasing concern (Gates, Gillespie, & Succop, 2011). Nurses in all specialty areas must guard their personal safety while providing direct patient care. Little data are available on the violence potential in correctional nursing. Other specialties such as emergency, long-term care, and psychiatric nursing report significant levels of physical and verbal abuse by patients (Jacobson, 2007; Pich et al., 2010).

Many of the safety principles recommended for traditional health care facilities (Joint Commission, 2010) are standard procedure in the correctional environment. Controlled access to facilities, scanning for weapons, and inspecting bags are a part of correctional security practices, as are conducting employee and staff background checks. Most correctional facility orientation programs include training in personal safety, facility safety processes, and staff responses to potentially unsafe situations. Nurses must continually guard personal safety and avoid complacency while working in the corrections environment.

From the Experts ...

"In 2010, an inmate arrested for simple burglary, with no prior arrests, killed one of our nurses in booking. Several other nurses and deputies had interacted with this man and no one saw this act of violence coming. A loose item on a desk was all it took. Looking at staff and inmate safety proactively, intentionally, and systematically must be everyone's responsibility."

Katherine Heinen, RN, MS
Martinez, CA

STAFF SAFETY
Safety First

Nurses starting in this specialty come from many practice settings, but few have been oriented to consider personal safety as primary to patient needs. Even in an emergency situation, the environment must be secured before focus can be directed to delivering life-saving treatment. In many ways, a correctional setting mirrors an in-combat military setting from a safety perspective. A primary role of corrections officers is to keep staff and inmates safe from physical harm. Unfortunately, nurses often receive very little education on personal safety during initial nursing education. Concern for personal safety must be a top priority when working in the corrections environment.

Personal Safety

Correctional nurses should always be vigilant for personal safety and comply with facility security procedures. Nurses use all senses, in particular sight and hearing, when monitoring personal security.

Visually scan a work area or travel route within the facility for signs of safety threat. It is optimum to be within sight of a security officer who is monitoring the area. If required to travel in "blind spot" areas of the facility, a video monitor or mirror should allow for visibility around a corner or secluded area. Do not move into any area in the facility that is not able to be visually scanned prior to entry.

Hearing is also an important sense to have on alert while working in the corrections environment. A sound alarm is a simple and effective security alert. Voice is the most basic mechanism to sound alarm. Always monitor distance to the next security point or custody officer. Be sure your voice will carry to that distance. Certain security codes may be activated to indicate a personal threat. Personal or body alarm devices have also become popular and come in a variety of sizes and formats.

Consider using the "sixth sense" when monitoring personal safety while on duty in a correctional facility. If a situation does not "feel" right, leave immediately or request additional resources. Cues to personal safety threat can be subtle and defy verbalization. Work through the issue rather than trying to overcome the fear. Be vigilant at all times. Each nurse has a responsibility to monitor personal safety and activate safety procedure when there are indications of jeopardy.

Physical countenance can aid safety. Walk in a controlled and confident manner. This establishes personal presence and reduces vulnerability. Ask for an escort or walk in teams if the destination is unfamiliar. There is safety in numbers. Nurses who must travel into less secure areas should be escorted by an officer or at least move within the facility with a second staff member. Work with custody to determine an optimum transit schedule for regular duties such as satellite medication administration or sick call locations outside the primary medical unit. In addition, always let others in the medical unit know a destination and expected return. Fellow staff should always know the whereabouts of other staff members.

From the Experts . . .

"I always tell my staff, as their manager I am personally responsible for their safety and their return home to their family at the end of the day. We cannot lose focus on where we work. It is important to let someone know where you are at all times or when leaving the building."

Carolyn Cook, RN, CCHP
Birmingham, AL

Consideration should be given to apparel choices when working in a correctional environment. In a predominantly young male environment, visual cues based on dress or demeanor can be misunderstood. Always dress modestly and functionally. Most correctional facilities have dress codes to guide clothing selection. Avoid necklaces (choking threat) and pins (can be used as a sharp). Do not wear sleeveless or low-necked tops. Choose loose-fitting, low-keyed outfits. Some facilities ban colors that are similar to inmate dress, such as khaki and denim.

Environmental Safety

Several components of the correctional environment maintain staff and inmate safety. Recently built facilities incorporate design features to maximize visibility in housing, treatment, and outdoor areas. In addition, visibility may be enhanced by mirrors, cameras, watch stations, and towers. Visual monitoring is supported by wall alarms in some settings.

Arrange exam rooms to prevent entrapment of staff members (OSHA, 2004). The inmate-patient should not come between the staff member and the room exit. Only needed equipment should be accessible. Storage units in patient areas should be locked and keys secured with staff members. Patients should not be left unattended in rooms or have access to equipment. This is especially true with dental equipment, which involves many sharps.

Security Policies and Procedures

As part of the security community, correctional nurses also follow safety policy and procedures developed by facility management. Most sites orient new nurses to these procedures and expect careful attention to all security processes. Nurse adherence to security processes affects not only individual safety, but also safety of all staff members and inmates.

Know the security codes used for staff violence. A code number or color may be used to indicate the need for a rapid response in an area of the facility. This code may be initiated by contact with a corrections officer, wall alarm, or hand-held communication device. Make it standard practice to know the safety response process and how to activate it from any location or transit route.

Security Checkpoints

Abide by all security procedures, including checking in with officers at established checkpoints entering and within the facility. Most facilities have an identification check at the entrance and a log-in process. Whether manual or electronic, the log-in/log-out process is a safety mechanism. Should a security issue arise, the command center needs to know the location of all staff members to provide for safe exit. Although rare, disasters or hostage situations require accounting for all individuals and planning for removal and treatment.

Confidential Information

Correctional nurses may be privy to information about security procedures such as scheduled cell searches or inmate pat-downs. Never share this information with patients or discuss them with colleagues in an inmate's presence. These security procedures must remain unannounced for maximum security benefit.

   Also keep personal information confidential. Do not disclose information about life, family, or personal schedule with or in front of inmates. Limit socializing to secure areas such as a staff lounge or locked nurses' station.

Contraband

Minimization and removal of contraband is a key environmental safety component. Even with strict entry searches, weapons, drugs, and cell phones frequently enter the facility, causing a safety hazard. Many common personal care items can be crafted into effective weapons. Officers will regularly perform sweeps of housing units to confiscate these items. Nurses assist in maintaining personal safety by alert attention and reporting of any observed contraband.

Medical Contraband

Many everyday items used in the delivery of health care can be turned into a weapon or bring a high price on the prison black market. Careful security of medications and health care instruments is paramount to maintaining a safe environment. A standard system for counting, and controlling all sharps such as syringes, needles, dental instruments and even finger-stick lancets should be maintained. Medications and sharps are attended at all times or locked away from sight and patient access. Even simple items such as alcohol wipes and paper clips can be misused in the wrong hands. Inmates may attempt to obtain these items from new staff members and then use this act as blackmail to obtain other, more serious items.

Key Control

A variety of keys are required to provide health care in a secure setting. All care delivery areas should have locked access. In addition, higher risk areas and materials will involve further key access. Narcotics and sharps are traditionally secured with a second key. Unit procedures should establish the whereabouts of security keys. Keys should not be left in plain sight or unattended in unlocked drawers.

Access Control

Limit inmate access to public rooms and hallways. If possible, have separate patient and staff rest rooms. Keep offices and supply rooms locked at all times. Do not allow inmate workers into locked areas without an escort. Use heightened awareness when in inmate-accessible rooms. Follow personal safety procedures in these areas.

PROFESSIONAL BOUNDARIES

A professional boundary is an important concept for both nurse and patient safety. Professional boundaries frame the scope of nursing practice. Correctional nurses, like those in long-term or disability care settings, may provide nursing services to a community of patients over an extended period of time. The frequency of day-to-day contact can lead to overfamiliarity, which may jeopardize staff safety. In addition, small county facilities and those in rural settings have increased likelihood of prior personal relationship between nurse and inmate-patient. This may lead to a blurring of the professional boundary and jeopardized safety. An understanding of professional boundaries leads to a safe and healthy framework of practice in a vulnerable clinical setting like corrections.

Professional boundaries in traditional practice settings focus on "the space between the nurse's power and the client's vulnerability" (p. 3) (NCSBN, 1998). While this is also true in corrections, an added factor emerges with the higher potential for manipulation with inmate patient populations. That segment of the patient population pursuing medical services for secondary gain could encourage a breach in professional boundaries where the nurse is in the vulnerable position. Staying within the Zone of Helpfulness will reduce the likelihood of professional boundary breach in correctional nursing practice (Figure 4.1).

Setting professional boundaries allows for a safe connection between the nurse and the patient based on the patient's health needs rather than any personal needs or motives of either party (Holder & Schenthal, 2007). Consider each patient encounter in the correctional setting from the perspective of therapeutic relationship. The goal of any contact is the advancement of health and reduction of illness for the patient. Boundary violations emerge when other goals are consciously or unconsciously pursued in the nurse–patient interaction. Certain behaviors are common to boundary violations (Exhibit 4.1). Watch for these signs in personal practice and the practice of care team colleagues.

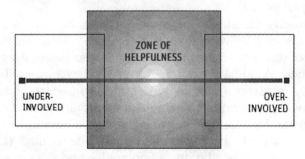

Every nurse-client relationship can be plotted on the continuum of professional behavior illustrated above.

FIGURE 4.1 Continuum of professional behavior.

Source: From National Council of State Boards of Nursing (1998, p. 4). Used with permission.

EXHIBIT 4.1
Signs of Boundary Violations

- Role reversal
- Secrecy
- Double binds
- Personal benefit rather than patient benefit in an encounter

Source: Adapted from Holder and Schenthal (2007).

When viewed from the perspective of staff and patient safety, it is the responsibility of every nurse to monitor personal and colleague adherence to professional practice boundaries. Continual awareness, cognizance of individual feelings and behaviors, observance of other professional behaviors, and always acting in the best interest of the patient are classic guiding principles advocated by the National Council of State Boards of Nursing (1998).

Patient

An understanding of the unique sociologic characteristics of the inmate-patient population can assist in guarding against professional boundary violations. Although some inmate-patients are honest and transparent in their interactions with staff members, a significant number have habituated manipulative and dishonest behaviors in their dealings in the world. Correctional nurses must develop skills to therapeutically interact with the patient population while guarding their personal and professional safety. Continuous validation of inmate statements about their health condition, their situation within the facility, and their personal medical history is important in delivering effective nursing care.

Manipulation

Inmate manipulation processes are well documented in the corrections professional literature. Although nurses have a different relationship to the inmate population than custody officers, awareness of these principles increases staff safety in the medical unit. For example, career criminals have perfected lying and other manipulative behaviors. They may lack remorse and can be very clever even if not well educated. Some of their interactions will be attempts to gain advantage in the health care relationship (Cornelius, 2009).

The manipulative inmate is a patient observer of human nature; looking for a vulnerable victim among officers and staff alike. He or she is willing to spend a significant amount of time observing and testing a victim before drawing them into a dangerous situation. Personal characteristics that indicate a possible victim can be observed in body language. A nurse who appears insecure, indecisive, nervous, weak, or with low self-esteem is vulnerable to manipulation and can fall prey to a manipulative inmate. In addition, staff members who appear complacent in their job duties may be able to be manipulated and blackmailed (Cornelius, 2009). Inmates target staff members who dress sloppy, sleep on duty, watch television, or take part in other inappropriate activities during work hours.

The manipulative inmate is also a good listener. Complacent staff share personal information while on duty. This personal information can be used by the inmate to gain trust, establish a personal relationship, and exploit a weakness in future interactions. Care must be taken to eliminate personal information from conversations with and around inmates. Rapport is better established by discussing impersonal but casual topics such as sports or movies with inmate-patients.

Once a target is selected from among staff members, the manipulative inmate begins to test the staff victim in small ways leading to a "turnout" where the staff member is cornered and blackmailed into taking actions at the inmate's bidding (Cornelius, 2009). The testing can be very subtle and staff members are often unaware of what is going on, convinced that the inmate is what he says he is and is being helpful and agreeable as a patient. Table 4.1 outlines the usual progression of an inmate manipulation. Correctional nurses must be ever vigilant of the potential for manipulation while remaining therapeutic in the nurse–patient relationship. Case Example 4.1 provides opportunity to apply this information.

CASE EXAMPLE 4.1

An inmate tells the nurse in sick call that he needs tramidol for his back pain and this is the only medication that will work. The nurse has been working in the medical unit for 6 weeks and this is her third encounter with this inmate. He leans closer to her and whispers, "You are the only nurse that really gives a damn around here. I know you will help me with this. I can't stand this pain much longer." What is the best response and actions for the nurse to take?

Inmate Anger

Another area of staff safety concern is the angry outburst of a patient pushed beyond his capacity for self-control. Anger management is often lacking in this patient community and correctional nurses must guard against potential violence from this source.

The best action is to prevent anger from escalating to violence. The nurse's demeanor in a nurse–patient interaction can diffuse potential anger from developing. Classic de-escalation techniques involve communication and interpersonal skills (Nau, Halfens, Needham, & Dassen, 2009). Correctional nurses balance the needs to appear and act assertive while not presenting an overly aggressive or overly servile demeanor. Table 4.2 presents the continuum of personal presentation with optimum de-escalation factors balanced between the extremes.

Several anger de-escalation techniques have been described for nurses dealing with angry and potentially violent patients (Exhibit 4.2). Extra personal space, double the usual handshake distance, is recommended both for calming the patient and providing a safety buffer for the nurse. Listening is an action that can reduce anger. Speech content and tone also affect degree of situation de-escalation. Responding to the concerns of the individual through mutual negotiation and shared problem solving can assist in a situation involving a rational patient (Cowen et al., 2003). In all cases, engage the assistance of available corrections officers if the patient is irrational and continues to be agitated or shows any signs of physical violence.

Care Team

Professional boundaries should also be considered when working within a care team. In this sphere, boundaries must be understood as they relate to scope of practice of team members. Both licensed and unlicensed staff are bound by the particulars of their job descriptions as to the functions and responsibilities to each other and to

TABLE 4.1   Inmate Manipulation Techniques

TECHNIQUE	DESCRIPTION	EXAMPLES	PREVENTION
Staff friendship	Patient personalizes comments and actions.	"You are the best nurse in this place." "I'm cleaning this floor especially for you." "You are the only one who cares."	Do not respond in kind. Do not accept personal conversation, touching, or offers of assistance. Tell the patient directly to stop and report actions according to facility policy.
Peer group alienation	Establishes a we -vs-them situation. Suggests rumors being spread by other staff members.	"How can the charge nurse say those things about you?" "I told the night shift nurse to stop complaining about you. You are a good nurse."	Disregard or validate any statement made by a patient about what another staff member said. Do not allow patients to divide staff. Keep in communication and on the same team.
Request for help	Request for sympathy in inmate's plight and help beyond standard nurse actions.	"Only you can help me with this issue." "I need to call my wife; she is sick with cancer and needs your help."	Stay within professional boundary of nursing action. Redirect patient to standard corrections policy. Be firm, fair, and consistent in responses to inmate requests.
Nudging	Testing by the inmate to see how far a staff member will deviate from rules. Usually minor in nature.	An "accidental" touching of a female breast. A request for a trivial item such as an alcohol wipe or rubber band.	Respond to even minor infractions according to facility policy. Do not allow deviation from even the smallest rules.
Turnout	Inmate uses previous relationship and "bending of rules" as leverage to pressure staff to more serious actions such as delivering contraband, sexual activity, or overlooking criminal actions in the facility.	"If you don't schedule my medical visit the same time as my friend in B block I'll have to tell about our secret touching in the exam room."	Even at this late time, turn the tables and report the activity. Do not go further into the situation. Get help from administration or management.

Source: Adapted from Cornelius (2009).

the patient population. In addition, licensed professionals must practice within the boundaries of their licensure and scope of practice. In the low-resource field of correctional health care, professionals may be challenged to stay within that scope in the demands of delivering both day-to-day and emergent health care behind bars.

TABLE 4.2 Aggressive, De-Escalating, and Servile Attitudes and Behaviors

TOPIC	AGGRESSIVE	DE-ESCALATING	SERVILE
Behavior toward the patient	Arrogant	Valuing the client	Servile
Dealing with the patient's concerns	Making the patient insecure	Reducing fear	Making unrealistic promises
Attempting to understand	Indifferent to causes of aggression	Enquiring about patient's queries and anxiety	Not communicating about causes
Degree of assertiveness	Commanding	Providing guidance to the patient	Intimidated
Style of negotiation	Uncompromising	Working out possible agreements	Making unreasonable concessions
Degree of composure	Acting hectically	Remaining calm	Feeling offended
Proportion of safety	Risky	Securing own safety	Overcautious

Source: Adapted from Nau, Halfens, Needham, and Dassen (2009).

EXHIBIT 4.2
De-Escalating Techniques

- A relaxed and comfortable stance
- Adequate personal space
- Calm, quiet, and slower speech
- Active listening
- Clarifying and reflecting on cause of anger
- Negotiation and shared problem solving
- Positive affirmation

Source: Adapted from Cowen et al. (2003).

Although nurses working in a traditional setting have many safeguards for their practice scope, such as management and educator support and like-profession leadership, correctional nurses are not always as fortunate. Some correctional nurses report directly to correctional managers who may not understand the varying scopes of practice for physicians, dentists, nurse practitioners, registered nurses, and licensed practical nurses. A correctional nurse can be asked to perform a task or make a diagnostic decision that is beyond the scope of practice for the licensure status in that state. This jeopardizes patient safety and the nurse's continued licensure. All team members must fully understand the scope of practice for each type of care provider. Written job descriptions delineating responsibilities within each respective professional's scope of practice also help maintain patient safety.

Corrections Staff

As mentioned earlier, corrections staff and management need a solid understanding of the nursing scope of practice so as not to make requests for or expect service provisions beyond safe practice. This can be particularly difficult when correctional officers misunderstand the ramifications of such tasks as medical review for escalating force. Nurses reviewing a medical record for any condition making pepper spray or a restraint chair contraindicated are not diagnosing mental or physical illness nor are they approving use of force. Clear written policies that spell out nurse actions and interventions in custody operations are vital.

Another boundary concern when working with correctional staff is the clear delineation of health care from custody. Nurses cannot occupy both roles within an inmate community. Nurses are care providers and not control enforcers. Provision of patient care is jeopardized when inmates view nurses taking custody actions in their role as a nurse. Correctional nurses engage custody officers to maintain control and deal with corrective actions with the inmate population.

Response to a Violent Incident

Enact staff debriefing and counseling should the unthinkable happen and a staff assault take place. Violence in the workplace leads to negative stress, decreased work productivity, and decreased quality of patient care (Gates, Gillespie, & Succop, 2011). In addition, fear of future assault and posttraumatic stress disorder can have a longstanding impact on staff who have sustained or witness a physical or verbal attack (Gerberich et al., 2004). A leave of absence or position reassignment may be needed following a violent incident.

PATIENT SAFETY

Patient safety has been a hallmark of nursing practice since the beginnings of the profession. It is a defining characteristic of professional practice. The safety thread is woven throughout the standards of correctional nursing practice (ANA, 2007). Although always foundational to correctional health care accreditation processes, more explicit reference to patient safety has only been identified recently (NCCHC, 2008). This trend is reflective of the patient safety movement in traditional health care settings. A recent study indicates nearly 80,000 annual preventable deaths (Reed & May, 2011). While death estimates are made based on traditional settings, it is safe to say that medical error leads to significant mortality and morbidity in the correctional setting, as well. Correctional nurses are positioned to make improvements to patient care that can reduce the risk of patient harm.

An expert panel was convened to apply patient safety principles to the correctional health care setting (Stern, Griefinger, & Mellow, 2010). Proposed standards for patient safety were developed based on guidelines already published by nationally recognized safety groups such as the Agency for Healthcare Research and Quality (AHRQ), Centers for Disease Control and Prevention (CDC), Healthcare Effectiveness Data and Information Set (HEDIS), National Commission on Correctional Health Care (NCCHC), and the Physician Practice Patient Safety Assessment (PPPSA). Ongoing revisions and refinements to these published standards are based on input from practitioners in the field when the proposed standards have been presented at national meetings. The most recent list of primary patient safety standards for correctional settings was provided by the primary facilitators of the group and is shown in Table 4.3. These proposed standards provide a foundation for building a solid patient safety program. Correctional nurses are involved in the

TABLE 4.3 Proposed Standards for Patient Safety in Prisons

PROPOSED STANDARDS FOR PATIENT SAFETY IN PRISONS	
SHORT TITLE	**PROPOSED SAFETY MEASURE**
Access to and Availability of Care	
Access to prenatal care	Pregnant female patients receive prenatal care within first trimester or within 14 days of incarceration.
Access to postpartum care	Postpartum female patients receive care within 7 weeks of delivery. Absent specific indicators for sooner follow up.
Culture of Safety	
Culture of safety from the top	Practice has a written statement in appropriate governing document emphasizing patient safety as a priority.
Active safety leadership by chief pharmacist and chief nurse	Chief pharmacist and chief nurse have active role on administrative leadership team and are accountable for medication management systems performance and patient safety related to nursing, respectively.
Preventable adverse event reporting	System is in place for reporting of all preventable adverse events (events in which a preventable error led to patient harm). Examples include (but are not limited to) patient receiving wrong medication resulting in an adverse reaction; development of a pressure sore in an infirmary patient; invasive procedure performed on wrong patient; patient sustaining a preventable fall.
Action taken on all reported errors (preventable adverse events and near misses)	System is in place to analyze and address all reported errors.
Shift from employee remediation to system improvement	System is in place to assure that when a preventable adverse event is discovered, practice addresses it in a framework (e.g., Just Culture) that seeks first to discover and fix what is wrong not who is wrong; punishment is reserved for instances of individual willfulness neglect. System includes appropriate policies, staff training, and executive monitoring of staff sanctions.
Grievance response and review	All health care grievances, formal and informal, are addressed by health care personnel. System is in place to analyze and address system issues.
Personnel	
Staff trained on patient safety	Human factors and key principles of error reduction (e.g., standardization, use of constraints, redundancy) are reviewed with all health staff during orientation and during each performance evaluation.
Patient safety is everyone's job	Organization has written statements in the documents appropriate to that organization (e.g., governing documents, mission statement, ethics statement, job description, post orders) reflecting, for both health and custody personnel, each staff member's responsibility in patient safety, including roles in team, error reporting, etc.

(continued)

TABLE 4.3 *(continued)*

PROPOSED STANDARDS FOR PATIENT SAFETY IN PRISONS	
SHORT TITLE	**PROPOSED SAFETY MEASURE**
Staff fatigue and burnout	System is in place to monitor unscheduled leave use.
Staff vacancy	System is in place to monitor ease of recruitment and retention statistical data (e.g., turnover rate, vacancy rate, agency use to fill positions).
Adequate nursing staffing	A staffing plan is in place sufficient to safely care for all patients (as measured by achieving goal safety levels).
Annual competency assessment of nonpractitioners	Practice maintains system to annually assess nursing and support staff competency appropriate for services and procedures performed, including devices and associated protocols/ guidelines. Competency is verified before staff is permitted to perform associated care function or train others.
Annual competency assessment of practitioners	Identical to previous standard, but applicable to physicians, nurse practitioners, and physician assistants.
Medication Management	
Up-to-date medication list	Complete medication history (including over-the-counter medications) is obtained and documented on every patient upon: change in medication, change of primary practitioner, or change in level of care (e.g., to and from infirmary or community hospital).
Medication list available	Medication list is available to all professional staff caring for patient at time of care.
Medication references	Up-to-date, standardized medication reference resource is available to all prescribers at the point of prescribing.
Medications in pregnancy	All female patients of childbearing age have documented negative pregnancy test or other notation before medications known to have significant teratogenic risk or contraindicated in pregnancy are prescribed.
Computerized practitioner order entry system	Prison has this system.
Medication properly labeled	All medications kept by patients on their person show patient name and identification number, prescriber, medication name, strength, dose, frequency, number of pills or time frame, lot number, date dispensed, expiration date.
Medication list to patient on release	Patients are provided up-to-date list of all medications they are receiving on release.
Handling of medications for external use	Topical medications (e.g., benzoin, podophylline) are labeled "For External Use Only" and are separated from internal-use medications in all storage areas.

(continued)

TABLE 4.3 *(continued)*

PROPOSED STANDARDS FOR PATIENT SAFETY IN PRISONS	
SHORT TITLE	**PROPOSED SAFETY MEASURE**
Handling of multidose injectables	All opened multiple-dose vials of injectable medications (e.g., lidocaine, dexamethasone, prochlorperazine, vitamin B12) labeled with date opened and include date on which unused product should be discarded (no later than 30 days after opening).
Check expiration dates	All medications, reagents, and other products that expire are routinely checked (at least quarterly) by designated staff member and are appropriately discarded once expired.
Transitions and Communication	
Critical info read back	For verbal or telephone orders or for telephonic reporting of critical test results, communication is verified by having receiving person record and read back completely.
Dangerous abbreviations	Staff may not use abbreviations on list of prohibited abbreviations, acronyms, symbols, and dose designations.
Correct patient name on tests	Standardized policies, processes, and systems are in place to ensure accurate labeling of radiographs, laboratory specimens, and other diagnostic studies, so that the right study is labeled for the right patient at the right time.
Specialist consultation timeliness	Internal and external consultations with specialists (employee or contractor, on-site or off-site) are completed within time frame ordered. Note: if the primary care practitioner modifies date needed, new date determines whether consultation is completed on time.
Specialist consultation followed	Consultant recommendations are followed or a documented clinical rationale from primary care practitioner exists for an alternative, medically appropriate plan of care.
Test and consultation tracking	Tests are tracked (what sent, where, when, when expected back, action taken if results are overdue); when results are received, they are seen by appropriate clinician and posted to medical record. Mechanism exists to report critical results, even in absence of requestor (e.g., vacation, after hours).
Nonmedication reconciliation	Nonmedication information (e.g., allergies, mobility limitations, language or communication limitations, and other disabilities) is reconciled whenever patient transitions from one primary provider or health care setting to another (e.g., infirmary to general population, prison to community, prison to hospital, prison to another prison).
Patient Involvement	
Informed consent	When written informed consent is obtained, it is by a clinician credentialed to order the intervention and contains explanation of risks and alternatives and patient describing back to the clinician key information heard, in one's own words.

(continued)

TABLE 4.3 *(continued)*

PROPOSED STANDARDS FOR PATIENT SAFETY IN PRISONS	
SHORT TITLE	**PROPOSED SAFETY MEASURE**
Informed refusal	Any written refusal of treatment is an informed refusal and is only obtained (at a time interval appropriate to the intervention) by clinicians privileged to order or refer for the intervention. Note: excludes noncritical single refusals of staff-administered medications.
Patient-tailored decisions	Care plans take patient's cultural and social environment (e.g., work, release plan) into account.
Health-adjusted correctional environment	Correctional environment is adjusted to special health needs of inmate (e.g., adding air conditioning).
Interpreters	Interpretation services are available for clinical encounters; interpreters should be qualified/certified; should not be custody staff or other prisoners except in emergencies.
Patient notification of results	Results of tests are communicated to the patient within 2 weeks of receipt; practice confirms and documents that patient received results.
Obtain advance directives	Practitioners seek advance directives for patients admitted to an infirmary who do not already have such directives.
Advance directives available	For those with advance directives, written documentation of patients' preferences are prominently displayed in medical record.
Specific Conditions	
Chronic disease registry	Practice maintains chronic disease registry, either free standing or within an electronic health record.
Access to care after acute mental health problem	During a recent period (can be any relevant period chosen by the system, typically a year), percentage of patients discharged from a prison acute mental health care bed getting follow-up visit with mental health staff within 1 day of discharge.[a]
Hand hygiene	Organization complies with category I recommendations in the CDC's hand hygiene guidelines.
Chronic disease monitoring	The following nationally accepted guidelines are followed for chronic disease management: (1) guidelines published by NCCHC; (2) correctional consensus psychiatric guidelines; (3) all patients receiving certain high-risk medications for ≥ 180 days receive appropriate lab test monitoring annually (or more often if clinically indicated).[b]
Warfarin monitoring	All patients on warfarin are tracked for appropriate International Normalized Ratio levels.
Pressure sore prevention	Written protocols are in place for prevention and management of pressure sores among nonambulatory patients.

(continued)

TABLE 4.3 *(continued)*

PROPOSED STANDARDS FOR PATIENT SAFETY IN PRISONS	
SHORT TITLE	**PROPOSED SAFETY MEASURE**
Pregnancy methadone	Patients admitted who are pregnant and opioid dependent, including those on methadone maintenance, will receive adequate opioid dosing to prevent withdrawal during pregnancy.

[a]The panel chose not to prescribe the threshold percentage that systems should achieve. Rather, at this early point in the use of patient safety standards in corrections, members felt systems should be at liberty to establish their own thresholds. They hoped that over time systems would gradually raise their own threshold or that as this standard was adopted by accreditation or professional organizations, these organizations would set a threshold. [b]For patients taking angiotensin-converting enzyme inhibitors, angiotensin receptor blockers, digoxin, or diuretics, the following are monitored: serum potassium, serum creatinine, and blood urea nitrogen; for patients taking carbamazepine, phenobarbital, phenytoin, or valproic acid, the serum concentration of the drug is monitored.

Source: M. Stern, R. Greifinger, personal communication, November 28, 2011.

assimilation and implementation of all patient safety standards. Several of the themes from the findings of this expert panel, however, are of special concern and bear more attention.

Culture of Safety

A primary component of most patient safety recommendations is the development of a culture of safety. A major challenge to improving patient safety is developing a work culture that overtly encourages and supports reporting of patient care errors and risks. More often a culture of silence exists in health care, and particularly the correctional setting, as practitioners fear punishment, negligence claims, and disciplinary action if an error is reported. In addition, the militaristic framework of correctional administration can lead to institutional ban or immediate dismissal if an error is revealed.

If errors are hidden or ignored, however, opportunities are missed to improve systems and processes and reduce future risk of patient harm. A culture of safety establishes improvement of care systems as the primary goal rather than punitive actions against individuals involved in the error (Morris, 2011). Although individuals may be at fault for errors and patient injury, the investigation of an incident begins with seeking the root causes of the event including, in particular, faulty or nonexistent systems or processes. Individual actions in the error are also investigated but balanced by a primary investigation of system issues. Critical organizational learning develops and care improvements are made when causes of error are investigated in all sectors. Research over the last few decades in traditional health care settings has unveiled several key components of a culture of safety which are listed in Exhibit 4.3.

Transitions and Communication

The oft-mentioned fragmentation of correctional health care services brought on by a challenging delivery setting makes communication among care providers of utmost importance. Communication has been found to be a root cause of a majority of adverse events in acute care settings (The Joint Commission, 2011). Systems must

EXHIBIT 4.3
Dimensions of a Patient Safety Culture

- Information exchange with other settings
- Teamwork
- Work pressure and pace
- Staff training
- Office processes and standardization
- Communication openness
- Patient care tracking/follow up
- Communication about error
- Leadership support for patient safety
- Organizational learning

Source: Adapted from Agency for Healthcare Research and Quality (n.d.).

be in place to standardize communication among team members, across shifts within a facility, and at all hand-off points along the care continuum (Nadzam, 2009).

In addition to standardized systems, attention must be given to the context, format, and delivery of clinical information. Communication is as much how information is delivered as what information is delivered (Nadzam, 2009). Structuring handoff and emergency decision-making conversations to present key information is one method for improvement. SBAR (Situation, Background, Assessment, Recommendation) has been used effectively in many care settings to guide communication and improve delivery of crucial information (Table 4.4).

Attention to nonverbal communication cues can also improve clinical communication. Communication among care professionals that is demeaning, condescending, or contains sexual overtones can decrease effectiveness, putting patient care in jeopardy. In addition, gender and culture impact communication style and format, risking misinterpretation leading to clinical error (Scalise, 2006). Actions that foster collaboration and shared decision-making among team members can improve outcomes and increase patient safety (AACN, 2005).

Finally, initiating communication among care professionals to avert error is a concern when focusing on patient safety. Avoiding an impending error requires intervention. Health care staff are often reluctant to initiate conversation about a potential safety situation. Nurses regularly see fellow staff members cutting corners, making

TABLE 4.4   Elements of SBAR Communication Structure

COMPONENT	COMMUNICATION
Situation	State what is happening at the present time that has warranted the communication
Background	Explain circumstances leading up to this situation. Put the situation into context for the listener
Assessment	Explain the analysis of what the problem is
Recommendation	Provide a recommendation for correction of the problem

Source: Adapted from Haig, Sutton, and Wittington (2006).

mistakes, or exhibiting incompetence; however, most remain silent (Maxfield et al., 2005). Encouraging the initiation of conversations about seven categories of concerns can reduce medical error and improve patient safety (Exhibit 4.4).

EXHIBIT 4.4
Seven Crucial Conversation Topics

- Broken rules
- Mistakes
- Lack of support
- Incompetence
- Poor teamwork
- Disrespect
- Micromanagement

Source: Adapted from Maxfield et al. (2005).

Patient Involvement

Consumer advocacy groups have been vocal for some time about the need for patient involvement in care decisions in the traditional setting (Leape, 2008). Although the correctional health care patient is bound by additional environmental constraints, active patient involvement in the care plan can reduce medical error risk in this setting as well. Full disclosure and patient partnering improves patient compliance and provides additional safeguards against error. An active, involved patient asks questions and validates treatment changes, a particular need in the fast-paced, high turnover world of correctional health care.

To improve safety, explain the plan of care and solicit active participation in the plan with every patient. Patient knowledge of medication actions and side effects is also important. Although exact dates of transports for medical procedures or diagnostic tests cannot be shared for risk of elopement, general timeframes for services encourage patient involvement. Correctional nurses can partner with their patients to improve safety and enhance implementation of the plan of care.

NATIONAL PATIENT SAFETY GOALS: APPLIED TO CORRECTIONS

The Joint Commission established National Patient Safety Goals (NPSGs) in 2002 for a variety of traditional settings. These goals have been revised and refined over the last decade. The goals for the hospital setting have application for correctional health care and will be used to frame a discussion of key patient safety issues for correctional nurses.

Patient Identification and Surgery Mistakes

Correctional nurses interact with large groups of patients over short periods of time when providing mass care such as medication administration or tuberculin skin testing. Inmates in some settings wear similar attire or can have similar sounding names. Pressure to rapidly provide care within the security schedule can lead to patient identification errors. Safety processes are necessary to avoid misidentification through the consistent use of armband or checking the ID card before administration of medication or treatment. NPSG standards require the use of at least two patient identifiers, such as name and birth date, to ensure delivery of correct medications and treatments.

Surgery is infrequently performed in correctional health care but warrants a mention here as it relates to patient identification. Many surgical errors in acute care are traced to misidentification of person or body part. Care must be taken that the right patient is receiving the right procedure in the correctional setting, as well. As more short procedures such as liver biopsy and skin cancer removals become common in ambulatory care settings such as a prison health care unit, identification procedures need to be in place to reduce risk.

Staff Communication

Staff communication, addressed earlier in this chapter, is a continuing theme in patient safety programs. The complex system in which nurses must deliver care, coupled with the wide variety of communication interactions among care providers involving high numbers of patient situations, creates many opportunities for miscommunication. NPSG standards emphasize the importance of getting test results to the right staff member in a timely fashion. Critical value test results must be dealt with immediately. However, the majority of lab tests in correctional settings are completed off-site. Communication with diagnostic facilities is fraught with problems. Labs may not be able to call the health care unit directly. Appropriate staff may be unavailable when needed. Medical staff may be off-site or working at a satellite setting when needed. The Joint Commission (2011) recommends a written standard for communication of critical blood test and diagnostic results. In some settings this may mean a written contract with the laboratory spelling out the steps taken to reach the appropriate medical provider with critical lab value results.

Medication Safety

Medication administration is a time-consuming nursing function in corrections. Time spent in medication administration can exceed time spent in all other nursing activities (Burrow, Knox, & Villanueva, 2006). Indeed, many facilities have designated nurses who spend their entire shift administering medication. Medication that individuals in the general U.S. population would self-administer must be secured in the medical unit and administered by health care staff in a correctional setting. Many medications, including some over-the-counter preparations, have high value in the prison black market and require restricted access for patient and staff safety.

Systems for medication delivery have common elements (Exhibit 4.5). Preventable error can take place at any point in the chain. Current National Patient Safety Goals for safe medication administration focus on communication of medication information and proper labeling. Deaths from medication error are most frequently linked to a wrong dose or wrong drug (AHRQ, 2008). Safe communication and labeling practice can reduce the potential for these errors.

All basic medication safety components of nursing practice are in effect when administering medication in jails and prisons. The safety movement over the last decade has made additions to the classic 5 rights of medication administration. Right

EXHIBIT 4.5
Medication Distribution System Elements

- Prescribing
- Order communication
- Product labeling, packaging, and nomenclature
- Compounding
- Dispensing
- Distribution
- Administration
- Patient education
- Monitoring outcome

Source: Adapted from AHRQ (2008).

patient, medication, dose, route, and time have been given three more components (Exhibit 4.6). By including a need for correct documentation, reason, and response to the medication, nurses can decrease the risk of medication error.

The Institute for Healthcare Improvement (IHI) disseminates a wide variety of best practices regarding key patient safety risks in medication delivery systems.

EXHIBIT 4.6
The Eight Rights of Medication Administration

1. Right patient
   - Check the name on the order and the patient.
   - Use two identifiers.
   - Ask patient to identify himself/herself.
   - When available, use technology (e.g., bar-code system).
2. Right medication
   - Check the medication label.
   - Check the order.
3. Right dose
   - Check the order.
   - Confirm appropriateness of the dose using a current drug reference.
   - If necessary, calculate the dose and have another nurse calculate the dose as well.
4. Right route
   - Again, check the order and appropriateness of the route ordered.
   - Confirm that the patient can take or receive the medication by the ordered route.
5. Right time
   - Check the frequency of the ordered medication.
   - Double-check that you are giving the ordered dose at the correct time.
   - Confirm when the last dose was given.

(continued)

EXHIBIT 4.6 *(continued)*

6. Right documentation
   - Document administration AFTER giving the ordered medication.
   - Chart the time, route, and any other specific information as necessary. For example, the site of an injection or any laboratory value or vital sign that needed to be checked before giving the drug.
7. Right reason
   - Confirm the rationale for the ordered medication. What is the patient's history? Why is one taking this medication?
   - Revisit the reasons for long-term medication use.
8. Right response
   - Make sure that the drug led to the desired effect. If an antihypertensive was given, has one's blood pressure improved? Does the patient verbalize improvement in depression while on an antidepressant?
   - Be sure to document your monitoring of the patient and any other nursing interventions that are applicable.

Source: From Bonsall (2011), used with permission.

These practices will be discussed as they relate to three key medication delivery processes in corrections—direct observation, self-administration, and pre-pour medication administration.

Medication Delivery Models

Directly administering prescribed medications to patients is the primary method for medication administration in correctional facilities. This process may be termed direct observation therapy (DOT), Watch-Take, medication (med) line or pill line. Medications are administered in a common area such as from a medication cart or medication room. General population inmates come to or are escorted to this location and present themselves to the nurse one-by-one to receive a single dose of prescribed medication. The patient is identified, medications poured and delivered, and the patient is viewed swallowing the medication. A mouth check is performed, usually by a corrections officer, to affirm the medication was swallowed. Health care staff are concerned that the prescribed medication regimen is maintained, while, custody staff are concerned that medication is not being hoarded for other purposes such as black market commerce or self-harm.

Med lines in large institutions can be very time consuming and may involve several staff members. Every effort should be made to reduce the potential for medication error in the structuring of the delivery system. Medication records and medication cards and bottles are most often kept in alphabetical order by patient name and drug name to speed location and accuracy. Strict maintenance of an efficient ordering of records and medications decreases the risk of administering a wrong medication.

Patient identification is also an important component of safe medication administration. All patients should present themselves with a form of identification that corresponds to the medication record. Picture identification is the most secure method but may not be possible, especially in the jail setting where inmate turnover is frequent. Most safety standards recommend two forms of identification (The Joint

Commission, 2011). This may consist of an institution identifier number and full name or birth date.

Other safety mechanisms are recommended by Institute of Healthcare Improvement (n.d.) include having allergy information at the site of administration and a medication reference available. Pharmaceutical advances and treatment protocols change quickly. Nurses cannot rely on their prior education and experience to keep current in this area of practice. In addition, having dose calculation aids available is also an important safety mechanism. While having the information directly on the drug label is most advantageous, writing calculation information directly on the medication administration record (MAR) or on the medication blister pack is also an option.

Pharmacy services can have a great effect on the safety of medication administration in corrections. Nurses do not always have input into the selection of pharmaceutical service providers. Recommended safety mechanisms of interest when making provider decisions include providing pharmacy-based dosing so that nurses are only rarely required to make on-site dose calculations such as partial pills or pouring doses of liquid medication. The IHI (n.d.) also recommends the use of pretyped medication records, orders, and flowsheets. These can be provided by an appropriately equipped pharmaceutical service. Most frequently, medications are provided by pharmacy services in 30-dose blister-pack cards with drug information and the patient's identifiers affixed. Efforts to increase the lettering size of medication name and patient name can assist in correct medication storage and delivery.

Because most correctional facilities do not have on-site pharmacy services, many maintain a supply of stock medications to allow initiation of certain medication regimens while awaiting order fulfillment. In addition, a back-up pharmacy should be available for the emergent delivery of the rare medication that is needed but not in stock.

A stock medication system can be a patient safety risk if not carefully maintained according to safety principles. The types and amounts of medications in stock should be kept to a minimum. This reduces security risk and chances for misuse. A large stock of medication requires additional staff time in maintaining supplies and checking expirations. Added expense incurrs when large supplies of unused medication expire before needed. The IHI (n.d.) also recommends that various strengths of medication availability be avoided. A variety of strengths of a single medication in stock can lead to dose errors in administration. Drugs that look or sound alike should be separated and clearly labeled with the name. Some units underline the differences in the name to emphasize the differences for staff when selecting medication for administration.

Removing any discontinued medication immediately also decreases the risk of medication error. Nurses have been known to hoard medications in the mistaken belief that this practice can speed medication delivery during challenging times such as weekend, nights, and holidays. However, the use of medications ordered for one patient for the treatment of another can be considered medication dispensing and not within the scope of nursing practice (Burrow, Knox, & Villanueva, 2006).

Inmate-patients may also self-administer medication, either in a nurse-supervised setting, such as insulin administration, or unsupervised when given keep-on-person (KOP) medications. Each facility determines which medications are safe for inmates to carry with them based on the population characteristics and past experience. The need for consistent administration may also be taken into account when determining which medications can be self-administered medication. For example, tuberculosis medication administration is rarely left to the discretion of the patient, as consistent dosing over a long period of time is necessary for maximum effect.

Involving the patient in administering his or her own medications can improve patient safety and assist with developing independent health habits. Patient education on drug and food interactions is important, as is information about medication effects and side effects. Confirm that the patient understands conditions that require medical attention and the process for obtaining more medication when the supply is dwindling. In many correctional facilities keep-on-person medication is provided for a 30-day period and must be reordered prior to the last dose to allow for shipment time. Systems need to be in place to monitor reordering of these medications. In addition, correctional staff need a system for regularly monitoring use of KOP medications in the inmate population. KOP medication should be patient-specific and only found with the patient for which it is ordered. Random checks of self-administration can be performed by having selected patients bring their KOP medications to a nursing sick call or clinic line to determine if the medication is being self-administered properly. Too little or too much medication left on a blister card during the check may indicate that the patient would benefit from education and counseling regarding inappropriate use or noncompliance.

The most risky method of medication administration is to pre-pour individual patient medication into cups or envelopes for later administration. Every effort should be made to avoid this risky practice. Many of the usual safeguards in a standard medication administration process are circumvented by setting up medications in advance of administration. Several situations in a correctional facility may compel nursing staff to pre-pour medications. The most likely scenario is the need to administer medications cell-side without sufficient time or the ability to transport medications in an administration cart sometimes seen in segregation units. In addition, periods of facility lock down may present unusual circumstances that must be handled so a pre-pour method is used during the emergency as safely as possible.

When pre-pouring medications is necessary, carefully evaluate the situation and creatively seek solutions that maintain patient safety principles. Of primary importance is the need to have the same nurse prepare and administer the medications. Nurses should not administer medications prepared by another. In addition, prepare medications immediately before administration. Medications should not be prepared hours before administration and definitely not prepared by one shift to be administered by another. Best practices in safe medication administration (IHI, n.d.) indicate that drugs should be labeled once they are out of original containers and a double-check process should be in place for particularly risky medications such as narcotics, insulin, and anticoagulants. Pre-pour medication administration is a particularly good time to involve patients in the medication check process. Compliant patients can be asked to validate that they are receiving the medication they are expecting. If a patient questions the medication being given, a double check of order and/or medication record is warranted.

Nurses frequently involved in medication administration have an opportunity for regular interaction with a large portion of the inmate community. Although interaction is brief, observations about health status, medication therapeutic effects, and side effects can be made. A therapeutic relationship, developed over time, allows a nurse administering medication to become the vanguard of the health care unit in the inmate community. Nurses can recommend that inmates initiate a sick call appointment or make note of potential inmate medical needs to communicate to other health care team members. In this way, intervention can take place before a regular chronic care appointment if conditions warrant, thus providing a safety buffer. Case Example 4.2 provides an opportunity to apply this information.

CASE EXAMPLE 4.2

A maximum security prison has been locked down for two days due to an outbreak of gang violence in the yard. Nurses must pass medications cell-side, as there is no inmate movement. Access to tiers is by narrow stairway and many hallways do not accommodate medication carts. Extra nurses are scheduled to deal with time-consuming cell-side mediation passes. What are your thoughts about how to increase efficiency and maintain timely administration during the lockdown? What patient safety principles are maintained with your approach? Are any of these principles breached?

SUMMARY

Safety is a primary objective in correctional nursing practice. Vigilance is continually needed for personal safety and the safety of the work team and patients. Unlike traditional care settings, nurses working in jails and prisons must first confirm that the environment is safe before rendering nursing care, even when emergency treatment is necessary. This requires a paradigm shift in response practices. Patient safety is also a major component of correctional nursing care. No other team member has greater opportunity to impact patient safety in this setting. Patient safety principles established for traditional care settings applied to the correctional environment can significantly reduce the chances for error and patient harm.

DISCUSSION QUESTIONS

1. Describe the personal safety principles that are in place in your work setting. What additional mechanisms could be added?
2. Share two possible professional boundary violations specific to your correctional work setting. How should nurses handle these situations?
3. List medication administration safety-risk points based on your current delivery system. Suggest ways to improve patient safety during this process.

REFERENCES

Agency for Healthcare Research and Quality (AHRQ). (2008). *Patient safety and quality: An evidence-based handbook for nurses.* AHRQ Publication No. 08-0043. Agency for Healthcare Research and Quality, Rockville, MD. Retrieved from http://www.ahrq.gov/qual/nurseshdbk

Agency for Healthcare Research and Quality (AHRQ). (n.d.) *Medical office survey on patient safety culture: Items and dimensions.* Retrieved from http://www.ahrq.gov/qual/mosurvey08/medoffitems.pdf

American Association of Critical Care Nurses (AACN). (2005). *Standards for the establishing and sustaining of healthy work environments*. Retrieved from http://www.aacn.org/WD/HWE/Docs/HWEStandards.pdf

American Nurses Association (ANA). (2007). *Corrections nursing: Scope & standards of practice*. Silver Spring, MD: Author.

Bonsall, L. M. (2011). *8 rights of medication administration*. Retrieved November 4, 2011, from www.nursingcenter.com/Blog/post/2011/05/27/8-rights-of-medication-administration.aspx

Burrow, G. F., Knox, C. M., & Villanueva, H. (2006). Chapter 29: Nursing in the primary care setting. In M. Puesis (Ed.), *Clinical practice in correctional medicine* (2nd ed.). St. Louis, MO: Mosby Elsevier.

Cornelius, G. (2009). *The art of the con: Avoiding offender manipulation* (2nd ed.). Alexandria, VA: American Correctional Association.

Cowen, L., Davies, R., Estall, G., Berlin, T., Fitzgerald, M., & Hoot, S. (2003). De-escalating aggression and violence in the mental health setting. *International Journal of Mental Health Nursing, 12*, 64–73.

Gates, D. M., Gillespie, G. L., & Succop, P. (2011). Violence against nurses and its impact on stress and productivity. *Nursing Economics, 29*(2), 59–67.

Gerberich, S. G., Church, T. R., McGovern, P. M., Hansen, H. E., Nachriener, N. M., Geisser, M. S. et al. (2004). An epidemiological study of the magnitude and consequences of work related violence: The Minnesota Nurses' Study. *Occupational and Environmental Medicine, 61*(6), 495–503.

Haig, K. M., Sutton, S., & Whittington, J. (2006). SBAR: A shared mental model for improving communication between clinicians. *Journal on Quality and Patient Safety, 32*(3), 167–175.

Holder, K., & Schenthal, S. (2007). Watch your step: Nursing and professional boundaries. *Nursing Management, 38*(2), 24–30.

Institute for Healthcare Improvement (IHI). (n.d.). *Improve core processes for administering medications*. Retrieved July 18, 2011, from http://www.ihi.org/knowledge/Pages/Changes/ImproveCoreProcessesforAdministeringMedications.aspx

Jacobson, J. (2007). ANJ reports: Violence and nursing. *American Journal of Nursing, 107*(2), 25–26.

Leape, L. L. (2008). Scope of problem and history of patient safety. *Obstetrics and Gynecology Clinics of North America, 35*, 1–10.

Maxfield, D., Grenny, J., McMillan, R., & Patterson, K. (2005). *Silence kills: The seven crucial conversations for healthcare*. Retrieved from http://www.silenttreatmentstudy.com/silencekills/SilenceKills.pdf

Morris, S. (2011). Just culture—Changing the environment of healthcare delivery. *Clinical Laboratory Science, 24*(2), 120–124.

Nadzam, D. M. (2009). Nurses' role in communication and patient safety. *Journal of Nursing Care Quality, 24*(3), 184–188. Retrieved from: http://www.jcrinc.com/Learning-Community-Nadzam-Deborah

National Commission on Correctional Health Care (NCCHC). (2008). *Standards for health services in prisons*. Chicago, IL: Author.

National Council of State Boards of Nursing (NCSBN). (1998). *Professional boundaries: A nurse's guide to the importance of appropriate professional boundaries*. Chicago, IL: NCSBN. Retrieved from https://www.ncsbn.org/ProfessionalBoundariesbrochure.pdf

Nau, J., Halfens, R., Needham, I., & Dassen, T. (2009). The de-escalating aggressive behavior scale: Development and psychometric testing. *Journal of Advanced Nursing, 65*(4), 1956–1964.

Occupational Safety and Health Administration. (2004). *Guidelines for preventing workplace violence for health care & social service workers*. Retrieved from http://www.osha.gov/Publications/OSHA3148/osha3148.html

Pich, J., Hazelton, M., Sundin, D., & Kable, A. (2010). Patient-related violence against emergency department nurses. *Nursing and Health Science, 12*(2), 268–274. Doi: 10.11/j.1442-2018.2010.00525.x

Reed, K., & May, R. (2011). *Healthgrades patient safety in American hospitals study*. Denver, CO: Health Grades, Inc. Retrieved from http://www.healthgrades.com/business/img/HealthGrades-PatientSafetyInAmericanHospitalsStudy2011.pdf

Scalise, D. (2006). Clinical communication and patient safety. *Hospitals & Health Networks/AHA, 80*(8), 49.

Stern, M. F., Greifinger, R. B., & Mellow, J. (2010). Patient safety: Moving the bar in prison health care standards. *American Journal of Public Health, 100*(11), 2103–2110.

The Joint Commission. (2010). *Sentinel event alert: Preventing violence in the health care setting.* Retrieved from http://www.jointcommission.org/assets/1/18/SEA_45.PDF

The Joint Commission. (2011). *2011 hospital national patient safety goals.* Retrieved from http://www.jointcommission.org/assets/1/6/HAP_NPSG_6-10-11.pdf

FIVE

Alcohol and Drug Withdrawal

Susan Laffan

To provide nursing care to incarcerated individuals who use or abuse alcohol and drugs, it is important to understand the widespread use of these substances. Newly admitted jail detainees and inmates have high rates of alcohol and opioid dependence. More than 65% meet *DSM-IV* criteria for alcohol, drug abuse, and addiction (The National Center on Addiction and Substance Abuse at Columbia University, 2010). According to the Bureau of Justice Statistics 2010 Special Report, the number of jail inmate deaths related to drug/alcohol use totaled 566 between 2000 and 2007 (Noonan, Sabol, & Li, 2010). Alcohol withdrawal is the syndrome with the highest mortality rate, although withdrawal from opiates and depressant drugs such as benzodiazepines can also prove life threatening (NCCHC, 2008).

These statistics emphasize the need for correctional nurses to give special attention to drug and alcohol withdrawal. Although nurses in all correctional settings must be concerned with potential substance withdrawal, those providing care in jails, prison reception centers, and juvenile detention facilities have greater likelihood of encountering individuals who are only recently restricted from access to substances of abuse. Correctional nurses must understand how to assess and manage substance withdrawal syndromes.

GENERAL PRINCIPLES OF SUBSTANCE WITHDRAWAL MANAGEMENT

The statistics on the use and abuse of both alcohol and drugs are overwhelming and paint the picture as to why correctional nurses need to be diligent with assessments, initiation of protocols, treatment, intervention, and reassessment. The correctional nurse's most important responsibility in handling substance abuse is identifying individuals who may withdraw from any substances, whether they are legally prescribed, illicit, or additive substances. Once these inmates are identified, the proper medical treatment can be initiated. Ongoing reassessments are critical for determining if the treatment ordered is appropriate and benefiting the patient.

Withdrawal and Detoxification

Withdrawal refers to the characteristic signs and symptoms that appear when a substance that causes physical dependence is abruptly stopped or greatly reduced. *Detoxification* is the process by which an individual is "gradually withdrawn from a drug by the administration of decreasing doses of the drug on which the person is physiologically dependent, of one that is cross-tolerant to it, or of one that medical research has demonstrated to be effective" (NCCHC, 2008, p. 104).

Symptoms vary widely based on the individual's level of withdrawal, the body's dependence on the substance, the type of substance causing the withdrawal, and if the individual is withdrawing from other substances as well. The goals of treatment include safely reducing severity of withdrawal symptoms, preventing seizures and delirium, facilitating the transition to rehabilitation services, and preventing complications. Implementation of safe, effective detoxification and withdrawal protocols begins with training of both medical and correctional staff. It is important that care providers regard substance disorders the same as any chronic illness, such as diabetes, or as emergent as any other life-threatening condition, such as a heart attack or stroke.

Correctional facilities' policies and procedures should address the following withdrawal and detoxification concerns:

- New arrival medical screening
- Situations requiring medical referral or provider notification
- Procedure for transferring an inmate to an offsite hospital
- Medical director-approved nursing protocols
- Special housing arrangements and observation units
- Clinical documentation in the health record including use of flow sheets and narrative notations
- Communication between correctional and medical staff
- Alcohol and drug withdrawal training for health care and correctional staff.

Recognizing Withdrawal

The key to substance withdrawal management is the recognition of potential or actual withdrawal symptoms. In the correctional setting, patients may not fully disclose use of alcohol and/or drugs for fear that information would be used against them legally; therefore, establishing an effective nurse–patient relationship is vital to the evaluation process. Reassurance that information discussed regarding alcohol and substance use and/or abuse will only be used for their medical treatment, and not be used as evidence or information obtained for legal proceedings, can help build that relationship.

All correctional staff must be knowledgeable in the signs and symptoms, recognition, protocols, and treatment of substance disorders. It is important for staff to be familiar with current trends in alcohol and drug use particular to the demographic area served, such as the abuse of prescription drugs (Oxycontin), or the use of heroin versus marijuana. Nursing staff must recognize the signs and symptoms of alcohol, sedative/hypnotic, and opioid withdrawal, including their time course,

EXHIBIT 5.1
Key Interview Questions to Evaluate Substance Use

Do you currently use any type of alcohol or drugs?
    If "no": has the individual used in the past?
What type?
    alcohol: beer/wine/liquor
    drugs: illegal vs. prescription (dosage)
             name of each drug
             route of drug (oral/smoke/inhaled/intravenous)
How much/many?
How often?
Date and time last used?
Have you ever had withdrawal symptoms or seizures/"shakes" when alcohol/
drug is stopped?
Have you ever been hospitalized for medical treatment of withdrawal
symptoms?

Source: Laffan (2007).

and be aware of the potential consequences of inadequate treatment, including death (Modesto-Lowe & Fritz, 2003).

Effective questioning at intake screening can help assess for alcohol and drug use and should include frequency of use, quantity used, duration of use, and last use, and—most importantly—disclosure of any history of prior episodes of withdrawal syndromes (Center for Substance Abuse Treatment, 2006). The assessment process begins immediately, from the first encounter with the patient during the receiving screening. Questions to ask during intake screening are provided in Exhibit 5.1. As important as the information gathered from the individual is, the observations of appearance (e.g., sweating, tremors, anxious, disheveled appearance), behavior (e.g., disorderly, appropriate, insensible), and state of consciousness (alert, responsive, lethargic). The interviewer's observations may be the key in determining the plan of care for the individual and the recognition of an imminent emergent event.

From the Experts ...

"In assessing patients at intake, it is imperative nurses have excellent assessment skills, knowledge of disease processes, and observation skills. This is especially true with drug and alcohol withdrawal, as this is a critical component in keeping patients safe. Early recognition, monitoring, and treatment will improve outcomes and decrease morbidity and mortality in patients with this specific medical problem."

B. Sue Medley-Lane, RN, CCHP
Pompano Beach, FL

Standardized assessment tools can assist with withdrawal screening for alcohol and drug use. These tools can be incorporated into the intake screening process. The National Institute on Alcohol Abuse and Alcoholism (2005) refers to several different types of screening tools for alcohol use and alcohol-related problems. Recommended tools include CAGE (Exhibit 5.2) and AUDIT (Figure 5.1). The CAGE questionnaire has also been modified to include drug abuse behavior (Brown & Rounds, 1995).

EXHIBIT 5.2
CAGE Alcohol Abuse Assessment Tool

Two positive responses are considered a positive test
C—Have you ever felt you should *cut down* on your drinking?
A—Have people *annoyed* you by criticizing your drinking?
G—Have you ever felt bad or *guilty* about your drinking?
E—*Eye opener:* Have you ever had a drink first thing in the morning to steady your nerves or to get rid of a hangover?

Source: Adapted from the National Institute on Alcohol Abuse and Alcoholism (2005).

Please circle the answer that is correct for you

1. How often do you have a drink containing alcohol?

| Never | Monthly or less | Two to four times a month | Two to three times per week | Four or more times a week |

2. How many drinks containing alcohol do you have on a typical day when you are drinking?

| 1 or 2 | 3 or 4 | 5 or 6 | 7 to 9 | 10 or more |

3. How often do you have six or more drinks on one occasion?

| Never | Less than monthly | Monthly | Two to three times per week | Four or more times a week |

4. How often during the last year have you found that you were not able to stop drinking once you had started?

| Never | Less than monthly | Monthly | Two to three times per week | Four or more times a week |

5. How often during the last year have you failed to do what was normally expected from you because of drinking?

| Never | Less than monthly | Monthly | Two to three times per week | Four or more times a week |

6. How often during the last year have you needed a first drink in the morning to get yourself going after a heavy drinking session?

| Never | Less than monthly | Monthly | Two to three times per week | Four or more times a week |

7. How often during the last year have you had a feeling of guilt or remorse after drinking?

| Never | Less than monthly | Monthly | Two to three times per week | Four or more times a week |

8. How often during the last year have you been unable to remember what happened the night before because you had been drinking?

| Never | Less than monthly | Monthly | Two to three times per week | Four or more times a week |

9. Have you or someone else been injured as a result of your drinking?

| No | Yes, but not in the last year | Yes, during the last year |

10. Has a relative or friend, or a doctor or other health worker been concerned about your drinking or suggested you cut down?

| No | Yes, but not in the last year | Yes, during the last year |

The Alcohol Use Disorders Identification Test (AUDIT) can detect alcohol problems experienced in the last year. A score of 8+ on the AUDIT generally indicates harmful of hazardous drinking. Questions 1–8 = 0, 1 2, 3, or 4 points. Questions 9 and 10 are scored 0, 2, or 4 only.

FIGURE 5.1 Alcohol Use Disorders Identification Test (AUDIT).

Source: Taken from the National Institute on Alcohol Abuse and Alcoholism, 2005. Used with permission.

Inmates with substance disorders can be categorized into three groups for the purposes of nursing intervention: (1) Those who do not require immediate medication but need continued monitoring; (2) Those who require immediate medication but lack other risk factors; and (3) Those at high risk who require medication and intensive monitoring.

The first group of individuals may have admitted to using alcohol or drugs prior to incarceration but do not display patterns of addiction to any substance. These individuals do not have any signs or symptoms of withdrawal, yet need to be monitored and reassessed to ensure that withdrawal symptoms do not manifest at a later date or time.

The second group of individuals admitted to using alcohol or drugs on a regular basis and are already experiencing signs of withdrawal. These individuals must be monitored closely for worsening of condition, despite the fact that medication is being provided specifically to treat the substance disorder.

The third group of individuals admitted to high amounts of *chronic* substance use, have had severe withdrawal symptoms in the past, are hemo-dynamically unstable, or are experiencing a change in mental status. These individuals must be closely monitored, with the use of cardiac monitors, medication (either PO or IV), and one-on-one nursing care. Inmates experiencing severe, life-threatening intoxication (overdose) or withdrawal should be transferred immediately to an acute care facility for treatment. Individuals at risk for progression to more severe levels of withdrawal should be kept under constant observation by qualified health care professionals or health-trained correctional staff.

Monitoring Withdrawing Inmates

There are a few general considerations that correctional nurses need to keep in mind when dealing with an inmate withdrawing from any substance. Observation and reassessment is the key. For individuals placed on a "watch," observations are usually done by correctional staff; however, it is important that nurses also evaluate these individuals on a regular basis. An inmate's signs and symptoms will determine how often a nurse should perform evaluations. Proper and appropriate placement of the individual within the correctional facility is important so the individual can be closely monitored. It is important to note that correctional facilities may differ in the exact location where observation cells are located, based on the layout of the facility and the medical/correctional staffing patterns within the facility.

One area of concern during substance withdrawal is the potential for aspiration. Correctional facilities should be deliberate in placing withdrawing inmates in safe, secure housing where they can be continually monitored. Nurses should check all emergency equipment at the beginning of each shift to ensure proper working order.

Personal safety—of the withdrawing inmate, fellow prisoners, and facility staff—is also a real concern in every case involving substance withdrawal. Individuals withdrawing from substances can have many behavioral signs and symptoms that could become dangerous to self or others, such as confusion or the phenomenon of "super-human strength."

Emergency Protocols

Emergency management of drug and alcohol withdrawal includes recognition, assessment, treatment, and/or referral to the most appropriate facility to administer care for that individual. Emergency treatment may include the initiation of physician-approved protocols and/or sending the individual to an acute care facility for more comprehensive treatment and monitoring.

Correctional nurses must be familiar with the medical resources available to them in the particular correctional facility in which they work. If they receive any information or observe any signs and symptoms suggesting substance overdose, the nurse must have the ability to quickly assess whether the particular correctional facility can supply the necessary care. Correctional facility medical departments vary widely across the United States. The correctional nurse has to know when a needed treatment is outside the scope of their practice or cannot be performed onsite due to lack of staff and/or equipment. When inmate transfer is required to obtain necessary medical care, all facility transfer protocols must be followed to ensure safety and security.

Some parameters that may warrant an inmate's urgent transfer to an offsite medical facility include:

- The patient has comorbid health problems, such as heart disease
- The patient has altered mental status
- The patient is not responding to the current course of treatment/medication
- The patient exhibits extremely high or low vital sign recordings, or drastic changes in vitals on re-assessment
- The patient exhibits signs of dehydration (nausea/vomiting/diarrhea; poor skin turgor, dry mucus membranes)
- The facility has medical staffing issues (i.e., facility not having 24-hour nursing coverage).

Individualized Treatment Plans

The development and implementation of an individual treatment plan is vital in providing the appropriate care and treatment. The correctional nurse must combine the information gathered from the individual, clinical observations, assessments, and measurable data (such as vital signs) to determine the appropriate plan of care for each individual. Follow-up and reevaluations that compare assessments and observations from different interviews are key to determining a change in a patient's status, indicating either a positive response to the treatment or that the treatment is not yielding the desired effects. Not obtaining the desired effects of treatment may lead to a poor outcome for the individual. Accurate documentation of all findings, initiation of protocols, contact with any providers, treatment provided, and reassessment of any intervention or treatment must be recorded for continuity of care.

Each category of drugs or alcohol produces a varying array of signs and symptoms. It is extremely important for the correctional nurse to be aware that individuals may have more than one substance in their body; therefore, there can be endless combinations of signs and symptoms. The key to recognizing deterioration in an individual's health status is the consistent reevaluation of that individual.

ALCOHOL WITHDRAWAL

Severe alcohol withdrawal carries one of the highest mortality rates of the withdrawal syndromes and is a serious concern (NCCHC, 2008). An individual who is withdrawing from alcohol can deteriorate rapidly if not properly monitored. Symptoms associated with ineffectively treated alcohol withdrawal progress over time. Table 5.1 shows common symptoms along a withdrawal timeline.

TABLE 5.1 Symptoms of Untreated Alcohol Withdrawal

TIME AFTER LAST DRINK	SYMPTOMS OF WITHDRAWAL	PEAK	DURATION
6–12 hours	Anxiety, agitation, fever, hypertension, nausea/vomiting, tachycardia, tremors	24–36 hours	48 hours
6–48 hours	Seizures	Varies	Varies
48–72 hours	Hallucinations	Varies	Varies
3–5 days	Delirium tremens	Varies	Varies

Source: Adapted from Campbell-Bright (2008).

Using standardized diagnostic criteria and assessment formats helps maintain consistency of treatment and is recommended by accrediting agencies (ACA, 2002, 2010; NCCHC, 2008). The Clinical Institute Withdrawal Assessment-Alcohol Revised (CIWA-Ar) is a nationally recognized evaluation tool for alcohol withdrawal monitoring (Bayard, McIntyre, Hill, & Woodside, 2004). The tool evaluates the following 10 symptoms—nausea and vomiting, auditory disturbances, anxiety, disorientation, tremors, visual disturbances, agitation, skin temperature, tactile disturbances, and headache (Figure 5.2). It provides a consistent evaluation of alcohol withdrawal symptoms over time. Institutions can develop protocols establishing at what score a provider should be contacted for additional evaluation and treatment orders.

Common medications used in the treatment of alcohol withdrawal treatment include Ativan, folic acid, Haldol, Librium, multivitamins, thiamine, and Valium (National Guidelines Clearinghouse, 2006). The actual medication(s), dosages, frequency, and duration are dependent on the protocols approved by the physician or direct physician orders.

DRUG WITHDRAWAL

In addition to alcohol, correctional nurses are confronted with several other substance withdrawal categories as listed here:

- Benzodiazepines: Xanax, Librium, Klonopin, Valium, Ativan, Serax, Restoril, Halcion
- Cannabis: Marijuana
- Hallucinogens: Ecstasy, MDA (Love Drug), LSD, PCP, psilocyben mushrooms; bath salts
- Inhalants: amyl and butyl nitrates, nitrous oxide, spray paint, hair spray, lighter fluid, duster spray
- Opiates: heroin, morphine, hydrocodone, hydromorphone, oxycodone, codiene
- Stimulants: cocaine, amphetamine, methamphetamine, Ritalin, Adderall, Concerta.

Benzodiazepine Withdrawal

Benzodiazepines are most commonly used to treat insomnia and anxiety. This class of drugs produces central nervous system (CNS) depression. The most common benzodiazepines are listed in Table 5.2.

The correctional nurse should recognize and monitor the signs and symptoms of benzodiazepine withdrawal. The most frequent withdrawal symptoms are anxiety, insomnia, restlessness, agitation, irritability, and muscle tension (Krishnamurthy,

Clinical Institute Withdrawal Assessment of Alcohol Scale, Revised (CIWA-Ar)

Patient:_____ Date: _____ Time: _____ (24 hour clock, midnight = 00:00)

Pulse or heart rate, taken for one minute:_____ Blood pressure:_____

NAUSEA AND VOMITING -- Ask "Do you feel sick to your stomach? Have you vomited?" Observation.
0 no nausea and no vomiting
1 mild nausea with no vomiting
2
3
4 intermittent nausea with dry heaves
5
6
7 constant nausea, frequent dry heaves and vomiting

TACTILE DISTURBANCES -- Ask "Have you any itching, pins and needles sensations, any burning, any numbness, or do you feel bugs crawling on or under your skin?" Observation.
0 none
1 very mild itching, pins and needles, burning or numbness
2 mild itching, pins and needles, burning or numbness
3 moderate itching, pins and needles, burning or numbness
4 moderately severe hallucinations
5 severe hallucinations
6 extremely severe hallucinations
7 continuous hallucinations

TREMOR -- Arms extended and fingers spread apart. Observation.
0 no tremor
1 not visible, but can be felt fingertip to fingertip
2
3
4 moderate, with patient's arms extended
5
6
7 severe, even with arms not extended

AUDITORY DISTURBANCES -- Ask "Are you more aware of sounds around you? Are they harsh? Do they frighten you? Are you hearing anything that is disturbing to you? Are you hearing things you know are not there?" Observation.
0 not present
1 very mild harshness or ability to frighten
2 mild harshness or ability to frighten
3 moderate harshness or ability to frighten
4 moderately severe hallucinations
5 severe hallucinations
6 extremely severe hallucinations
7 continuous hallucinations

PAROXYSMAL SWEATS -- Observation.
0 no sweat visible
1 barely perceptible sweating, palms moist
2
3
4 beads of sweat obvious on forehead
5
6
7 drenching sweats

VISUAL DISTURBANCES -- Ask "Does the light appear to be too bright? Is its color different? Does it hurt your eyes? Are you seeing anything that is disturbing to you? Are you seeing things you know are not there?" Observation.
0 not present
1 very mild sensitivity
2 mild sensitivity
3 moderate sensitivity
4 moderately severe hallucinations
5 severe hallucinations
6 extremely severe hallucinations
7 continuous hallucinations

ANXIETY -- Ask "Do you feel nervous?" Observation.
0 no anxiety, at ease
1 mild anxious
2
3
4 moderately anxious, or guarded, so anxiety is inferred
5
6
7 equivalent to acute panic states as seen in severe delirium or acute schizophrenic reactions

HEADACHE, FULLNESS IN HEAD -- Ask "Does your head feel different? Does it feel like there is a band around your head?" Do not rate for dizziness or lightheadedness. Otherwise, rate severity.
0 not present
1 very mild
2 mild
3 moderate
4 moderately severe
5 severe
6 very severe
7 extremely severe

AGITATION -- Observation.
0 normal activity
1 somewhat more than normal activity
2
3
4 moderately fidgety and restless
5
6
7 paces back and forth during most of the interview, or constantly thrashes about

ORIENTATION AND CLOUDING OF SENSORIUM -- Ask "What day is this? Where are you? Who am I?"
0 oriented and can do serial additions
1 cannot do serial additions or is uncertain about date
2 disoriented for date by no more than 2 calendar days
3 disoriented for date by more than 2 calendar days
4 disoriented for place/or person

Total **CIWA-Ar** Score _____
Rater's Initials _____
Maximum Possible Score 67

FIGURE 5.2   Clinical Institute Withdrawal Assessment of Alcohol Scale.

Source: The CIWA-Ar is not copyrighted and may be reproduced freely.

Dickinson, & Eickelberg, 2011a). Less frequent symptoms can include nausea, diaphoresis, blurred vision, and nightmares. Onset of these conditions depends on the duration of action of the actual medication. For example, short-acting benzodiazepines, such as lorazepam or temazepam, will show withdrawal symptoms within 24 hours of cessation while long-acting benzodiazepines, such as diazepam, may not show withdrawal symptoms for up to 5 days of last ingestion (Krishnamurthy et al., 2011a).

From the Experts ...

"When I first started in corrections 26 years ago, it was much easier to identify and place patients on the right withdrawal protocols. Over the years, we've noticed such an increase in patients with polysubstance abuse that it is a much more difficult task to determine just the right treatment protocol to utilize. Nurses must be diligent to properly assess patients with this in mind, and to ensure that monitoring continues well past the initial receiving screening."

Kathryn J. Wild, RN, MPA, CCHP
Santa Ana, CA

TABLE 5.2   Benzodiazepine Medications

GENERIC NAME	TRADE NAME	EQUIVALENT DOSE (MG)	HALF-LIFE (H)
Alprazolam	Xanax	0.5–1	6–15
Chlordizaepoxide	Libruim	25	24–48
Clonazepam	Klonopin	1–2	30–40
Clorazepate	Tranxene	7.5–15	30+
Diazepam	Valium	10	20–50
Estazolam	ProSom	1	10–24
Flurazepam	Dalmane	15–30	50–200
Lorazepam	Ativan	1–2	10–20
Oxazepam	Serax	10–30	5–10
Temazepam	Restoril	15–30	3–20
Triazolam	Halcion	0.25	1–5
Zolpidem	Ambien	10–20	2–5

Source: Adapted from Weaver (2009).

Benzodiazepine withdrawal is rarely life threatening and treatment focuses on management of symptoms such as fluid volume maintenance, treatment of nausea and diarrhea, and possible prescription of substitution medication to manage severe anxiety. Rapid high-dose withdrawal such as may occur on entry into correctional facilities, can precipitate seizure activity. Short-term use of barbiturates, such as phenobarbital, may be initiated to curtail complications from benzodiazepine withdrawal (Krishnamurthy et al., 2011a).

Cannabis Withdrawal

Cannabis (marijuana) intoxication produces relaxation, euphoria and altered sensory perception (Krishnamurthy et al., 2011c). Although a withdrawal syndrome has been reported with as little as a week of use, symptoms are mild and manageable. Typical marijuana withdrawal symptoms and/or resulting conditions include anorexia, anxiety, irritability, restlessness, and sleep disturbance. Treatment is supportive only and may only rarely involve mild sedation for unusually severe agitation or restlessness (Carlson & Kennedy, 2006).

Hallucinogen Withdrawal

Hallucinogenic substances are capable of distorting an individual's perception of reality. Substance-induced hallucinations are most often visual, but they can also manifest as a sense of peace, a feeling of panic, or a fear of dying or going insane. Among these drugs are Ecstasy, LSD, Peyote buttons, psilocybin, bath salts, MDMA, and rohypnol; common street names for these substances include— cactus, big chief, magic mushroom, shrooms, god's flesh, pearly gates, heavenly blue, acid, cube, California sunshine, blue dots, and sugar (National Institute of Drug Abuse, 2011).

Withdrawal symptoms may include agitation, confusion, tremors, hyper-flexia, ataxia, rigidity, dilated pupils, fever, and diaphoresis (Macher, 2010). A withdrawal syndrome has not been identified for hallucinogens, although up to 10% may have symptoms such as fatigue, irritability, and mood disorders (Krishnamurthy et al., 2011c).

Inhalant Withdrawal

Inhalants are breathable chemical vapors or gases that produce psychoactive (mind-altering) effects when abused or misused (National Inhalant Prevention Coalition, n.d.). Intoxication with solvents, aerosols, and gases often produces a syndrome most like that of alcohol intoxication but only lasting 15 to 45 minutes. Commonly used inhalants include amyl and butyl nitrates, nitrous oxide, spray paint, hair spray, and lighter fluid (National Institute of Drug Abuse, 2011). Intoxication with inhalants is self-limiting and rarely requires medical attention. Withdrawal can cause occasional tachycardia and diaphoresis, but symptoms requiring treatment are rare (Krishnamurthy et al., 2011c). However, correctional nurses should be aware that, while very rare, use of inhalants has resulted in severe complications due to oxygen displacement or "freezing" of lung tissue.

Opiate Withdrawal

Opiates (such as heroin, morphine, hydrocodone, hydromorphone, oxycodone, and codeine) are a classification of drugs that are either derived from the opium poppy, or that mimic the effect of an opiate (a synthetic opiate or opioid). Opiate drugs are narcotic sedatives that depress activity of the central nervous system, reduce pain, and induce sleep. Early opiate withdrawal symptoms include agitation, anxiety, muscle aches, increased tearing, insomnia, and sweating. Late withdrawal symptoms include abdominal cramping, diarrhea, dilated pupils, nausea, and vomiting. Symptoms usually start within 12 hours of last opiate/opioid usage and within 30 hours of last methadone exposure (see Table 5.3).

The Clinical Opioid Withdrawal Scale (COWS) is a nationally recognized assessment scale that targets the main withdrawal symptoms of nausea/vomiting, diarrhea, myalgias, anxiety, and insomnia (Figure 5.3). Using a consistent evaluation measure over time allows nurses to determine when withdrawal symptoms are lessening or worsening, requiring changes in treatment plans.

TABLE 5.3 Opioid Intoxication and Withdrawal Signs and Symptoms

OPIOID INTOXICATION	OPIOID WITHDRAWAL
Bradycardia	Tachycardia
Hypotension	Hypertension
Hypothermia	Hyperthermia
Sedation	Insomnia
Pinpoint pupils (meiosis)	Enlarged pupils (mydriasis)
Hypokinesis (slow movement)	Hyperflexia (abnormal heightened reflexes)
Slurred speech	Diaphoresis
Head nodding	Piloerection (gooseflesh)
Euphoria	Increased respiratory rate
Analgesia	Lacrimation (tearing)
Calmness	Muscle spasms
	Abdominal cramps, nausea, vomiting, diarrhea
	Bone and muscle pain

Source: National Guideline Clearinghouse (2006).

Opioid withdrawal is uncomfortable for patients but generally not life threatening (Carlson & Kennedy, 2006). No single approach to detoxification is guaranteed to be best for all patients. The withdrawal symptoms—agitation, anxiety, tremors, muscle aches, hot and cold flashes, nausea, vomiting, and diarrhea are not life threatening, but are extremely uncomfortable. The intensity of the reaction depends on the dose and speed of withdrawal (Harvard Mental Health Letter, 2004).

Opiate withdrawal treatment involves supportive care and medications. Medication may include loperamide (Imodium) for diarrhea, clonidine (Catapres) to control autonomic symptoms of withdrawal, dicyclomine hydrochloride (Bentyl) to treat abdominal cramps, hydroxyzine (Atarax) or promethazine (Phenergan) for nausea and vomiting, methocarbamol (Robaxin) to treat muscle cramps and joint pain, and trazadone (Desyrel) to treat depression and anxiety. In addition, methadone or buprenorphine may be prescribed as a substitute for the withdrawing opioid and then tapered to minimize withdrawal symptoms (Krishnamurthy, Tetrault, & O'Connor, 2011b). Case Example 5.1 applies information from this section.

CASE EXAMPLE 5.1

An 18-year-old male, during intake screening, admits to a history of five bags of IV heroin use daily. He last used heroin 6 hours prior to arrival and exhibits fresh track marks on both arms. He complains of nausea and cramps upon arrival. He continues to complain of nausea and has had witnessed vomiting and diarrhea. Based on information in this chapter, what assessment, safety, and treatment measures should be put in place?

Patient's Name:	Date:	Time:
Reason for this assessment:		

1. Resting pulse rate: _____ beats/minute Measured after the patient is sitting or lying for one minute. 0 Pulse rate 80 or below 1 Pulse rate 81–100 2 Pulse rate 101–120 4 Pulse rate greater than 120	**7. GI upset**: *over last half hour* 0 No GI symptoms 1 Stomach cramps 2 Nausea or loose stool 3 Vomiting or diarrhea 5 Multiple episodes of diarrhea or vomiting
2. Sweating: *over past half hour not accounted for by room temperature or patient activity.* 0 No reports of chills or flushing 1 Subjective reports of chills or flushing 2 Flushed or observable moisture on face 3 Beads of sweat on brow or face 4 Sweat streaming off face	**8. Tremor**: *observation of outstretched hands* 0 No tremor 1 Tremor can be felt, but not observed 2 Slight tremor observable 4 Gross tremor or muscle twitching
3. Restlessness: *observation during assessment* 0 Able to sit still 1 Reports difficulty sitting still, but is able to do so 3 Frequent shifting or extraneous movements of legs/arms 5 Unable to sit still for more than a few seconds	**9. Yawning**: *observation during assessment* 0 No yawning 1 Yawning once or twice during assessment 2 Yawning three or more times during assessment 4 Yawning several times/minute
4. Pupil size 0 Pupils pinned or normal size for room light 1 Pupils possibly larger than normal for room light 2 Pupils moderately dilated 5 Pupils so dilated that only the rim of the iris is visible	**10. Anxiety or irritability** 0 None 1 Patient reports increasing irritability or anxiousness 2 Patient obviously irritable, anxious 4 Patient so irritable or anxious that participation in the assessment is difficult
5. Bone or joint aches: *if patient was having pain previously, only the additional component attributed to opiate withdrawal is scored* 0 Not present 1 Mild diffuse discomfort 2 Patient reports severe diffuse aching of joints/ muscles 4 Patient is rubbing joints or muscles and is unable to sit still because of discomfort	**11. Gooseflesh skin** 0 Skin is smooth 3 Piloerection of skin can be felt or hairs standing up on arms 5 Prominent piloerection
6. Runny nose or tearing: *not accounted for by cold symptoms or allergies* 0 Not present 1 Nasal stuffiness or unusually moist eyes 2 Nose running or tearing 4 Nose constantly running or tears streaming down cheeks	**Total Score:**_____ [The total score is the sum of all 11 items.] Initial of person completing assessment:_____

Score: 5–12=Mild; 13–24 = Moderate; 25–36 = Moderately severe; >36 = Severe withdrawal

Source: Adapted from Wesson et al. 1999. Reprinted with permission.

Note: For each item, circle the number that best describes the patient's signs or symptoms. Rate just on the apparent relationship to opiate withdrawal. For example, if heart rate is increased because the patient was jogging just prior to assessment, the increased pulse rate would not add to the score.

FIGURE 5.3   Clinical Opioid Withdrawal Scale (COWS).

Stimulant Withdrawal

Stimulants such as cocaine, amphetamines, and methamphetamine produce a variety of effects by enhancing the activity of the central and peripheral nervous systems, particularly increasing catecholamine neurotransmitter activity (Krishnamurthy et al., 2011c). Stimulant use causes enhanced alertness, awareness, endurance, productivity, heart rate, blood pressure, and the perception of a diminished requirement for food and sleep. Abrupt cessation of a stimulant, such as when a user enters the correctional system, can lead to depression, anxiety, fatigue, increased appetite, and difficulty concentrating.

Treatment of stimulant withdrawal focuses on managing symptoms. Supportive therapy can include rest, exercise, and a healthy diet (Krishnamurthy et al., 2011c). In addition, increased concern for suicidal tendency is warranted and should be monitored (Carlson & Kennedy, 2006). Case Example 5.2 applies information from this section.

CASE EXAMPLE 5.2

A 21-year-old female is arrested for possession of methamphetamines. She admitted to using methamphetamines that day prior to her arrival to the jail, and she complained of feeling dizzy and weak. She is unable to stand or sit still during the intake process and was observed pacing and shaking. She stated to correctional officers, "I have to go to the hospital because I am overdosing." The inmate was put in an observation cell in the booking area. When she was moved to another cell, a clear wrapper fell from her uniform pants. She collapsed and was taken to the hospital by car two hours later. Assessment findings on arrival to the hospital: P 140, R 44, BP 80/42, PO 94% on room air, T 105.6 rectal. She suffered continuous seizures and three cardiac arrests, and was pronounced dead 22 hours after arrival to the hospital. What is missing from the care delivered to this patient?

SPECIAL NEEDS INMATES
Pregnant Women

Opiate addiction in pregnancy is a concern, as abrupt discontinuation of medication can endanger the fetus, causing miscarriage or premature labor (Carlson & Kennedy, 2006). Methadone maintenance therapy should be continued throughout the pregnancy to maintain fetal health and is recommended by correctional accrediting agencies (ACA, 2002, 2010; NCCHC, 2008).

The Elderly

Owing to the natural aging process of the body, the elderly are at an increased risk for co-occurring medical conditions. Medical complications are a serious risk for substance withdrawal, because elderly patients cannot as easily tolerate rapid heart rate, severe swings in blood pressure, or acute psychosis produced by the withdrawal process. The elderly also may be at a greater risk for drug interactions, since they may be receiving medications to treat other problems. Potential for falls also should be evaluated in the context of withdrawal from or interaction with prescribed medications (Winkel & Bair, 2008).

Mental Health Issues

Drugs and alcohol can mask mental health symptoms an inmate may be experiencing. During and after withdrawal, mental illness can emerge unexpectedly. Individuals can be at a high risk for suicide or self-harm as the numbing effects of these substances are eliminated (Paton & Jenkins, 2002). Additional treatment may be necessary, from the mental health perspective, such as counseling and psychotropic medication.

Correctional nurses should be alert to the emergence of symptoms of mental illness in withdrawing patients and initiate appropriate evaluation and treatment.

ONGOING MANAGEMENT OF SUBSTANCE ABUSE

The correctional nurse should not only be familiar with the need for ongoing treatment and education, but also appreciate the importance of continued support for the individual once withdrawal is successfully completed. As important as it is to initiate an established protocol, perhaps even more critical is regular reevaluation/reassessment of the efficacy of the selected interventions and treatments. Negative outcomes can result from changes in the patient's condition that are not recognized and acted upon. The correctional nurse may refer the individual to the facility's social service department or chaplain for further guidance. To facilitate continued support, correctional nurses should have a current list of resources available so that they can refer individuals to rehabilitation programs within the correctional facility and in the community. Counseling services as well as rehabilitation facilities, drug courts, and reentry programs are other considerations in long-term management of substance abuse. There also are established self-help groups such as Alcoholics Anonymous (AA) and Narcotics Anonymous (NA), as well as rehabilitation facilities, drug court, and reentry programs, which may be helpful inside and outside of the correctional setting.

One of the most important factors in long-term management of substance abuse is patient education, which, to be effective, must be ongoing with each individual during each interaction—from formal to informal—including verbal encounters with individuals, provision of written materials regarding particular substance abuse issues, and referral into programs available. Patient education should be tailored to the patient's individual education level and readiness to listen/accept the information being provided. Successful education elicits acceptance and acknowledgment of the need for rehabilitation programs.

SUMMARY

The high prevalence of inmates who have used drugs, alcohol, or any combination of these, coupled with the high rate of incarceration, means that correctional nurses must be vigilant in assessing for potential life-threatening events. Correctional nurses need to be at the forefront of providing care to these individuals, so it is important for correctional nurses to have extensive knowledge about withdrawal syndromes. Because inmates may not be forthcoming with accurate information about their substance use, correctional nurses must be prepared to ask for specific information about substance use, observe inmates for symptoms suggestive of withdrawal, and listen carefully to concerns voiced by inmates and correctional staff. Improper management of individuals who are experiencing withdrawal symptoms can lead to poor outcomes for addicted inmates, which can include severe physical symptoms and death.

DISCUSSION QUESTIONS

1. Compare your facility's withdrawal screening process with information from this chapter. What changes would you suggest?

2. How are nurses in your facility trained to manage withdrawal from common substances used by the inmate population?
3. Differentiate signs and symptoms of the various drug withdrawal syndromes.

REFERENCES

American Correctional Association. (2002). *Performance-based standards for correctional health care in adult correctional institutions.* Alexandria, VA: Author.

American Correctional Association. (2010). *2010 Standards supplement.* Alexandria, VA: Author.

Bayard, M., McIntyre, J., Hill, K. R., & Woodside, J. (2004). Alcohol withdrawal syndrome. *American Family Physician, 69*(6), 1443–1450.

Brown, R. L., & Rounds, L. A. (1995). Conjoint screening questionnaires for alcohol and drug abuse. *Wisconsin Medical Journal, 94,* 135–140.

Campbell-Bright, S. (2008, July 22). "Alcohol Withdrawal Assessment and Treatment." On-line power point program. *Clinical Specialist, Medicine ICU.*

Carlson, H. B., & Kennedy, J. A. (2006). The treatment of alcohol and other drug withdrawal syndromes in persons taken into custody. In M. Puisis (Ed.), *Clinical practice in correctional medicine* (2nd ed.). Philadelphia: Mosby Elsevier.

Center for Substance Abuse Treatment. (2006). *Detoxification and substance abuse treatment, treatment improvement protocol (TIP0Series 45 (DHHS publication no. (SMA) 06-4131).* Rockville, MD: Substance Abuse and Mental Health Services Administration.

Harvard Mental Health Letter. (2004, December). *Treating opiate addiction, Part 1, detoxification and maintenance.* Retrieved from www.health.harvard.edu/mental

Krishnamurthy, A., Dickinson, W. E., & Eickelberg, S. J. (2011a). Management of sedative–hypnotic intoxication and withdrawal. In C. A. Cavacuiti (Ed.), *Principles of addiction medicine: the essentials* (pp. 212–222). Philadelphia, PA: Wolters Kluwer.

Krishnamurthy, A., Tetrault, J. M., & O'Connor, P. G. (2011b). Management of opioid intoxication and withdrawal. In C. A. Cavacuiti (Ed.), *Principles of addiction medicine: The essentials* (pp. 223–228). Philadelphia, PA: Wolters Kluwer.

Krishnamurthy, A., Wilkins, J. N., Danovitch, I., & Gorelick, D. A. (2011c). Management of stimulant, hallucinogen, marijuana, phencyclidine, and club drug intoxication and withdrawal. In C. A. Cavacuiti (Ed.), *Principles of addiction medicine: The essentials* (pp. 229–244). Philadelphia, PA: Wolters Kluwer.

Laffan, S. (2007). *Withdrawal and the detoxification process: A nursing care perspective, Conference Session.* Updates in Correctional Health Care, Orlando, FL.

Macher, A. M. (2010, November/December). Abuse of club drugs—Ecstasy. *American Jails,* pp. 67–73.

Modesto-Lowe, V., & Fritz, E. M. (2003). Recognition and treatment of alcohol use disorders in U.S. jails. *Psychiatric Services, 54,* 1413–1414.

National Commission on Correctional Health Care (NCCHC). (2008). *Standards for health services in jails.* Chicago, IL: Author.

National Guideline Clearinghouse. (2006). *Practice guideline for the treatment of patients with substance use disorders.* Retrieved from http://guidelines.gov/content.aspx?id=9316

National Guideline Clearinghouse, Substance Use Disorders, 8/14/2006, www.guideline.gov, 18.

National Institute of Drug Abuse. (2011). *Commonly abused drugs chart.* Retrieved from http://www.drugabuse.gov/drugs-abuse/commonly-abused-drugs/commonly-abused-drugs-chart

National Inhalant Prevention Coalition. (n.d.) Retrieved from http://www.inhalants.org/guidelines.htm

National Institute on Alcohol Abuse and Alcoholism. (2005). *Alcohol alert number 65.* Retrieved from http://pubs.niaaa.nih.gov/publications/aa65/AA65.htm

Noonan, M., Sabol, W., & Spencer, L. (2010). *Bureau of justice statistics special report: Mortality in local jails 2000–2007 (NCJ 222988).* US Department of Justice (DOJ). http://www.ojp.usdoj.gov.

Paton, J., & Jenkins, R. (2002). *Mental health primary care in prison. UK Edition.* World Health Organization Collaborating Center for Research and Training for Mental Health. Retrieved from http://www.prisonmentalhealth.org/

The National Center on Addiction and Substance Abuse at Columbia University. (2010). *Behind bars II: Substance abuse and America's prison population*. New York, NY: The National Center on Addiction and Substance Abuse at Columbia University. Retrieved from http://www.casacolumbia.org/articlefiles/575-report2010behindbars2.pdf

Weaver, M. F. (2009). Treatment of sedative–hypnotic drug abuse in adults, 17.1.

Wesson, D., Lind, W., & Jara, G. (1999). *Buprenorphine in pharmacotherapy or opioid addiction: Implementation in office-based medical practice. Translating the experience of clinical trials into clinical practice*. San Francisco, CA: California Society of Addiction Medicine.

Winkel, V., & Bair, B. (2008). Substance use disorders in older adults. *Clinical Geriatrics, 16*(7), 25–29.

SIX

Chronic Conditions

Patricia Voermans

With more than 2 million persons in the United States imprisoned in federal and state prisons and jails, understanding the types of chronic conditions and prevalence among the correctional population is important to address the needs of this growing population (NCCHC, 2002). Inmate populations are predominantly young male individuals with an average age of less than 35 years, an age generally expected to be relatively healthy, yet there is growing evidence that a number of chronic diseases are more prevalent among this group than the general population (Binswanger, Krueger, & Steiner, 2009; Wilper et al., 2009).

The disproportionate disease burden is attributed in part to factors associated with the minority composition of the prison and jail population. In 2006, African American male incarceration rates in prisons and jails was 4.8% compared to 1.9% of Hispanic men and 0.7% of Caucasians. African American women were incarcerated at four times the rate of Caucasian female individuals and 2 times more than Hispanic women (Sabol, Minton, & Harrison, 2007). Social determinants such as ethnicity and income are associated with health status and health care access. Ethnic minorities from poor backgrounds report a higher prevalence of chronic diseases, lack of access to health care, and unhealthy behaviors compared to the national norm. Also, self-reported health habits and chronic diseases were higher among these groups than others in a national survey regarding diabetes, hypertension, cardiovascular diseases, obesity, and cigarette smoking (CDC, 2011a). Factors influencing health such as trauma, excessive alcohol and substance abuse, poor diets, and limited medical care prior to incarceration are also common among inmates (Wilper et al., 2009).

Longer sentences are producing a rapidly growing segment of older inmates that will continue to increase (Rickard et al., 2007). An inmate is considered chronologically 10 years older than their nonincarcerated peers and considered elderly at 50 years of age. The likelihood of developing a chronic disease increases with aging and may be more common among elderly inmates (Smyer & Burbank, 2009). Health care costs of these older prisoners are four times higher than caring for younger prisoners. The context of the correctional environment with exposure to excessive noise and lack of control over routines may also exacerbate comorbid conditions (Bishop & Merten, 2011). Prisons and jails are ill prepared to address the health needs associated with age-related changes among older inmates, such as nutrition, hydration, vision, mobility, and hearing (Reimer, 2008).

Wilper et al. (2009) found over one-third of inmates in federal prison, state prisons, and local jails suffered a chronic medical condition and, based on age standardization, had higher rates of diseases from viral infections, diabetes, hypertension, and persistent asthma compared to the general population. Using the National Health Interview Survey (NHIS), Binswanger (2010) found that the most common chronic conditions among inmates aged 34–49 in prisons and jails were; obesity (47%), hypertension (24.7%), arthritis (23.1%), asthma (13.9%), and hepatitis (12.9%).

CHRONIC DISEASE MANAGEMENT

National medical consensus groups have developed treatment guidelines for specific chronic diseases, including hypertension, dyslipidemia, diabetes, and asthma, that are aimed at reducing morbidity and mortality. The National Commission on Correctional Health Care (NCCHC) and the American Correctional Association (ACA) endorsed these guidelines and developed standards requiring prisons and jails to develop systems of care for addressing chronic diseases that are consistent with national recommendations. Both organizations audit institutional performance to these specific standards during their accreditation surveys (ACA, 2003; NCCHC, 2008). One of the largest prison systems, the Federal Bureau of Prisons (FBOP) has developed very detailed chronic disease monitoring guidelines that incorporate the NCCHC and ACA recommendations. These guidelines are posted online at http://www.bop.gov/news/medresources.jsp.

There are compelling reasons to improve chronic disease care in prisons and jails. An educated patient engaging in self-care can reduce morbidity, health care costs, and benefit the communities to which the majority of inmates return. During incarceration, patient accessibility provides a unique opportunity to address significant health needs for successful treatment outcomes because care can potentially be consistent and monitored with periodic follow up.

However, providing chronic disease management programs in prison and jail environments is challenging in the face of a focus on security rather than health care and with limited resources. Little is known about the effectiveness of disease management in corrections, but evidence suggests management of chronic diseases among prisoners is often poor. "Among inmates with a persistent medical problem, 13.9% of federal inmates, 20.1% of state inmates, and 68.4% of local jail inmates had received no examination since incarceration" (Wilper et al., 2009, p. 669). Efforts are underway to address chronic care in prisons. The California prison system, under a mandate of receivership to improve care, is adapting a chronic care model used in nonincarcerated settings to prevent complications in patients with uncontrolled asthma (Chang & Robinson, 2011). According to Dr. David Burnett, medical director (personal communication, September 27, 2011), the Wisconsin Department of

Corrections (WDOC) embarked on development of a chronic care model in 2002. In addition to treatment guidelines for chronic diseases, performance measures similar to HEDIS (Health Effectiveness and Data Information Set) were developed and measured. Through the continuous quality improvement process, care improved as demonstrated by these performance measures and had a positive impact on cost control.

The Nurse's Role in Chronic Disease Management

A multidisciplinary team consisting of physicians, nurses, and other health professionals is essential for effective chronic disease management programs. Correctional nurses have a key role in the team by coordinating and managing chronic disease care. Nurses are often the first to assess the patient's health status on intake and in episodic care. They intervene when patients develop adverse events such as hypoglycemia or asthma exacerbations and are gatekeepers in referring problems to the advanced practitioner. Nurses have a collaborative role in assuring patient access to care and gathering necessary information for decision making by members of the team. They are also the primary source for patient education and support the patient in self-care to achieve chronic disease treatment goals.

Patient Education

Patient teaching is one of the most important roles for nurses in patient care and a standard of practice (ANA, 2007). Studies show education can help the patient cope with the emotional and practical aspects of the impact of chronic disease on quality of life by influencing positive behavior modification.

Patient education and counseling are cornerstones to achieve an optimal function and manage pain. The patient's motivation is foremost in achieving management goals. Therefore, a nursing assessment of the patient's knowledge of disease process and personal expectations is important for planning. The patient may have a knowledge deficit, ineffective coping mechanisms, or unrealistic expectations for treatment.

Motivating patients to change behavior is a major goal in chronic disease management. Teaching about the disease processes and treatment goals may influence the patient to make more informed choices. However, providing knowledge alone will not necessarily result in behavior change. Health behavior is complex with many variables, such as the patient's attitude, self-efficacy, and perceived benefit or attributes of the behavior, that will determine the likelihood of change. The patient's attitude is influenced by a trusting relationship with the nurse and a belief the treatment goals will make a positive personal difference.

Challenges in providing patient education in corrections include lack of resources, environment, cultural differences, literacy skills, and the absence of

From the Experts . . .

"Patient education is the key to controlling and preventing chronic illnesses in the correctional environment."

Christine Edmund RN CCHP
Orlando, FL

family involvement. Literacy levels among the U.S. prison population are generally lower than among the nonincarcerated population according to a national literacy study. Findings indicated proficiency varied among this group and were directly dependent upon educational attainment and demographic composition (Greenberg, Dunleavey, Kutner, & White, 2007). Often patients do not understand essential health information such as discharge instructions. The patient is either given too much information or provided education materials that are not understandable. Messages should be short, simple, and to the point (Aldridge, 2004).

Nursing skills necessary for effective teaching are knowledge of subject matter and effective communication methods. Success also involves partnering with the patient in developing goals. It is important to identify cultural influences in this diverse population and include these influences in teaching strategies. Communication that is patient centered, by asking open-ended questions, rather than provider centered can be effective and build trust with the patient (Hartley & Repede, 2011).

Collaborative Care

Continuity of medical regimen is critical for effective chronic disease management, yet evidence suggests it is lacking among those entering correctional facilities. Up to 36% of inmates taking prescription medications for an active medical problem stopped the medication when entering a local jail (Wilper et al., 2009). Verification of prescribed medications can be difficult. Newly incarcerated inmates may not remember the drug, pharmacy, or prescriber. The use of alias names poses challenges in retrieving health information from outside providers. Initiation of medications may be delayed due to lack of assessment and lack of screening procedures for chronic diseases. Patient adherence to prescribed treatment during incarceration can be spotty because of knowledge deficit and lack of motivation. Patient compliance may be difficult to monitor due to complicated health delivery systems, frequent intrasystem transfers, and lack of tracking methods. A number of prisons and jails have no electronic record systems and must rely on paper tickler systems.

Institutional challenges include systems issues contributing to inconsistent or late medication delivery, lack of privacy with medications for diseases such as HIV, administration times that interfere with leisure activities, and medication that is not available because of limited formularies or other resources. Drugs such as narcotics, muscle relaxants, and other mood altering substances can be subject to abuse. Inmates may feign symptoms to seek certain drugs for secondary gain.

Security Interface

Restrictive correctional environments produce many obstacles to achieving optimal patient health goals in chronic disease management. Trying to balance patient care with security needs can be very frustrating for the nurse because of limits that affect patient/nurse relationships. The nurse is put in a position of negotiating boundaries of care with security, which can lead to conflicts with custody staff and impede the effectiveness of care delivery and the nurse's objectivity (Weiskopf, 2005). One correctional expert suggests that promoting institutional change may be more influential than prevention messages in chronic disease prevention in prisons. Changes that positively affect health include eliminating smoking, providing heart-healthy diets, and increasing exercise options (Puisis & Appel, 2006).

MANAGEMENT OF SPECIFIC CHRONIC DISEASES
Asthma

Asthma is one of the most common chronic diseases in the United States and can have a significant impact on a person's quality of life. Asthma prevalence is higher among female individuals than among male individuals and higher among children than among adults. Asthma prevalence in the United States was 14.8% among poor multiracial populations compared to 7.8% in the general population (CDC, 2011b).

Asthma is a chronic inflammatory disease of the airways associated with variable degrees of airway obstruction and characterized by symptoms of wheezing, coughing, and chest tightness. It is believed to develop from environmental factors and genetic predisposition. Environmental factors include dust pollens, molds, cockroach infestations, mites, animal dander, air pollution, and tobacco smoke. Bronchoconstriction occurs usually in response to a stimulus resulting in airway edema with inflammation, mucus accumulation, and limitation of airflow. It is reversible or partially reversible either spontaneously or with medication. The airway reaction is associated with an exaggerated immunoglobulin E (IgE) response to allergen triggers such as dust, pollen, and molds. Other stimuli such as cold air, stress, and sensitivity to aspirin and nonsteroidal anti-inflammatory drugs can also induce bronchospasm (National Heart, Lung, and Blood Institute [NHLBI], 2007).

Asthma severity is based on symptom frequency and categorized in steps from mild (Step 1) to severe (Step 6). Treatment decisions are based on symptom severity and adjusted in a stepwise approach to manage asthma (NHLBI, 2007). Control is a major goal of management. According to the NCCHC (2011a) guidelines, asthma symptom control should be assessed at each follow-up as good, fair, or poor. These designations correspond to NHLBI (2007) and GINA (2010) guidelines specifying levels of control as: controlled, partly controlled, and/or uncontrolled.

Nursing Management

The history and description of patient symptoms help determine the diagnosis and level of asthma severity. Necessary data collection includes questioning the patient about past hospitalizations, previous asthma attacks, and frequency of exacerbations. Conditions such as allergies, sinusitis, rhinitis, upper respiratory infections, and gastroesophageal reflux are associated with the disease and important to the patient database. Also important to developing a care plan is monitoring the patient's use of medication, including inhalers, corticosteroids, and querying use of other medications, such as aspirin, that could precipitate an attack. Correctional nurses should question the patient about their functional health patterns such as activity level, fatigue, sleep intolerance, coughing episodes, breathlessness, and coping issues. Nursing diagnoses associated with asthma may include ineffective airway clearance, impaired gas exchange, activity intolerance, and anxiety.

The clinical manifestations of asthma can be variable. The patient may present with wheezing, complaining of breathlessness, cough, and chest tightness often after exposure to allergens or irritants. Symptoms can occur at various times, but coughing at night is frequent. A thorough lung assessment for adventitious respiratory sounds such as wheezing, crackles, rhonchi, and diminished sounds as well as use of accessory muscle is critical to the nursing assessment. There are validated tools such as the Asthma Control Test, Asthma Control Questionnaire, and Asthma Therapy Assessment Questionnaire that can be used in patient assessments to assess the level of control (GINA, 2010). Other assessments should include a skin inspection for cyanosis, diaphoresis, and listening to heart sounds, as tachycardia may result from overuse of albuterol inhalers. Pulmonary function studies such as spirometry are recommended to diagnose and monitor asthma. A spirometer is a hand-held device that is used for diagnosis and a standard of practice in office settings. Incorporating the use of this tool in correctional settings may reduce the need for or frequency of off-site specialty care (Puisis & Appel, 2006). Changes in signs and symptoms may indicate an exacerbation. Severe exacerbations need close monitoring. Shortness of breath, wheezing, cough, trouble speaking, and an increased respiratory rate may indicate changes in airway clearance and impaired gas exchange. Additional testing such as oxygen saturation or peak flows may be indicated. Assess the skin for cyanosis, pallor. Assess functional patterns; activity tolerance may be impaired with decreased oxygenation. Persons with exacerbations can become extremely anxious. Developing coping strategies such as meditation or visualization as part of the plan of care could be helpful. Administer oxygen and additional therapies as ordered. Be alert to the possible need for hospitalization (Pruitt & Lawson, 2011).

Patient Education

Asthma control is more likely to be successful if the patient learns self-management skills. Nurses provide asthma patient education as well as monitor various treatments such as medications, inhaler use, spirometry testing, peak flow meters, and compliance with therapy. Patients with moderate and severe asthma need an individualized action plan that specifies when to take action, how to self-monitor using peak flow meters, and how to recognize symptoms.

The patient should receive a demonstration of their prescribed inhaler at an initial visit and their technique evaluated at subsequent visits thereafter. The nursing care plan must also include monitoring medication compliance, medication side effects, techniques for using self-assessment tools such as peak flow meters, and actions to avoid environmental triggers. Education about medication actions, side effects, and how and when to take them is critical to positive treatment outcomes. Patient teaching includes techniques for inhaler use and reassessment at each visit. Requiring return demonstrations is crucial to verify the patient can use these devices appropriately.

Collaborative Care

Diagnosis is based on the patient's reports of symptoms and objective measures of pulmonary function studies. A self-action management plan that lists the patient's medications, when to use, and the danger zones should be developed with the patient (NHLBI, 2007). Peak flow meters can be a helpful tool in patient self-management. The variations in readings from normal can alert the patient to an impending exacerbation.

Additional goals include maintaining the patient's functional status and limiting or preventing negative effects from pharmacotherapy. Rescue medications such as albuterol, a short-acting beta agonists (SABA), are used as quick relief from symptoms. Preventive inhaled corticosteroids (ICS), oral corticosteroids for exacerbations and severe asthma, and leukotriene receptor antagonists may be used. Spacers are needed in some cases to ensure the medications are delivered effectively for those patients who may not be able to appropriately coordinate the inhaler with breaths (NHLBI, 2007).

Many times patients stop using ICS because they are feeling well and believe it does not do anything for them. Tachycardia can result from excessive use of albuterol. Patients with exercise-induced asthma take albuterol or cromolyn before engaging in exercise to prevent an asthma episode. Inhalers can also be used as contraband and monitoring the number used is important for determining control as well. Excessive inhaler use should be brought to the attention of the practitioner.

An asthma action plan defines control as the patient feeling good and has a peak flow at 80% or above their personal best (see Figure 6.1). This is labeled the green zone. When the patient develops symptoms and has a peak flow less that 80%

DEPARTMENT OF CORRECTIONS
Division of Adult Institutions
DOC-3446 (Rev. 6/03)

WISCONSIN

OFFENDER NAME		DOC NUMBER	STAFF SIGNATURE	
ASTHMA SEVERITY		PERSONAL BEST PEAK FLOW	DATE PREPARED	

MY DAILY ASTHMA MEDICATION IS

NAME	TYPE	NAME	TYPE
DIRECTIONS:		DIRECTIONS:	
NAME	TYPE	NAME	TYPE
DIRECTIONS:		DIRECTIONS:	
NAME	TYPE	NAME	TYPE
DIRECTIONS:		DIRECTIONS:	

☺ **The Green Zone:** All clear...*I should be here everyday.*

My peak flow is: _____ (80-100% of personal best)
- I am able to do my usual activities.
- I can sleep without having symptoms.
- I have few if any symptoms during waking hours.

I should:
- Continue my maintenance inhalers as outlined above.
- Continue my rescue inhaler as needed.

☺ **The Yellow Zone:** Caution...*this is not where I should be.*

My peak flow is: _____ (50-80% of personal best)
- My symptoms may be mild or moderate.
- I am not able to do my usual activities.
- My symptoms may keep me awake at night.

I should:
- Use my rescue inhaler 2 to 4 puffs every 20 minutes up to 1 hour, or use my nebulizer every 20 minutes for up to 1 hour. Recheck my peak flow after 1 hour. If I am still in the Yellow Zone, I will repeat my rescue inhaler (2 to 4 puffs) or nebulizer (1 treatment) every 4 to 6 hours, continue checking my peak flows, and send a note to the health care system if I am not back in the green zone within 24 hours.
- Increase my maintenance inhaler (_____) to _____ puffs _____ times a day.
- Other things to do: _____

☹ **The Red Zone:** Medical Alert...*this is an emergency!!*

My peak flow is: _____ (Less than 50% of personal best)
- My symptoms are severe.
- I am having difficulty breathing even at rest.
- The muscles in my neck/chest are pulled tight.
- My symptoms are worse after 24 hours in the Yellow Zone

I should:
- Use my rescue inhaler 4 to 6 puffs every 20 minutes up to 1 hour, or use my nebulizer every 20 minutes for up to 1 hour. Recheck my peak flow after 1 hour
- **Ask an officer to contact the health care system NOW!** *I may need emergency treatment if my breathing does not improve.*
- Increase or start my prednisone or other prescribed steroid pill at _____ tablets.
- Other things to do: _____

DISTRIBUTION: Copy – Care Plan Section of Medical Record

FIGURE 6.1 Asthma self-management care plan.

Source: Wisconsin Department of Corrections. Used with permission.

but above 60% of their personal best, the plan identifies specific actions to take, such as increasing rescues or ICS inhale use, and who to call. The red zone, 60% or less of their personal best, is dangerous and the time for immediate action. Emergency actions may include administration of oxygen, use of rescue inhalers, and systemic corticosteroids (NHLBI, 2007).

Overcrowding, old buildings, lack of air quality control, and lack of air-conditioning in hot, humid weather pose risks for the asthmatic. Special housing assignments such as locating the patient near health services or placing them in a smoke-free environment may be necessary, especially for those with severe persistent asthma (Puisis & Appell, 2006). Annual influenza immunizations are important to prevention (NHLBI, 2007).

Security Interface

Security staff must be educated about symptoms associated with respiratory distress and the need to facilitate immediate access to medical care when a patient reports difficulty breathing. The NCCHC (2011a) guidelines recommends inhalers and spacers be kept in cells with the patient. However, not all prisons and jails permit inhalers to be kept on person, especially in segregated settings. A contingency plan must be developed to assure quick access to care should an asthma attack occur. On occasion, chemical agents are used by security staff in crisis situations. Health services is usually the point of contact to inform officers about patients who may be adversely affected by chemical agents and will be the first contact if the inmate develops adverse effects. Case Example 6.1 applies information from this section.

CASE EXAMPLE 6.1

A 23-year-old male individual is brought to health services because he is having trouble breathing. A review of his medical record indicates he is being seen in the chronic care clinic every three months for asthma. He had been evaluated the previous morning and no problems were noted. He has an albuterol inhaler prescribed every 4 to 6 hours as needed for shortness of breath or wheezing and an ICS inhaler to be taken twice a day. His vital signs are: T. 99.1 F; BP 126/78; P 100; R. 22 and his peak flow readings are 75% of his baseline level. Name three behaviors and/or environmental factors that could account for this change in status in one day. What additional subjective and objective information is needed to plan care?

Arthritis

Arthritis increases with aging; as many as 50% of individuals 65 years and older have osteoarthritis (O/A). Adults with arthritis and obesity are more likely to be physically inactive compared to nonobese individuals with arthritis, and the presence of arthritis may also become a barrier for an individual to engage in physical activity because of the discomfort (CDC, 2011c). The disease process involves remodeling of joint surfaces. As the disease progresses, joint cartilage becomes thin and rough, spaces narrow and bony surfaces rub together, synovial fluid escapes, and bone spurs develop at tendon and ligament attachment sites. The destruction of cartilage results in the weight-bearing joints being unable to withstand the load. Stiffness and mild-to-severe discomfort and disability is a common symptom. It occurs after periods of rest, especially early in the morning, and resolves within 30 minutes after moving about. In O/A, affected joints are asymmetrical. The most commonly affected joints are the digits of the hands, hips, knees, cervical, and lower lumbar areas (NIH, 2011).

There is no cure for arthritis. Evidenced-based osteoarthritis treatment recommendations are focused on two primary causes of arthritis; obesity and lack of exercise. However, weight management and exercise is often ignored, instead analgesic and/or inflammatory medications are the mainstay of treatment (Hunter, Thuina, & Hochberg, 2011). In correctional institutions, health staff can encourage a patient individually to exercise, but exercise equipment, group activities that promote exercise, and freedom to engage in a variety of exercise programs may be very limited or absent.

Nursing Management

Nursing care planning includes improving pain control and maintaining function. A comprehensive patient history should include questions about previous injuries, specific joints involved and joint pain, the patient's current functional status, mobility, use of adaptive equipment, and coping mechanisms. Assessment components of the physical examination include weight and body mass index (BMI), visualization of joints for deformities and range of motion, presence of crepitus, a determination of muscle strength, presence of muscle atrophy, and tenderness to palpation. Identify triggers or activities that cause pain and develop a care plan with therapeutic interventions that encourage the patient to use prescribed medications for pain relief and assistive devices for ambulation and maintaining activities of daily living. Encourage the patient to perform isometric, passive, and active range of motion exercises (Gulanick & Myers, 2011a). Identify safety needs such as appropriate housing, need for a low bunk or lower tier, and allowable adaptive equipment are essential to effective management.

Nurses schedule and coordinate periodic follow-up to evaluate pain control, functional status, review the patient's use of medications, check for side effects, review laboratory values, and carefully document findings. Identify real or perceived barriers to compliance and use the data to make readjustments in the plan of care. This information is also used to guide treatment decisions by the interdisciplinary team.

Patient Education

Pain management is a major focus of therapy and optimal treatment outcomes are more likely if the patient is knowledgeable about medication purpose, dose, and side effects. Heat and cold applications can be helpful in relieving discomfort but pose a challenge in the corrections environment. Devices available such as electrical heating pads or tubs for warm baths may not be available and the patient may be limited to using towels or washcloths for these applications. Patients can be instructed to place a damp towel in a microwave, if available, but cautioned to test the towel before application to prevent a burn.

Teaching patients how to use adaptive equipment such as canes, walkers, crutches, and braces correctly and safely is an important function for nursing. Independent nursing interventions include teaching patients about proper alignment, safe body mechanics, and hot and cold therapies. Stretching exercises can have positive impact by decreasing pain and maintaining mobility. Some institutions offer yoga which is tremendously helpful in establishing balance and increasing flexibility.

The patient who cannot walk or jog because of major joint impairment may work out on a stationary bike as an alternative.

Collaborative Care

Patient management goals include (1) maintaining or improving joint function (2) using joint protection measures to improve or activity tolerance (3) achieving independence in self-care (4) using pharmacologic and nonpharmacologic strategies to manage pain satisfactorily (Arthritis Foundation, 2011; Roberts, 2004).

Physical activity has been proven to reduce pain and improve physical function among persons with arthritis (CDC, 2011c). Standard exercise recommendations specify walking or biking 30 minutes, 3 days or more a week. Impaired mobility such as the fear of falling, joint stiffness, or pain may significantly impact the patient's participation in exercise and cause functional limitations (CDC, 2011c).

Classes of medication often used for arthritis analgesia include acetaminophen, salicylates, nonsteroidal anti-inflammatory drugs (NSAIDs), intra-articular corticosteroid injections, muscle relaxants, and narcotics. All can result in toxicities if taken excessively and patients should be cautioned not to exceed the daily recommended doses. Acetaminophen intake should not exceed 4 g/day. ASA and NSAIDS can have significant effects on the gastrointestinal system. The patient should be educated to take the medicine with food and report any blood in stools. Aspirin may pose a danger for stroke in patients with poorly controlled hypertension. Managing chronic pain in corrections is also complicated because of the potential for abuse and secondary gain. Muscle relaxants and narcotics are highly coveted and especially prone to misuse as contraband. Therefore, the correctional nurse has a great responsibility to monitor patient use of medications for patient and security reasons.

Substances such as topically applied capsaicin can be helpful in some cases because they interfere with the local transmission of pain. The patient must be instructed not to use with an external source of heat to prevent burns. An alternative therapy, glucosamine, is sometimes used but has questionable effectiveness.

Rest and immobilization of an arthritic joint may be necessary at times as a method of joint protection. The joint should always be positioned in a functional position but never for a prolonged time because of the potential for joint stiffness. Additional measures include avoiding forceful repetitive movements and stress positions, use of assistive devices when needed, weight loss, instructions in good body mechanics, and help in balancing or pacing daily tasks (Roberts, 2004).

Low-impact exercises are recommended to increase joint function and decrease joint pain and stiffness. A physical therapy consultation may be helpful in developing an exercise regimen specific to the patient's need. Exercise for patients in segregation status is especially challenging because of the small confinement space and generally limited out-of-cell time. In-cell exercises of calisthenics, stretching, and in-place walking are possible although not easily adopted by inmates.

Security Interface

Collaboration between health care and security staff is critical to ensure the patient has access to any ordered adaptive devices and exercise equipment such as treadmills and bikes. Security levels, inmate movement, and equipment location influence availability of exercise programs. Older inmates or those with limited mobility may not be able to access an upper level or a distant building for exercise. Wheelchair use, special housing, or low bunks may need to be provided. Low bunks are highly sought after by inmates and may be the subject of numerous health requests because medical authorization is often required. Healthcare staff should develop guidelines based on medical need to reduce the risk of inappropriately providing or withholding permission. In general, nursing interventions are key in working with the patient and custody to identify locations, times, and equipment the patient can access to reinforce any recommended physical therapy or exercise programs.

Diabetes

The American Diabetes Association (ADA) estimated diabetes prevalence among prisoners to be lower than the general population, 4.8% of the 2.3 million of the incarcerated population (ADA, 2010). However, a recently published national survey comparing federal, state, and jail inmates to the U.S. population found a higher prevalence when standardizing for age, as follows; 11.1% of federal, 10.1% of state, and 8.1% of jail inmates (Wilper et al., 2009).

Type 1 comprises about 5% of all diabetics. The disease can occur at any age, although it is more common under the age of 30. At the time of disease onset the patient is no longer producing endogenous insulin due to the destruction of B islet cells believed to be due to an autoimmune process. Symptoms include frequent urination, excessive thirst, extreme hunger, unusual weight loss, and extreme fatigue and irritability (ADA, 2011).

Type 2 accounts for 90% of all diabetes, has a gradual onset, and generally occurs later in life, usually after age 35 or 40. It is greater in some ethnic populations, especially Native Americans. Endogenous insulin is still being produced but insufficient for the body's needs or is poorly utilized. Another mechanism involved is an inappropriate production of glucose in liver that may interfere with glucose regulation. The disease is believed to have a genetic component that produces insulin resistance, but is also associated with modifiable lifestyle factors of inactivity and obesity. Symptoms may include frequent infections, blurred visions, cuts and bruises that are slow to heal, and tingling or numbness in the hands or feet. Often persons have no symptoms (ADA, 2011).

Gestational diabetes can develop during pregnancy and is usually detectable at 24–28 weeks. The percentage of women who develop the disease is about 4% and they are at increased risk for cesarean delivery, neonatal complications, and perinatal death. Treatment of women with gestational diabetes requires specialized care and management. Women who develop gestational diabetes have a 35%–60% chance of developing diabetes in the next 10–20 years (CDC, 2011d).

Acute complications of diabetes include hypo- and hyperglycemia. Both are potentially serious complications requiring immediate treatment. Hypoglycemia, low blood glucose, is defined as a blood glucose level less than 60 mg/dL and can result from illness, missed meals, or inappropriate doses of medications. Symptoms often include tremors, diaphoresis, confusion, weakness, and visual disturbances that will lead to loss of consciousness, seizures, coma, and death, if untreated. Severe hypoglycemia is a medical emergency but can be quickly reversed with the administration of 10–15 g of a fast-acting carbohydrate such as orange juice, milk, or glucose tablets. If unconscious, a third party may be needed to administer 1 mg of glucagon sublingually, subcutaneously, or intramuscularly. Some patients can feel early symptoms of hypoglycemia and take action, others cannot. Any episode of severe hypoglycemia requires follow-up by the medical staff (ADA, 2010). Diabetic acidosis is a physiologic state where insulin becomes deficient with resultant hyperglycemia that if untreated results in electrolyte imbalances and can lead to acidosis and ketosis. If the hyperglycemia is accompanied by nausea and vomiting, the patient may be in diabetic ketoacidosis, which is life threatening. Early symptoms include lethargy, then dry skin as dehydration worsens. Rapid breathing occurs to blow off carbon dioxide and a sweet fruity breath may be detected. Coma and death will occur without immediate treatment (ADA, 2010).

Nursing Management

As in the general population, early identification of the disease is imperative, as prompt intervention decreases risks of acute complications and the need for off-site care (FBOP, 2010; NCCHC, 2011b). The ADA (2010) screening recommendations for all diabetic inmates entering prisons and jails are:

- Reception screening should occur within *1–2 hours* to identify all inmates with diabetes currently using insulin therapy or at high risk for hypoglycemia. Obtain capillary blood glucose (CBG) and urine ketone test (as clinically indicated) on all insulin treated patients, obtain immediate CBG on those patients exhibiting signs/symptoms consistent with hypoglycemia, and continue usual meal schedule and medication administration.
- Intake screening should occur within *2–4 hours* and include a comprehensive history to identify the type of diabetes, duration, presence of complications, family history, and pertinent behavioral patterns.
- Intake physical examination should occur within *2 hours– 2 weeks*, including laboratory tests to assess glucose levels, HgA1c, lipids, urine for ketones, and chemistries to assess kidney and liver function.

Additional information about hospitalizations, frequency of hypoglycemic episodes, functional health patterns, and both prescribed and over-the-counter medication use are important for care planning. Efforts should be taken to verify prescriptions and past medical history to continue medication and nutrition therapy without interruption.

Ongoing chronic care appointments are scheduled according to clinical need, usually every 3–6 months. Between visits, the nurse has a major role in monitoring the diabetic patient, including:

- Assessing the patient's knowledge of treatment strategies, periodic blood pressure checks, and weight
- Compliance with medications, diet, and exercise
- Blood glucose readings and episodes of hypoglycemia or adverse events
- Obtain ordered laboratory tests and report abnormalities
- Identify real or perceived barriers to compliance
- Coordinate follow-up and periodic reassessments
- Schedule annual dental, foot, dilated eye exam, and annual influenza immunization (ADA, 2010).

CBG is necessary to monitor blood glucose and to adjust medications accordingly. Type 1 diabetics usually need to perform CBG 3–4 times daily, while well-controlled Type 2 diabetics may need to monitor only once daily. Testing must be immediately available for the patient when experiencing symptoms of hypo- or hyperglycemia. In correctional settings the process to perform this function varies. Security procedures may require the patient to come to a central location to check blood glucose. In facilities where patients are permitted to use a glucose meter, the nurse is responsible to teach and validate the patient's skills to assure accurate readings. Results are usually recorded on flow sheets and available for review at chronic clinic visits. Infection control measures for cleaning the machine and disposal of lancets and syringes are also necessary teaching points for the patient.

Another very challenging but critical function in corrections involves coordinating medications with timing of meals, snacks, and insulin, especially short-acting insulin to prevent episodes of hypoglycemia. Considerations include meal time, access to insulin administration in relation to the meal, inmate movement time, actions to take in a lockdown situation where meals may be delayed, and contingency plans to provide food such as a sack lunch or snack if insulin was given and the meal was delayed (FBOP, 2010; NCCHC, 2011d).

From the Experts ...

"The chronic care nurse ensures that all necessary tests, including periodic tests, are done timely and are available for provider to review, visits are scheduled according to guidelines, and co-morbidity is identified and managed. The frequency of contact between the nurse and patient provides the avenue to monitor compliance with diet, medications, exercise, and other instructions. There is a very low rate of unscheduled visits or sick call visits when the care of a diabetic is well coordinated by the nurse."

Oluyemi M. Awodiya, MBA, RN, CCHP
Wilmington, DE

Regular exercise is an important component of management to lower blood glucose and control weight. In some situations the nurse may need to facilitate exercise by providing a written pass for use of the equipment or movement to a building that houses exercise equipment.

An at-risk patient must have a plan to manage episodes of hypoglycemia and hyperglycemia, including recognition of signs and symptoms, a source of quick-acting glucose, and access to immediate medical care.

In some institutions, patients are allowed to draw up their insulin, but administration of the medication is always conducted under some security or nursing supervision. There have been cases where patients have taken inappropriate doses for various reasons, such as self-harm or to get out of the facility on an emergency basis. Patients who have declining visual or motor skills may not be able to accurately draw up and administer their own insulin.

Diabetics are at great risk for infections that could result in amputations. Patients need to know how to protect their feet and examine them frequently for any sores or infections. In some cases, the nurse may need to facilitate toenail clipping where the patient has physical limitations, advanced circulatory compromise of their feet, or in institutions that do not allow inmate use of clippers. Nurses may also be responsible for obtaining special shoes for diabetics and assessing the patient for symptoms of neuropathy.

Patient Education

Components of patient teaching include, disease process and how to prevent chronic complications such as foot ulcers, survival skills regarding acute complications of hypo- and hyperglycemia, nutrition and diet, self-monitoring of blood glucose, how to take medications, personal hygiene, sick day management, exercise, and follow-up monitoring.

Limited food choices and physical inactivity along with commissaries offering snacks high in refined sugar, salt, and fat make dietary modifications difficult (Puisis & Appel, 2006). Correctional nurses should provide education on food choices to self-select from a heart-healthy menu, snack time as clinically ordered, and choices that the inmates can purchase from the commissary.

Collaborative Care

Maintaining blood glucose levels near normal is defined as HbgA1c less than 7%. Additional goals include a preprandial glucose between 90–130 mg/dL, a postprandial glucose less than 180 mg/dL, and a blood pressure less than 130/80 Hg (ADA, 2010). Individuals at risk for hypoglycemia may require less stringent goals, particularly patients with a history of severe hypoglycemia, limited life expectancy, comorbid conditions, and the elderly (ADA, 2010). The Wisconsin Department of Corrections (WDOC), using the chronic care model, has been able to lower the number of diabetic patients who are in poor control (HbA1c greater than 9%). The number of patients in poor control is now 6%–10% of all diabetics (personal communications, D. Burnett, MD 9/27/2011). Insulin administration is challenging in prisons and jails. Meal times vary, with limited time to consume the meal and not always conducive to a schedule. There may be a long lapse between the evening meal and breakfast. Snack bags may be needed to prevent hypoglycemia. Knowledge of meal time is essential for coordinating insulin administration. The patient should be cautioned not to add drugs such as those obtained over the counter (OTC) without checking with their treatment provider because of potential effect on blood glucose levels.

Security Interface

All correctional staff should recognize symptoms of hypo- and hyperglycemia and know how to take appropriate emergency action (ADA, 2010). The nurse will be the first contact for advice when officers have questions about a diabetic patient. The nurse must ensure that the custodial staff has instructions for emergency care for diabetic patients at risk for hypoglycemia.

Cardiovascular Diseases

Heart disease was found to be the leading cause of deaths among inmates (42%) in local jails (Bureau of Justice Statistics, 2010) and one of the many chronic medical conditions possibly responsible for excess mortality from cardiovascular, liver disease, and liver cancer among former inmates (Binswanger et al., 2009). Correctional populations are comprised of a higher number of underserved minorities without prior access to primary healthcare. Persons without health insurance have poorer control of hypertension and LDL-C than those with health care access and a higher prevalence of disease morbidity and mortality (CDC, 2011e). African Americans have higher rates of mortality due to coronary artery disease. Hypertension is also more aggressive and prevalent among this group, with resulting target organ damage such as stroke and chronic kidney disease.

Guidelines for treating hypertension and hyperlipidemia are published in *The Seventh Report of the Joint National Committee on Prevention, Detection, Evaluation, and Treatment of High Blood Pressure (JNC 7)* and the *Adult Treatment Panel III (ATP III)* for hyperlipidemia. These guidelines contain treatment goals and lifestyle recommendations, and stress the need for a multidisciplinary approach to patient care. The NCCHC guidelines for hypertension (2011c) and hyperlipidemia (2011d) disease management in corrections support the use of these national practices in correctional settings and include specific strategies to apply the national practice guidelines in the correctional environment. See Tables 6.1 and 6.2 for lipid goals and Table 6.3 for blood pressure classifications.

Nursing Management

The goals of therapy are to reduce morbidity through blood pressure and lipid control using medications and lifestyle modifications including:

1. Assessing, monitoring, and control of disease severity to reduce cardiovascular risk
2. Patient education and self-management about the disease process, lifestyle modifications, and medication use
3. Mitigation of factors that increase blood pressure
4. Medications recommended by national guidelines

The comprehensiveness of the assessment is determined by the setting, length of sentence, and purpose. For inmates with longer sentences, an in-depth history and physical

TABLE 6.1 ATP Classifications of LDL, Total, and HDL Cholesterol (mg/dL)

LDL Cholesterol—Primary Target of Therapy	
<100	Optimal
100–129	Near Optimal/Above Optimal
130–159	Borderline High
160–189	High
≥190	Very High
Total Cholesterol	
<200	Desirable
200–239	Borderline High
≥240	High
HDL Cholesterol	
<40	Low
≥60	High

Source: National Heart, Lung, and Blood Institute, (2002, September). *Third report of the National Cholesterol Education Program (NCEP) Expert Panel on Detection, Evaluation, and Treatment of High Blood Cholesterol in Adults (Adult Treatment Panel III)*, (NIH) Publication No. 02-5215). Used with permission.

TABLE 6.2   ATP Classifications of Serum Triglycerides (mg/dL)

<150	Normal
150–199	Borderline high
200–499	High
≥500	Very high

Source: National Heart, Lung, and Blood Institute. (2002, September). *Third report of the National Cholesterol Education Program (NCEP) Expert Panel on Detection, Evaluation, and Treatment of High Blood Cholesterol in Adults (Adult Treatment Panel III)*, (NIH) Publication No. 02-5215). Used with permission.

examination should be done. When incarceration is of shorter duration, the focus is to address immediate needs (Puisis & Appel, 2006). Determining risk, a major focus of treatment guidelines, requires the collection of data regarding risk factors, including:

- Age (greater than 55 years for male adults and greater than 65 years for female adults)
- History of smoking
- Excess intake of dietary sodium
- Male gender
- Family history
- Obesity
- Sedentary lifestyle
- Excessive alcohol use
- Lower socioeconomic status and ethnicity (NHLBI, 2002).

Hypertension diagnosis, disease severity, and management are dependent on accurate blood pressure measurements (Exhibit 6.1). When inmates enter the correctional system, especially jails, they may have high blood pressure readings, a result of alcohol or illicit drug use. Therefore, repeat blood pressure measurement should be scheduled to improve accuracy (FBOP, 2009). Self-measurement of blood pressure is considered useful to improve adherence to therapy, evaluating "white-coat hypertension" and in supporting self-care. Although this is not a prevailing practice in correctional environments, if the practice is possible, it should be utilized. Correctional nurses need to be aware of the circumstances of blood pressure measurement. Blood pressure readings should not be taken on an arm through a cuff port. Lung or heart

TABLE 6.3   The Seventh Report of the Joint National Committee (JNC 7) Blood Pressure (BP) Classification

BP CLASSIFICATION	SYSTOLIC BP (MMHG)	DIASTOLIC BP (MMHG)	LIFESTYLE MODIFICATION
Normal	<120	<80	Encourage
Prehypertension	120–139	80–89	Yes
Stage 1 Hypertension	140–159	90–99	Yes
Stage 2 Hypertension	≥160	≥100	Yes

Source: National Heart, Lung, and Blood Institute. (2003, December). *The seventh report of the Joint National Committee on Prevention, Detection, Evaluation, and Treatment of High Blood Pressure (JNC 7 Express)*, National Institutes of Health (NIH) Publication No. 03-5233. Used with permission.

EXHIBIT 6.1
Criteria for Accurate Blood Pressure Measurements

The patient should be seated quietly for at least 5 minutes in a chair with feet on the floor, and arm supported at heart level.

An appropriate-sized cuff, one that has a bladder that encircles 80% of the arm is required.

The cuff should be calibrated and at least two measurements should be taken.

The initial BP should be taken on both arms to note any differences and subsequently checked when a high reading is obtained in one arm.

Source: Content adapted from the National Heart, Lung, and Blood Institute. (2003, December). *The seventh report of the Joint National Committee on Prevention, Detection, Evaluation, and Treatment of High Blood Pressure (JNC 7 Express).*

sounds may be difficult to hear because of noise. Patients may not respond to nursing queries if there is a lack of privacy or they are angry. Data from health care assessments that are collected in security cells or other locations where sound, privacy, or the placement of the patient can be inaccurate and compromise treatment.

The correctional nurse is the main point of contact with the patient, providing education and monitoring the patient's self-care. Collaborative nursing functions include obtaining laboratory information, coordinating appointments, and communicating with other team members. Key to each encounter for management of cardiovascular disease is a body mass index (BMI) or waist measurement and blood pressure reading.

Patient Education

Teaching patients how to select heart-healthy foods supports patient self-management and is preferable to a mandated diet. To help patients make wiser choices, nurses can review menus, canteen lists, and food labels with the patient to help them avoid or limit sodium, fat, and calories. Dietary manuals and teaching materials provided in the national guidelines may also be a resource for patient instruction. Table 6.4 provides information about lowering cholesterol through diet.

TABLE 6.4   Cholesterol Drop With Therapeutic Lifestyle Changes (TLC)

DROP YOUR CHOLESTEROL WITH TLC		
	CHANGE	LDL REDUCTION (%)
Saturated fat	Decrease to less than 7% of calories	8–10
Dietary cholesterol	Decrease to less than 200 mg/day	3–5
Weight	Lose 10 pounds if overweight	5–8
Soluble fiber	Add 5–20 g/day	3–5
Plant sterols/stanols	Add 2 g/day	5–15
Total		20–30

Source: Your Guide to Lowering your Cholesterol with TLC (2005)—taken from NIH NHLBI, Third Report of the National Cholesterol Education Program (NCEP) Expert Panel on Detection, Evaluation, and Treatment of High Blood Cholesterol in Adult Treatment Panel (ATP III); NIH publication No. 06-5235 p.16. Used with permission.

Exercise can help lower body weight, blood pressure, and lipid levels. For those who are new to physical activity, recommend light activity such as walking slowly. Thirty minutes of moderate-intensity exercise is recommended most days of the week. Examples of moderate-intensity activities include brisk walking (15-minute mile), biking on a stationary bike at 5 miles in 30 minutes, as well as some work such as gardening or cleaning. Emphasize that not all the exercise needs to be completed at one time and may be done in 10–15 minute intervals (NHLBI, 2005). Many inmates engage in weight training for increasing muscle mass and toning, however, this is not a substitute for the daily exercise.

Collaborative Care

Pharmacological therapy is the mainstay of treatment; however, adherence may be very poor due to side effects, motivation, and lack of knowledge. At times patients stop their medications because their last blood pressure reading was normal, not realizing that long-term treatment with medications is usually needed to maintain a normal blood pressure. Medication compliance can also be monitored by reviewing the number of blister packs issued through a keep-on-person (KOP) system or number of refusals during medication passes. Patient use of over-the-counter medications (OTC) is also important information to the treatment plan.

Security Interface

There are many challenges to the proper use of medical diets in the correctional environment. Patients may reject special diets if they have limited food choices and no alternatives to personal dislikes. Offering a master menu of a heart-healthy diet containing carbohydrate content for each meal may be the easiest and most cost-effective means to facilitate good outcomes. Commissary offerings should also include healthy food choices and include listings of carbohydrate contents of items (ADA, 2010). Case Example 6.2 is an opportunity to apply information from this section.

CASE EXAMPLE 6.2

A 30-year-old patient with hypertension has an elevated reading during a routine blood pressure check. He reports that he does not like being on medication and has not taken his antihypertensive medication for the last month. He states that if he works out and watches his diet he will be fine. What education would you include in his plan of care? What collaborative care functions could be included to help achieve compliance?

Epilepsy/Seizure Disorder

A study in a typical prison in the United Kingdom revealed that clinical management of epileptic seizure disorders was poor when compared to the National Institute for Clinical Excellence (NICE) standards of care (Tittensor, Collins, Grunewald, & Reuber, 2008). The prevalence and quality of care among prisoners with epilepsy in the United States is unknown.

An epilepsy diagnosis is defined as two or more unprovoked seizures and results in a change in behavior caused by a spontaneous, uncontrolled electrical

TABLE 6.5   International Classification of Seizures

Partial Seizures
A. Simple partial seizures (consciousness not impaired)
1. With motor symptoms 2. With sensory symptoms 3. With autonomic symptoms 4. With psychic symptoms
B. Complex partial seizures (with impaired consciousness)
1. Simple partial seizures followed by impairment of consciousness 2. With impairment of consciousness at seizure onset
C. Partial seizures evolving to secondarily generalized seizures
1. Simple partial secondarily generalized 2. Complex partial secondarily generalized 3. Simple partial evolving to complex partial evolving to generalized
Generalized seizures
A. Absence seizures (formerly called petit mal) B. Myoclonic seizures C. Clonic seizures D. Tonic seizures E. Tonic clonic seizures (formerly called grand mal) F. Atonic seizures (drop attacks)
Unclassified seizures

Source: Adapted from http://professionals.epilepsy.com/page/seizures_classified.html

discharge of neurons in the brain that interrupts normal body functions. Convulsions, muscle spasms, and loss of consciousness may occur. Seizures are usually unpredictable, brief (less than 5 min), and stop spontaneously. The International Classification of Seizures describes the two major categories, generalized and partial seizures, with subtypes (Table 6.5). Heredity may have a role in epilepsy but most cases are acquired after birth. In 70% of cases, no cause is apparent. If the seizure is not associated with other neurologic disease, it is called idiopathic. Some of the known causes of epilepsy are listed in Table 6.6.

Several surveys and studies indicate a relationship between stigma and seizure frequency and a resulting poorer quality of care for persons with epilepsy. Individuals with epilepsy may have increased social isolation due to misconceptions and fear about epilepsy and struggle to overcome poor self-esteem. Public education has decreased the negative image today, but persons with epilepsy who perceived higher levels of stigma had lower levels of self-efficacy in disease management (National Institute of Neurological Disorders and Strokes [NINDS], 2002, 2011).

Nursing Management

The focus of nursing care is observation and description of symptoms to assist with diagnosis, patient education, and patient safety. Nursing care includes:

1. Assessment to identify and describe seizure activity,

TABLE 6.6 Causes of Seizure Activity

CAUSES OF EPILEPSY	CAUSES OF NONEPILEPTIC SEIZURES
• Oxygen deprivation (e.g., during childbirth) • Brain infections (e.g., meningitis, encephalitis, cysticercosis, or brain abscess) • Traumatic brain injury or head injury • Stroke (resulting from a block or rupture of a blood vessel in the brain) • Other neurologic diseases (e.g., Alzheimer disease) • Brain tumors • Certain genetic disorders	• Alcohol withdrawal • Benzodiazepine withdrawal • Massive sleep deprivation • Excessive use of stimulants, cocaine, etc. • Psychogenic (conversion disorder, somatization, factitious disorder, malingering) • Acute head trauma (within 1 week) • Central nervous system infection or neoplasm • Uremia • Eclampsia • High fever • Hypoxemia • Hyperglycemia or hypoglycemia • Electrolyte disorder

Source: Content adapted from Kammerman and Wasserman (2001) and the CDC (2011f).

2. Educating about the disease and the therapeutic regimen, including medications and lifestyle adjustments, and
3. Identifying safety measures to prevent injury and potential comorbidities that could occur with falls, self-inflicted bites, prolonged hypoxic states with resulting neurological damage, and medication side effects (Gulanick & Myers, 2011a, b; Ozuna, 2004).

Seizures due to epilepsy must be differentiated from an isolated event that originates from a nonepileptic cause (Table 6.6). An objective assessment of a seizure includes the following detailed observations; a complete description including the time of onset, any events preceding the seizure such as aura, limbs and affected muscles, types of movements, and the length of time each phase lasted. Subjective information includes any headaches, aura, or mood swings before and after a seizure (Ozuna, 2004).

An inventory of the patient's current medication use, compliance with antiseizure medications, use of and/or overdose of drugs such as cocaine and amphetamines, and alcohol withdrawal is another major portion of the nursing health history. Jail admissions are of particular concern, when an inmate may have been without antiepileptic medications for several days and is at risk for seizures (Puisis & Appel, 2006).

Patient Education

Patient teaching about the disease process associated with their type of seizure, their prescribed medication, the importance of adhering to prescribed medication administration times, and all side effects is essential for effective treatment. Inform the patient about keeping appointments for ordered laboratory tests.

Increased seizures can occur in the presence of fatigue and stress. Therefore, education messages must also include measures to promote good health habits, eating regular meals, and reviewing relaxation techniques. Identify safety measures such as appropriate housing, restrictions of low bunk, low tier, job assignment, or providing a medical alert bracelet or other allowable identification. Discuss with the patient what information will be shared to assure necessary actions for first aid in the event of a seizure and still protect their health privacy. Advice about driving regulations should be provided for persons nearing discharge and a list of community resources for continuity of care.

Collaborative Care

Most useful to diagnosing epilepsy is a comprehensive health history and an accurate description of the seizures, including frequency and date of the last seizure (NINDS, 2011). In addition to a comprehensive health history and neurological examination, other tests such as an electroencephalogram (EEG), computed tomography (CT), or magnetic resonance imaging (MRI) may be indicated to diagnose epilepsy (CDC, 2011f; Scottish Intercollegiate Guidelines Network [SIGN] 2003).

Any seizure lasting longer than 5 to 10 minutes is a life-threatening condition and requires emergency response. Patients with seizures who also need emergent practitioner or emergency room evaluation include those with:

- No previous seizure history,
- Seizures lasting longer than 5 to 10 minutes,
- Seizure recurs without patient returning to normal consciousness,
- Failure to return to normal consciousness in a timely fashion after a seizure, and significant injury due to a seizure (CDC, 2011f; NINDS, 2002).

Psychogenic nonepileptic seizures (PNES), sometimes referred to as pseudo seizures, are events that appear to be epileptic seizures but are without the characteristic electrical discharges (NINDS, 2011). The term *pseudo* conjures up an image of the seizure not being real and that the patient is faking it. In most instances, PNES is due to a psychiatric disorder and the majority of these seizures are not volitional (Reuber et al., 2003). When a seizure event is believed to be psychological in origin, the patient should be referred for mental health services because they cannot be treated as epileptic seizures (NINDS, 2011). In the correctional environment, a concern exists that a patient could invent a seizure for secondary gain such as a low bunk, mood-altering medication, or special treatment. Approximately 10% to 30% of patients with nonepileptic seizures also have epilepsy (Glosser, 1988; Puisis & Appel, 2006; Reuber et al., 2003).

Seizures are treated in most epileptic patients with anticonvulsant medications. These medications are mood altering, and in the prison and jail settings can be illegally traded as contraband. Patients may also be strong-armed for them and therefore not effectively treated. Access and administration to these medications should be controlled (NINDS, 2011; Puisis & Appel, 2006).

Anticonvulsant medications are prescribed in increasing doses until the seizure is controlled or until toxic side effects occur. Monotherapy is sufficient in most cases but a second medication may be added if seizures are not controlled. Patients should be assessed by nursing at each follow-up visit for knowledge of, compliance with, and side effects of medications. Monitoring therapeutic drug levels may be necessary to confirm suspected toxicity and to check for patient compliance. Therapeutic levels are only guides and subtherapeutic levels are acceptable if the patient is without seizure activity. Medication doses are adjusted on the basis of clinical symptoms, not blood levels (Tittensor et al., 2008).

Pregnant women with epilepsy should be managed by a specialist and receive prenatal vitamins and folic acid to prevent fetal abnormalities. Hormonal changes can sometimes affect seizure activity and some anticonvulsant medications can cause harm to the fetus. Seizures leading to hypoxia in pregnant women could have devastating consequences for the fetus (CDC, 2011f; NINDS, 2011).

Security Interface

Custody staff having contact with an inmate who has a seizure disorder must have information about any restrictions or precautions with regard to housing, work, or programming assignments. This information should be provided by the nurse without divulging diagnostic details. Patients with epilepsy may not want others to know for fear of isolation or other stigma associated with the diagnosis.

Security staff should be taught the following first-aid measures for a seizure with loss of consciousness:

- Remain calm;
- If the patient is standing, help them to the floor and cushion the person's head
- Roll them to their side and keep their airway open. Use a jaw tilt if necessary to open the airway and loosen any tight clothing around the neck;
- Do not restrict the person from moving unless they are in danger;
- Never place an object in the patient's mouth, not even liquid or medicine. These could compromise their airway and cause choking or damage to the person's tongue, jaw, or teeth. Contrary to a widespread myth, people cannot swallow their tongue;
- Remove any sharp or solid objects the person might hit during the seizure; and
- Note the time of the seizure, how long it lasts, and what symptoms occurred to inform emergency or health staff (NINDS, 2011).

Security staff can become very alarmed when a seizure occurs and initiate emergency actions. However, information from custodial staff can also be biased depending on their interaction with the inmate. One correctional system reported an incident where security staff informed the nurse the inmate was faking a seizure and should be ignored. The inmate had a history of conflict with security staff. The patient, in fact, was having seizures. Caution must be taken by the nurse not to accept information without careful confirmation based on fact and actual observation. When in doubt about information obtained about the patient, it is best to err in favor of the patient's health and safety.

SUMMARY

The importance of chronic disease monitoring is recognized by correctional health professionals, but the effectiveness of delivery systems in these complicated environments is mixed. More work is needed to identify chronic disease care models that are effective in the correctional setting and benchmark with other correctional systems. Nursing is a key team player in operationalizing chronic disease care planning and monitoring as well as a major provider of patient education in correctional facilities. More research is needed to identify evidence-based nursing practices and support nurses in providing patient-centered, chronic disease care.

DISCUSSION QUESTIONS

1. Describe the prevalence of chronic diseases in the general inmate population. How does that compare with the patient population at your facility?
2. Compare the nursing involvement in chronic disease management in your facility with that described in this chapter. Are there ways to increase nurse involvement in patient education and collaborative management?
3. List resources for developing chronic disease care guidelines.
4. Describe security involvement in various chronic diseases discussed in this chapter. What are the key components of custody's role? Are there ways to improve officer involvement in your facility?
5. Select one of the chronic conditions discussed in this chapter. Review a medical record for a patient in your facility who has this condition. Identify examples of the key components of nursing care described in this chapter.

REFERENCES

Aldridge, M. (2004). Writing and designing readable patient education materials. *Nephrology Nursing Journal of the American Nephrology Nurses Association, 31*(4), 373–377. Retrieved from http://www.ncbi.nlm.nih.gov/pubmed/15453229

American Corrections Association (ACA). (2003). *Standards for Adult Correctional Institutions* (4th ed.). Alexandria, VA: ACA.

American Diabetes Association (ADA). (2010, January). Diabetes management in correctional institutions. *Diabetes Care, 33*(Suppl. 1), S75–S81.

American Diabetes Association (ADA). (2011). *Diabetes basics*. Retrieved August 23, 2011, from http://www.diabetes.org/

American Nurses Association (ANA). (2007). *Corrections nursing: Scope and standards of practice*. Silver Spring, MD: Author.

Arthritis Foundation. (2011). *Osteoarthritis causes*. Retrieved November 7, 2011, from http://www.arthritis.org/what-is-osteoarthritis.php

Binswanger, I. A. (2010, October 25). *Chronic medical diseases among jail and prison inmates*. Retrieved February 7, 2011, from http://www.corrections.com/news/article/26014

Binswanger, I. A., Krueger, P. M., & Steiner, J. F. (2009). Prevalence of chronic medical conditions among jail and prison inmates in the USA compared with the general population. *Journal of Epidemiology Community Health, 63*, 912–919.

Bishop, A. J., & Merten, M. J. (2011). Risk of comorbid health impairment among older male inmates. *Journal of Correctional Health Care, 17*(1), 34–45.

Bureau of Justice Statistics. (2010, July). Mortality in local jails, 2000–2007, *Special Report: Death in Custody Reporting Program*, NCJ 222988, revised October 26, 2010.

Centers for Disease Control and Prevention. (2011a, May 20). Surveillance of health status in minority communities—racial and ethnic approaches to community health across the U.S. (REACH US) Risk Factor Survey, United States 2009. *MMWR Recommendations and Reports, 60*(SS06), 1–41.

Centers for Disease Control and Prevention. (2011b, January 14). CDCs health disparities and inequality report: current asthma prevalence–United States, 2006–2008, *MMWR Recommendations and Reports, 60*(Suppl. 84), 84–86.

Centers for Disease Control and Prevention. (2011c, May, 20). Arthritis as a potential barrier to physical activity among adults with obesity—U.S., 2007 and 2009. *MMWR Recommendations and Reports 60*(19), 614–618.

Centers for Disease Control and Prevention. (2011d). *National diabetes fact sheet, diagnosed and undiagnosed diabetes in the United States, all ages, 2010*. Retrieved August 26, 2011, from http://www.cdc.gov/diabetes/pubs/pdf/ndfs_2011.pdf

Centers for Disease Control and Prevention. (2011e, February 4). Vital signs: Prevalence, treatment, and control of high levels of low-density lipoprotein cholesterol—United States, 1999–2002 and 2005–2008. *MMWR Recommendations and Reports 60*(4), 109–114.

Centers for Disease Control and Prevention. (2011f). *Public health and epilepsy.* Retrieved August 29, 2011, from http://www.cdc.gov/epilepsy/basics/public_health.htm

Chang, B., & Robinson, G. (2011, April). Chronic care model implementation in the California state prison system. *Journal of Correctional Health Care, 17*(2), 173–182.

Federal Bureau of Prisons (FBOP). (2009, April). *Management of lipid disorders, clinical practice guideline.* Retrieved June 26, 2011, from http://www.bop.gov/news/medresources.jsp

Federal Bureau of Prisons (FBOP). (2010, November). *Management of diabetes, clinical practice guideline.* Retrieved June 26, 2011, from http://www.bop.gov/news/medresources.jsp

Global Initiative for Asthma (GINA). *Global strategy for asthma management and prevention, 2010.* Available from: http://www.ginasthma.org/

Glosser, J. (1988, October). Psychogenic nonepileptic seizures: Theoretical considerations. *Neuropsychology Neuropsychological Behavioral Neurology, 11*(4), 225–235.

Greenberg, E., Dunleavey, E., Kutner, M., & White, S. (2007). *Literacy prison survey (NCES 2007-473). U.S. Department of Education.* Washington, DC: National Center for Education Statistics. Retrieved from http://nces.ed.gov/pubs2007/2007473.pdf

Gulanick, M., & Myers, J. (2011a). Musculoskeletal care plans. In *Nursing care plans* (7th ed., pp. 663–666). St. Louis, MO: Mosby Elsevier.

Gulanick, M., & Myers, J. (2011b). Neurological care plans. In *Nursing care plans* (7th ed., pp. 524–528). St. Louis, MO: Mosby Elsevier.

Hartley, M., & Repede, E. (2011, September). Nurse practitioner communication and treatment adherence in hypertensive patients. *The Journal for Nurse Practitioners, 7*(8), 654–659.

Hunter, D. J., Thuina, N., & Hochberg, M. (2011, January). Quality of osteoarthritis management and the need for reform in the US. *Arthritis Care & Research, 63*(1), 31–38.

Kammerman, S., & Wasserman, L. (2001, August). Seizure disorders: Part 1. Classification and diagnosis. *West Journal of Medicine, 175*(2), 99–103. Retrieved April 19, 2011, from http://www.ncbi.nlm.nih.gov/pmc/articles/PMC1071497/

National Commission on Correctional Health Care. (2002) *The health status of soon-to-be-released inmates: A report to congress* (Vol. I). Chicago: Author (available at http://www.ncchc.org/pubs_stbr.vol 1.html)

National Commission on Correctional Health Care (NCCHC). (2008). *Standards for health services in prisons.* Chicago, IL: Author.

National Commission on Correctional Health Care. (2011a). *Guideline for disease management in correctional settings: Asthma.* Retrieved August 28, 2011, from http://www.ncchc.org/resources/guidelines/Asthma2011.pdf

National Commission on Correctional Health Care. (2011b). *Guideline for disease management in correctional settings: Diabetes.* Retrieved August 28, 2011, from http://www.ncchc.org/resources/guidelines/Diabetes2011.pdf

National Commission on Correctional Health Care. (2011c). *Guideline for disease management in correctional settings: Hypertension.* Retrieved August 28, 2011, from http://www.ncchc.org/resources/guidelines/Hypertension2011.pdf

National Commission on Correctional Health Care. (2011d). *Guideline for disease management in correctional settings: Hyperlipidemia.* Retrieved August 28, 2011, from http://www.ncchc.org/resources/guidelines/Hyperlipidemia2011.pdf

National Heart, Lung, and Blood Institute. (2002, September). *Third report of the National Cholesterol Education Program (NCEP) Expert Panel on Detection, Evaluation, and Treatment of High Blood Cholesterol in Adults (Adult Treatment Panel III).* National Institutes of Health (NIH) Publication No. 02-5215. Washington, DC: U.S. Department of Health and Human Services. Retrieved August 28, 2010 from http://www.nhlbi.nih.gov/guidelines/cholesterol/atp3full.pdf

National Heart, Lung, and Blood Institute. (2003, December). *The seventh report of the Joint National Committee on Prevention, Detection, Evaluation, and Treatment of High Blood Pressure (JNC 7 Express).* National Institutes of Health (NIH) Publication No. 03-5233. Washington, DC: U.S. Department of Health and Human Services. Retrieved August 28, http://www.nhlbi.nih.gov/guidelines/hypertension/express.pdf

National Heart, Lung, and Blood Institute (NHLBI). (2005, December). *Your guide to lowering your cholesterol with TLC (2005)*, NIH publication No. 06-5235. Washington, DC: U.S. Department of Health and Human Services. Retrieved August 28, 2011, from http://www.nhlbi.nih.gov/health/public/heart/chol/chol_tlc.pdf

National Heart, Lung, and Blood Institute (NHLBI). (2007, October). *Guidelines for the diagnosis and management of asthma*, National Asthma Education and Prevention Program, Expert Panel Report 3, National Institutes of Health (NIH) Publication number 08-5846, pp. 1–60. Retrieved from http://www.nhlbi.nih.gov/guidelines/asthma/asthsumm.htm)

National Institute of Health (NIH). (2011). *Arthritis*. Retrieved November 7, 2011 at http://www.niams.nih.gov/Health_Info/Osteoarthritis/osteoarthritis_ff.asp

National Institute of Neurological Disorders and Strokes (NINDS). (2002, November). *Health disparities epilepsy planning panel*. Retrieved August 29, 2011, from Stigma http://www.ninds.nih/gov.news_and_events/proceedings/epilepsy_panel_2002.htm

National Institute of Neurological Disorders and Strokes (NINDS). (2011). Seizures and epilepsy: Hope through research. Retrieved November 6, 2011, from http://www.ninds.nih.gov/epilepsy/detail_epilepsy.htm

Ozuna, J. M. (2004). Nursing management, chronic neurologic problems. In S. M. Lewis, M. McLean Heitkemper, S. Ruff Dirksen, P. G. O'Brien, & J. Foret Gibbons (Eds.), *Medical surgical nursing: Assessment and management of clinical problems* (6th ed., pp. 1555–1563). St. Louis, MO: Mosby.

Pruitt, B., & Lawson, R. (2011, May). Assessing and managing asthma. *Nursing, 2011*, 46–52. www.nursing2011.com

Puisis, M., & Appel, H. (2006). Chronic disease management. In M. Puisis (Ed.), *Clinical practice in correctional medicine* (2nd ed., pp. 66–88). St. Louis, MO: Mosby Elsevier.

Reimer, G. (2008, July). The graying of the U.S. prisoner population. *Journal of Correctional Health Care, 14*(3), 202–208.

Reuber, M., Pukrop, R., Mitchell, A. J., Bauer, J., & Elger, C. E. (2003, November). Clinical significance of recurrent psychogenic nonepileptic seizure status. *Journal of Neurology 250*(11), 1255–1362.

Rickard, R. V., & Rosenberg, E. (2007 July). Aging inmates: A convergence of trends in the American Criminal Justice System. *Journal of Correctional Health Care, 13*(3), 150–162.

Roberts, D. (2004). Nursing management, arthritis and connective tissue diseases. In S. M. Lewis, M. McLean Heitkemper, S. Ruff Dirksen, P. G. O'Brien, & J. Foret Gibbons (Eds.), *Medical surgical nursing: Assessment and management of clinical problems* (6th ed., pp. 1555–1563). St. Louis, MO: Mosby.

Sabol, W. J., Minton, T. D., & Harrison, P. M. (2007). *Prison and jail inmates at midyear 2006* (Bureau of Justice Statistics Bulletin, NCJ 217675). U.S. Department of Justice, Office of Justice Programs. Retrieved July 5, 2011, from https://www.ojp.usdoj.gov/bjs/abstract/pjim06.htm

Scottish Intercollegiate Guidelines Network (SIGN). (2003, April). *A national clinical guideline: Diagnosis and management of epilepsy in adults*, (70). Retrieved August 29, 2011, from http://www.guideline.gov/content.aspx?id=5694heN&cpsidt=19963277

Smyer, T., & Burbank, P. M. (2009, December). The U.S. correctional system and the older prisoner. *Journal of Gerontological Nursing 35*(12), 32–37.

Tittensor, M. P., Collins, J., Grunewald, R. A., & Reuber, M. (2008, January). Audit of health care provision for UK prisoners with suspected epilepsy. *Seizure, 17*(1), 69–75. Retrieved August 27, 2011, from http://www.ncbi.nom.nih.gov/pubmed/17720553

Weiskopf, C. S. (2005, February). Nurses experience of caring for inmate patients. *Journal of Advanced Nursing, 49*(4), 336–343.

Wilper, A. P., Woolhandler, S., Wesley Boyd, J., Lasser, K. E., McCormick, D., Bor, D. H. et al. (2009). The health and health care of US prisoners: Results of a nationwide survey. *American Journal of Public Health, 99*(4), 666–672.

SEVEN

Dental Conditions

Catherine M. Knox

The first person an inmate sees for a dental complaint will usually be a nurse. This contact may take place at receiving screening, during the health appraisal, as a result of a request for service, or in an emergency. The nurse is expected to assess the patient and determine if the patient can treat the condition themselves with nursing advice and instruction, or if a referral is necessary. If the patient is to be referred, the nurse also determines how soon the appointment will take place. In addition, there are some populations in the correctional setting who have specialized needs for nursing attention to their oral care; these include diabetics, pregnant women, and adolescents.

INCIDENCE OF DENTAL CONDITIONS AMONG INCARCERATED PERSONS

Studies that describe the oral health of inmates coming to jails and prisons report that this population has great need for dental care. In the North Carolina prison system, 23% of the inmates admitted had extensive needs for dental care (needing three or more urgent procedures), more than half the reception population needed comprehensive examination for periodontal disease and corresponding treatment, and tooth decay was more prevalent among incoming inmates than the comparison community population (Clare, 1998). Another study conducted of new admissions to the Iowa state correctional system found dental decay at rates significantly higher than the general community. This study also reported that these inmates had significantly more decay than a survey done 13 years earlier (Boyer, Nielsen-Thompson, & Hill, 2002). According to the Centers for Disease Control and Prevention, African American and Mexican American adults have twice the amount of untreated dental decay as non-Hispanic Whites (Disparities in Oral Health, 2009). These same disparities, perhaps magnified, are seen in the corrections population (Boyer et al., 2002; Clare, Bolin, & Jones, 2006; Treadwell & Formicola, 2005; Williams, 2007). Other factors contributing to the prevalence of dental conditions among inmates are traumatic injury, alcohol use, tobacco use, and drug use (Conklin, Lincoln, & Tuthill, 2000; Cropsey, 2006; May, 2006; Metsch, 2002).

STANDARDS FOR DENTAL CARE IN CORRECTIONAL FACILITIES

While the need for dental care is quite high, the extent of dental services available varies from facility to facility. A study of prison systems reported substantial variation in levels of service provided (Makrides & Shulman, 2002). Some correctional facilities have a dental program that employs full-time dentists, dental assistants, and dental hygienists, while others may not have any dental services on site and refer all care to dentists in the community. Every facility, though, must have a provision for inmates to be screened for their dental needs and have a method to provide necessary dental care and treatment.

The requirement to provide dental care is contained within the requirement to provide health care that arises from the Eighth Amendment, protection from cruel and unusual punishment, established in *Estelle v. Gamble*, 429 U.S. 97 S. Ct. 285 (1976). A more specific description of minimally acceptable dental care is contained in *Dean v. Coughlin*, 623 F. Supp. 392 (S.D. N.Y. 1985). This ruling established that inmates shall receive same-day evaluations and treatment of dental emergencies, that a priority system be used to address dental needs based upon seriousness, follow-up care be provided, and that care is monitored via quality assurance and audit.

Standards for oral care required by the National Commission on Correctional Health Care (NCCHC) and the American Correctional Association (ACA), two of the organizations that accredit correctional facilities, include admission screening, instruction in oral hygiene and prevention, examination, and treatment according to a plan of care. These standards anticipate that nurses complete oral screening at admission, provide instruction in oral hygiene and prevention, assess, and triage requests for dental care. Nurses performing this work must have been trained by a dentist (American Correctional Association, 2002, 2010; NCCHC, 2008a, 2008b, 2011).

TRAINING AND GENERAL PRINCIPLES IN THE ASSESSMENT OF ORAL COMPLAINTS

The training content for nurses to conduct assessments of oral health should include normal anatomy, terminology used to describe the oral cavity, patient interview, and assessment techniques. Training should also include the identification of abnormal conditions for which patients are likely to request attention in the correctional setting, and guidelines for referral to a dentist or other medical professional. The NCCHC stipulates that such training must consist of more than a self-study program. This training may be obtained at conferences, through schools of nursing, and other continuing education venues, or may be provided according to a curriculum developed or approved by the dental director of the facility. Nurses report feeling more confident in their assessment skills after working with the dentist who sees inmate-patients from the facility. This hands-on experience is an excellent way to review the presentation and response to common dental problems as well as how and when to refer for a dental appointment.

From the Experts ...

"Spend time talking with your facility dentist. Look in the mouth with the dentist until you say ... Oh, I can handle that ..."

Shirley Hodge, RN
Pendleton, OR

The objective portion of the assessment of a dental complaint always includes taking the patient's vital signs. In addition to this equipment, the nurse will need a penlight, flashlight, or other good light source; a tongue depressor; 2 × 2 cotton gauze; and personal protective equipment. Besides observation, the nurse will palpate the tongue, teeth, oral mucosa, jaw, and cheek, and may use percussion on the teeth. An approach to nursing assessment of the oral cavity is outlined in Table 7.1. This information does not replace the information and training that nurses obtain from the responsible dentist at the facility or dentist in the community who will receive referrals from nurses at the correctional facility.

TABLE 7.1 Assessment of Dental Conditions

ASSESSMENT	NORMAL FINDINGS	ABNORMAL FINDINGS
Lips and buccal mucosa		
Exterior: Inspect the outer lips for symmetry of contour, color, and texture. Ask the patient to purse the lips as if to whistle.	Uniform pink color (darker, e.g., bluish hue, in Mediterranean groups and dark-skinned patients) Soft, moist, smooth texture Ability to purse lips Symmetry of contour	Pallor; cyanosis Blisters; generalized or localized swelling; fissures, crusts, or scales Inability to purse lips
Internal: Inspect and palpate the inner lips and buccal mucosa for color, moisture, texture, and the presence of lesions. Pull the lip outward and away from the teeth. Grasp the lip on each side between the thumb and index finger. Palpate any lesions for size, tenderness, and consistency.	Uniform pink color (freckled brown pigmentation in dark-skinned patients) Moist, smooth, soft, glistening, and elastic texture Excessive dryness (drier oral mucosa in elderly due to decreased salivation) Mucosal cysts; irritations from dentures; abrasions, ulcerations; nodules	Pallor; leukoplakia (white patches), red, bleeding
Teeth and Gums		
Ask the patient to open the mouth. Using a tongue depressor, retract the cheek. Use a light to view the surface	32 adult teeth Smooth, white, shiny tooth enamel Moist, firm texture to gums	Missing teeth; ill-fitting dentures Excessively red gums Spongy texture; bleeding;

(continued)

TABLE 7.1 *(Continued)*

ASSESSMENT	NORMAL FINDINGS	ABNORMAL FINDINGS
buccal mucosa from top to bottom and back to front. Repeat the procedure for the other side. Ask the patient to relax the lips and first close, then open, the jaw. Observe the number of teeth, tooth color, the state of fillings, dental caries, and tartar along the base of the teeth. Note the presence and fit of partial or complete dentures. Assess the texture of the gums by gently pressing the gum tissue with a tongue depressor.	No retraction of gums (pulling away from the teeth)	tenderness Receding, atrophied gums; swelling that partially covers the teeth Ill-fitting dentures; irritated and excoriated area under dentures
Tongue/Floor of the Mouth		
Inspect the surface of the tongue for position, color, and texture. Ask the patient to protrude the tongue and move side to side.	Central position, moves freely; no tenderness Pink color (some brown pigmentation on tongue borders in dark-skinned patients); moist; slightly rough; thin whitish coating	Deviated from center; excessive trembling; restricted mobility
Inspect the base of the tongue, the mouth floor, and the frenulum.	Smooth, lateral margins; no lesions	Smooth red tongue (may indicate iron, vitamin B12, or vitamin B3 deficiency) Dry, furry tongue, white coating
Palpate the tongue and floor of the mouth for any nodules, lumps, or excoriated areas. Palpate the tongue, using a piece of gauze to grasp its tip (stabilize it), and with the index finger of other hand, palpate the back of the tongue, its borders, and its base.	Smooth tongue base with prominent veins. Smooth with no palpable nodules.	Nodes, ulcerations, discolorations (white or red areas); areas of tenderness Swelling, ulceration Swelling, nodules
Palates and Oropharynx		
Inspect for color, shape, texture, and the presence of bony prominences. Depress tongue with a tongue depressor as necessary, and use a penlight for appropriate visualization.	Lighter pink hard palate, more irregular texture Irritations Bony growths on the hard palate Pink and smooth posterior wall	Discoloration (e.g., jaundice or pallor) Reddened or edematous; presence of lesions, plaques, or drainage Inflammation

Source: Adapted from Berman, Snyder, Kozier, and Erb (2008).

ORAL HEALTH SCREENING AND ASSESSMENT

Nursing personnel are employed at nearly every correctional facility and therefore are the most available members of the health care team to identify an inmate's need for dental care upon admission to the facility; to respond to emergencies that may involve trauma to the head and neck, including the oral cavity; to evaluate inmate requests for health care that concern a dental condition; and to arrange for needed dental services.

In addition to these types of encounters, periodic assessment of oral health is recommended for patients who are pregnant, have certain chronic medical or dental conditions, or are less able to care for their own oral hygiene. Nurses should perform the oral health assessment as part of the regular follow-up with these patients. Finally, nurses should include an oral health assessment of any patient admitted for inpatient care and address oral care in the nursing care plan.

Receiving Screening

The primary focus of oral health screening at intake is to identify any inmate whose condition requires the attention of a dentist more urgently than waiting until the dental examination normally takes place. Facility policy will stipulate when the inmate is to receive a comprehensive examination by a dentist. So, the nurse conducting intake screening needs to identify and refer any inmate with a condition that needs to be seen by a dentist sooner than when the routine dental exam will take place. Questions that should be asked during intake screening include: Are you currently undergoing a dental procedure or receiving dental treatment? Have you been hospitalized recently? What medications are you taking currently? Do you have any dental concerns? It is important that nurses completing intake screening have clear criteria for referral to a dentist, given that the routine dental exam may not take place for some time. Case Example 7.1 applies information from this section.

CASE EXAMPLE 7.1

The U.S. Bureau of Prisons policy requires that inmates received at long-stay facilities be examined by a dentist within 14 days of admission (U.S. Bureau of Prisons, 2005). An inmate who has arrived at a long-stay facility reports during receiving screening that he had been on penicillin for a week and understood that he was to have a tooth extracted at the facility he just came from. What does the nurse completing receiving screening need to do with this information?

Initial Health Assessment

The initial health assessment is the next routine health care encounter that takes place after admission to a correctional facility. The health assessment includes a more comprehensive patient history, vital signs, lab work, and a physical examination. The purpose of the health assessment is to establish a plan of subsequent care based upon the individual's health status and identified health problems. Nurses may be involved in taking the patient's history, collecting data, and performing the physical examination. This is another time that an inmate may give a history of symptoms and possibly treatment for dental or other oral health conditions. Patients who are pregnant, have cardiovascular disease or diabetes, are immunosuppressed, have mental illness, or any other disabling condition should be identified and a plan for management of their ongoing care developed, including oral care. Finally, the health assessment is also a good time for nurses to screen high-risk persons for oral cancer so that it can be treated early, when survival rates are better.

Medical Emergencies

Another type of encounter that may require nursing assessment of the oral cavity is an emergency or "man down" call. The symptoms of injury or disease that may evolve into a dental emergency include inability to breathe or swallow. These symptoms may be caused by infection or injury, neurological impairment resulting from disease or injury of the head, swelling and fever indicative of systemic infection, persistent severe pain and/or bleeding of the tooth, fractured teeth and laceration, or other traumatic injury of the oral cavity. Standard procedures for emergency first response also apply to dental emergencies.

Routine Requests for Health Care Attention

Nurses are responsible for receiving and responding to nonemergent requests for health care attention at sick call. Many of these requests will be for dental problems. The purpose of the nurse's assessment of oral health complaints is to determine the nature and severity of the dental problem, to determine and provide supportive care for the patient, and to arrange more definitive treatment as necessary. If the patient has already been seen by a dentist, there will be a priority-based plan of care in the record, which should be reviewed by the nurse during the assessment. The patient interview should also include questions about recent dental procedures and any post-procedure instructions given.

Many of the nonemergent requests for dental care are for treatment of tooth decay and gum disease, cleaning of teeth and gums, and prosthetics such as dentures and partials. These procedures are often considered routine and patients are put on a list to receive treatment as time allows. Nurses are expected to reassess any patient who submits subsequent requests because the patient's dental condition may have worsened and an urgent or emergent treatment referral is necessary.

The facility dentist should provide guidelines for nurses to refer and/or schedule patients for dental care. In the next section, the typical kinds of dental complaints nurses see in the correctional setting are described. The focus of the nursing assessment, usual treatment approach, and guidelines for referral are also discussed. Nurses who do not have guidelines for assessment, treatment, and referral may want to discuss the material in this chapter with the dentist at their facility and establish more definitive directions.

COMMON DENTAL CONDITIONS

The most common dental complaints that nurses will encounter in the correctional setting are trauma, infection, and pain. A typical encounter with a patient is provided in Case Example 7.2 and can be used to apply material discussed in this section. Protocol or algorithms are guidelines used by nurses to complete a focused assessment, treat, and arrange referral for the kinds of health concerns that are commonly seen in the correctional setting. Guidelines regarding dental conditions should be selected or

CASE EXAMPLE 7.2

A youth at a juvenile detention facility is brought to the clinic by correctional staff for an abrasion under the left eye. The correctional staff are concerned that the youth may have been in a fight. In the privacy of the exam room the nurse comments on the abrasion and asks about what happened. The youth reports that he was on his bunk in the dorm, sleeping, and had a dream he was running across a field and tripped in a hole. He awoke sprawled on the floor after falling off the top bunk. The nurse takes his vital signs, which are within normal range. What aspects of this patient's condition would you assess? What criteria will guide your decision about action(s) to take?

developed by nurses in conjunction with the dentist who provides services to inmates at the facility. The guidelines should also be reviewed and approved for use by the facility physician. In the absence of assessment protocol or if the condition is not covered by protocol, the nurse should conduct a general assessment by interviewing the patient, observing and describing the condition, and noting how it deviates from normal. General time lines for nurses' referral of dental conditions to a dentist or other provider can be found in Table 7.2 (Adu-Tutu, 2009).

Trauma

Lost or broken teeth, fractures of the jaw and/or facial structure, oral lacerations, and bleeding are examples of dental injuries that result from trauma. These injuries may come about accidentally or intentionally. The incidence of traumatic injury among inmates is high; their medical history often includes incidents of traumatic injury and there is considerable opportunity for accidental as well as intentional injury while incarcerated. Cell extraction, restraint, and other types of force are used in the correctional setting to maintain safety, yet these procedures also carry risk of injury (May, 2006).

Dental complaints that arise from injury to the head and neck are considered emergent and life threatening, especially if the patient has any of the following: loss of consciousness, difficulty breathing, diminished respiration, difficulty swallowing, nausea, or headache. If bleeding is present, check for presence of cerebrospinal fluid. The nurse should be prepared to provide an airway, respiratory support, and control bleeding until emergency personnel arrives (Adu-Tutu, 2009).

An accurate and complete patient history is important but it may be difficult to obtain, especially if there is loss of consciousness, inmate fear of reprisal, or if the inmate is trying to avoid disciplinary sanction. The nurse should consider other mechanisms of injury when the patient reports an accidental injury. If it aids in diagnosis and treatment, it may be worth verifying if there is any independent information about what may have happened (such as reports from correctional staff or security camera footage). The injury may be more serious than the patient's description of the incident, so an examination of the head and mouth is most important to thorough and responsive treatment.

Urgent contact with and referral to a dentist or a physician should be sought when a patient has a permanent tooth come out of the socket and the tooth is intact, a fractured tooth with moderate-to-severe pain, or a fractured jaw. Subsequent treatment will depend upon how recent the injury is and what the assessment data

TABLE 7.2 Referral Guidelines

CONDITION	CONTACT OR APPOINTMENT WITH DENTIST
At intake is on medication from another provider for recent dental procedure	Before the end of the shift
At intake reports having had a recent dental procedure that required follow-up appointment	Next business day
Post-extraction bleeding continues more than 3 hours with continuous pressure	Within the same shift
Two to 3 days after extraction still has pain and swelling	Within 72 hours
Dental injury resulting from injury to head or neck with any of the following: Loss of consciousness Difficulty breathing or swallowing Nausea Headache	Immediately
Avulsed tooth	Immediately
Fractured tooth with moderate-to-severe pain (3 or more on pain scale)	Before the end of the shift
Fractured jaw	Before the end of the shift
Laceration	Before the end of the shift
Generalized facial swelling with Temperature 101°C or more Pulse more than 100	Immediately
Localized swelling with fever less than 101°C	Within 24 hours
Severe pain (7–10 on pain scale) related to any dental condition	Within 24 hours
Moderate-to-severe pain (3–6 on pain scale) related to any dental condition	Within 72 hours
Any lesion of the oral cavity not improved in 1 week	Within 72 hours

Source: Adu-Tutu (2009).

include. The nurse should know the patient's tetanus and allergy status. The provider will direct the next steps in treatment, arrange for pain control, and prescribe diet modification. Orders may include x-rays and antibiotics, as well. These patients need to be advised on how to minimize further irritation of the tooth and/or socket, reduce swelling and immobilize the area, and given direction on use of over the counter products to control pain while healing.

Nurses should also make urgent contact with a dentist for any laceration of the face and/or oral cavity. The patient may or may not need suturing depending on what type of tissue is involved, how large the laceration is, and whether bleeding can be stopped after application of pressure, so it is very important to get direction from the treating dentist or physician. Once the dentist or physician has decided how the wound will be closed, other orders will include pain relief, tetanus, diet, and antibiotics. The patient may be advised to use salt water rinses to relieve tissue irritation and to use over-the-counter products for pain.

Early and immediate intervention may result in saving the tooth, preventing permanent disablement and/or disability, and alleviating pain. Failure to contact a provider in these conditions is a failure to advocate for the patient on the part of the nurse.

Infection

The teeth and supporting bone as well as in the gum and soft tissue of the mouth are all sites of possible infection, which may be highly localized and chronic or may be generalized and systemic. Many factors contribute to the potential for infection in the oral cavity, including poor oral hygiene, lack of dental treatment, pregnancy, puberty, changes in the production of saliva, tobacco use, drug use, and underlying medical conditions such as diabetes.

In severe cases of infection, vital signs and the general appearance of the patient are the main indicators of the need for an emergent referral to a dentist or medical provider. Any patient with facial swelling, a temperature over 101°F, and pulse greater than 100 most likely has a systemic infection or cellulitis and will need aggressive antibiotic therapy with possible incision and drainage (Adu-Tutu, 2009; Makrides, 2006; Makrides, 2009). Other signs of significant infection include increasing swelling, dehydration, rapid respirations, fatigue, considerable pain, and a wasted or sick look (Makrides, 2006). Facial hair may hide the extent of swelling, so it is important to palpate the area in addition to visual observation (Makrides, 2009). The nurse needs to consider the patient's problem list or history, since patients with underlying medical conditions that result in immunosuppression are at risk of infection that can be severe.

Patients with localized swelling and fever less than 101°F, who have normal respirations and no difficulty swallowing, need to be seen by a dentist or medical staff within the next 24 hours. These patients will likely be started on an antibiotic, so the nurse should be sure to inquire and check for allergies in advance of prescription and administration of medication. The patient should be observed closely over the next 2 days for the swelling to reduce. Supportive care includes a soft diet and over-the-counter pain medication. Once the infection is under control, the dental treatment plan treatment may include repair or extraction of the tooth and treatment of underlying gum disease. The dentist or medical provider should be contacted if the patient's condition deteriorates over the next 24 hours or if the patient does not improve within 48 hours.

A milder form of infection may manifest as an abscess in the tissue around the tooth resulting from tooth decay. Gingivitis is another infection that causes reddened, inflamed gums that bleed easily. Brushing and flossing with regular dental prophylaxis controls the growth of plaque, prevents loss of tooth surface and decay, and prevents the formation of calculus and resulting bacterial infection in the mouth. The inmate population has been described in several studies as having teeth and gum disease that exceeds rates of disease and decay in the general community (Boyer et al., 2002; Clare, 1998; Gilhooly, Simon, & Sells, 2001). Many inmates have had limited access to basic dental care before incarceration and may not have taken care of their teeth and gums by brushing and flossing (Conklin et al., 2000). Use of illegal drugs (methamphetamine, cocaine, and opiates) is also associated with higher rates of disease and decay in the oral cavity (Metsch, 2002). Methamphetamine, in particular, contributes to tooth decay and gum disease because its use is associated with reduced production of saliva, increased desire for intake of sugar, and grinding of teeth (Makrides, 2009).

Nurses seeing patients with complaints of inflammation, soreness, or gingivitis but with minimal pain or swelling should stress improved oral hygiene and refer the patient for a nonurgent or routine dental appointment. Interview the patient to get a thorough description and history of the problem and then examine the oral cavity to identify and describe the problem area. An accurate and thorough description of the problem assists dental staff to prioritize the patient for an appointment. Dental care may include tooth restoration, extraction, and deep cleansing of the periodontal area, known as root planing. Self-care recommendations until seen by the dentist include use of a salt water rinse to soothe tissue inflammation, perhaps use of toothpaste specific to sensitive teeth, and over-the-counter analgesics.

Patients may also complain of lesions in the soft tissue of the mouth or throat. It is important to approach the interview and examination in a general and methodical way rather than focus only on the area that the patient is concerned about. There are many possible conditions that may be the cause of an oral lesion; the nurse should be familiar with normal oral anatomy and by observation be able to identify and describe abnormal findings. Nurses should be familiar with the presenting features and referral recommendations of the dentist for oral cancer, herpes, candidiasis, gonorrhea, and canker sores. Generally, any lesion that does not improve in 1 week needs to be referred for further evaluation (Adu-Tutu, 2009).

Pain

Patients may or may not complain of pain in conjunction with the dental problem for which they are seeking attention. Assessment and documentation of the patient's description of pain and functional ability aids diagnosis and prioritization of referral urgency. Use of a standardized pain scale gives patients a yardstick to which they can compare their experience of pain and is a recommended communication tool between the patient and their providers. Recognizing that each patient experiences and interprets pain uniquely, the description of pain experienced is partly diagnostic of the degree to which the nerves in the root of the tooth are involved.

Patients with severe dental pain (7–10 on a 10-point scale) will have trouble sleeping and eating. Pain is described as constant but may vary in intensity depending upon position and activity. Other descriptions may include: pounding, throbbing, stabbing, and shooting pain. Patients with this kind of pain have trauma, decay, or infection that involves the nerves, tissue, and blood vessels in the root of the tooth and perhaps the connected bone. These patients need treatment by a dentist or medical provider started within 24 hours (Adu-Tutu, 2009). Treatment will consist of pain control and possible antibiotics with subsequent treatment of the underlying problem. Left untreated, the pain eventually subsides, but the patient will return again for health care attention, this time with an acute periodontitis or an abscess. These teeth will be very sensitive when chewing and to percussion (Makrides, 2006).

Patients with moderate to severe pain (3–6 on a 10-point scale) will describe an inability to concentrate and an interference with tasks. The pain is sensitive to temperature, certain substances (sugar), and/or pressure. The pain may be described as dull or tingling in sensation. This kind of pain is associated with decay or damage (fracture) that involves the dentin or middle layer of the tooth, which has less nerve exposure than the root of the tooth. These patients need an urgent appointment with a dentist and treatment initiated within 72 hours of the referral (Adu-Tutu, 2009).

MEDICAL CONDITIONS AND ORAL HEALTH
Cancer

Screening for oral cancer with the inmate population is very important. Cancer of the mouth is the sixth most common cancer and is becoming more common. It also has a low survival rate primarily because disease is not identified until late in its progression (Adu-Tutu, 2009; Makrides, 2009). Tobacco and alcohol use are each risk factors for oral cancer. The carcinogenic action of both tobacco and alcohol is synergistic, greatly increasing the risk of developing oral cancer (Brocklehurst, 2010). Over half of oral cancers are located on the tongue and pharynx (Makrides, 2009).

The inmate population reports high rates of alcohol and tobacco use (Conklin et al., 2000; Cropsey, 2006; May, 2006) and should be screened for oral cancer when they present with any dental complaints or respiratory symptoms, such as lesions, numbness, colds, or sore throats. While there are a limited number of studies of oral cancer screening, a Cochrane Review (Brocklehurst, 2010) recommends opportunistic screening by visual examination during regular health care encounters by qualified health care providers of persons who use alcohol and tobacco products. Nurses should refer to a dentist for examination and potential biopsy (Makrides, 2009) those patients who have:

- Lesions that are red or red with white with diffuse borders
- White patches that cannot be rubbed off the oral mucosa
- A lesion that does not improve within a week
- A lump or numbness in the mouth or jaw
- Hoarseness, difficulty chewing or swallowing

Clearly documenting the findings that result in the decision to refer for dental examination will assist the dentist in prioritizing the patient's appointment. A thorough assessment and accurate documentation of the lesion may save both the patient and the dentist a second visit. If the facility already makes use of a Polaroid or digital camera in clinical care, this may greatly assist in communicating the results of oral screening to the dentist.

Systemic Disease

The interaction between oral health and health generally was highlighted by the Surgeon General in the year 2000 (National Institute of Dental and Craniofacial Research, 2000). Since then, organizations and health care professionals have been engaged more fully in efforts to improve oral health (National Institute of Dental and Craniofacial Research, 2003). Correctional health professionals have recognized for some time that systemic diseases have oral signs and symptoms (e.g., HIV disease). There is more and more evidence that periodontal disease exacerbates certain systemic diseases.

Immunosuppressive Disease

Patients with diseases or conditions that result in immunosuppression are likely to present with candidiasis and/or hairy leukoplakia of the oral cavity. Neither of these conditions are seen when the immune system is intact, and, in some cases, identification of these by a dentist is the first sign of underlying disease (Oral Health in America: A Report of the Surgeon General, 2000). Other conditions of the mouth that arise with immunosuppression include canker sores (aphthous ulcers) and fever sores (herpes). Infections of the mouth in immunosuppressed patients can be overwhelming for the patient. The treatment plan for patients with immunosuppressing illnesses should anticipate the potential for any of these oral conditions and outline the steps to be taken by the patient for self-care and timeframes for referral if the condition must be addressed by a medical or dental professional. A useful handout with photos that describes mouth problems of patients with HIV that supports self-care can be found at http://www.nidcr.nih.gov/OralHealth/Topics/HIV/MouthProblemsHIV/default.htm.

Diabetes

Diabetes and oral health are linked in multiple ways. First, increased blood sugar levels caused by diabetes contribute to tooth decay and periodontal disease. Second, treating periodontal infection and reducing inflammation are associated with reduced levels of blood glucose. Third, the nerve and vascular complications of diabetes effect saliva production and healing of the oral cavity (Barnett, 2006; Makrides, 2006; Registered Nurses Association of Ontario, 2008).

The oral hygiene of diabetic patients should be assessed as part of the chronic care plan, their oral status addressed in treatment planning, and appointments for restorative and routine care made a priority. A standardized assessment tool is recommended primarily so that oral problems are identified early and treated. Nurses should advocate for and facilitate inclusion of oral health in managing care for these patients.

Pregnancy

Women who are pregnant also need special attention for their oral health. Changes in hormones and immune response during pregnancy increase dental plaque, which can result in gingivitis and periodontal infection (Barak, Oettinger-Barak, Oettinger, Machtei, & Peled, 2003). Periodontal disease is associated with adverse pregnancy outcomes including preterm/low birth weight, miscarriage, and preeclampsia (Dasanayake, Gennaro, Hendricks-Munoz, & Chhun, 2008; New York State Department of Health, 2006).

Another reason to pay attention to women's oral health during pregnancy is to reduce the incidence and severity of caries in the child (New York State Department of Health, 2006). Pregnancy is a time when women are highly receptive to information and counseling to change behaviors that adversely affect their children. This is a good time for the nurse to help mothers set in place habits that support good oral hygiene and regular dental care. The New York Department of Health has published a practice guideline for oral health care during pregnancy that includes comprehensive recommendations for health providers as well as useful posters, brochures, and teaching material for patients. It can be accessed at http://www.nyhealth.gov/publications/0824.pdf.

Women should be referred to the dentist early in the pregnancy so that a plan of both restorative and preventive care can be developed. Any pregnant woman who complains of gingivitis or other symptoms of periodontal disease should be referred more urgently to the dentist for care to reduce risk of adverse outcomes. Nurses should support and stress the safety and effectiveness of oral care and dental treatment during pregnancy.

ORAL HYGIENE AND HEALTH PROMOTION

Inmates in the correctional setting see nurses more often than any other health care provider. Nurses should know what oral hygiene practices experts recommend so that they give patients good advice on oral care and reinforce the plan for the patient's dental care.

Supporting Patient Self-Care

Oral Hygiene

The oral cavity requires more intensive daily care than any other part of the body. This is because dental plaque is constantly building; its growth can be disrupted, but it is never completely removed (National Institute of Dental and Craniofacial Research, 2000). Recommendations for individuals to take care of their oral health are listed in Exhibit 7.1.These have been adapted for use in correctional settings and may be provided as a patient handout or used by nurses in patient teaching.

Dry Mouth

Dry mouth, or xerostomia, is a bothersome symptom for patients. Patients may describe it as burning or soreness and have difficulty speaking, chewing, and swallowing. Dry mouth is a side effect of many medications; it also occurs in conjunction

---

EXHIBIT 7.1
Oral Health Recommendations for Individuals

- Use fluoride toothpaste. You only need to use a pea-sized amount of paste on your toothbrush.
- Brush teeth and gums at least twice a day.
- Floss between teeth after brushing; rinse with mouthwash.
- Avoid tobacco. Tobacco use in any form increases the risk for gum disease, oral and throat cancers, and oral fungal infection (candidiasis).
- Limit alcohol. Heavy use of alcohol is also a risk factor for oral and throat cancers. When alcohol is used as well as tobacco, risk of oral cancers is even greater.
- Avoid snacks full of sugars and starches. Limit the number of snacks eaten throughout the day.
- Eat five helpings a day of fiber-rich fruits and vegetables.
- Request ongoing dental care as recommended by your dentist. If you have any changes in your mouth, seek health care attention.
- Diabetic patients should work to maintain control of their disease because it also brings higher risk of gum disease.
- If you have "dry mouth," drink plenty of water, chew sugarless gum, and avoid tobacco and alcohol.

Source: Adapted from Centers for Disease Control and Prevention (2006).

with or as a result of aging, certain systemic diseases, and radiation treatment (Forrester, Nash-Luchenbach, & Tistler, 2004).

Patients can be reminded by the nurse to practice good oral hygiene and advised to avoid salty, sugary, spicy foods, caffeine, tobacco, and other substances that irritate oral tissue. Self-care advice includes drinking plenty of water, rinsing frequently with water or salt water with baking soda, chewing sugarless gum or sugar-free candy, and eating foods that are soft and nutritious (National Institute of Dental and Craniofacial Research, 2011).

Sensitive Teeth

Patients may also seek health care attention for sensitive teeth. This condition is most often caused by decay, fractures, or other erosion into the tooth with inflammation of the gums or a receding gum line. Patients should be encouraged to maintain or improve their oral hygiene practices and be advised to use toothpaste for sensitive teeth. The patient should also be informed that this type of toothpaste requires several applications before they will have less sensitivity and so should continue to use the product (American Dental Association, n.d.). Usually only after the patient has tried the desensitizing toothpaste will dentists consider additional steps. Patients should be advised by the nurse to carry out daily oral care as recommended in Exhibit 7.1 until seen by the dentist for a routine appointment.

Reinforcing Follow-Up Care

Patient interest in dental follow-up may subside after more acute symptoms such as pain have diminished. Yet, until the underlying problem has been addressed, the patient's condition will only deteriorate and an acute episode will return. Because access to dental care is so limited in correctional facilities, nurses would do well to facilitate and support the patient's adherence to the plan for oral hygiene and completing scheduled follow-up care as recommended by the dentist. A follow-up study of inmates incarcerated continuously for 3 years in North Carolina showed improvement in dental health (Clare, 2002). Helping patients make progress in completing recommended treatment better utilizes already limited dental resources and avoids more time consuming and expensive treatment later on.

Patient Education on Oral Care

Patient education about oral health and prevention is an expectation of both the ACA and NCCHC (American Correctional Association, 2002, 2010; NCCHC, 2008a, 2008b, 2011). This information must be provided to all inmates or detainees, not just those who are seeking health care attention. Correctional nurses role and responsibility for providing patient education is delineated in Standard 5B of the Scope & Standards of Corrections Nursing. The importance of targeted education in health teaching is stressed, stating that the corrections nurse "Uses health promotion and health teaching methods appropriate to the situation and the patient's developmental level, learning needs, readiness, ability to learn, language preference, and culture" (American Nurses Association, 2007, p. 26). Brochures, flyers, posters, newsletters, as well as other forms of electronic media can be used to disseminate information about oral health. There are many websites that provide information about oral health; some of these, such as the American Dental Association, are listed in Table 7.3. There are

TABLE 7.3   Dental Resources on the Web

NAME OF ORGANIZATION	WEB ADDRESS
The Academy of General Dentistry	http://www.knowyourteeth.com/family/
The Merck Manuals Online Medical Library Ear, Nose, Throat, and Dental Disorders	http://www.merckmanuals.com/ professional
New York State, Department of Health, Oral Health	http://www.nyhealth.gov/prevention/dental/
National Institute of Dental and Craniofacial Research, National Institutes of Health, Oral Health	http://www.nidcr.nih.gov/OralHealth/
Centers for Disease Control and Prevention, Division of Oral Health	http://www.cdc.gov/oralhealth/
Oral Health America	http://www.oralhealthamerica.org
Maternal and Child Health Library Georgetown University	http://www.mchlibrary.info/ KnowledgePaths/kp_oralhealth.html
National Maternal & Child Oral Health Resource Center	http://www.mchoralhealth.org/
The American Dental Association	http://www.ada.org/
Dry Mouth, developed by the Wm. Wrigley Jr. Company	http://www.drymouth.info/

also resources on some of these sites that can be used to facilitate patient access to ongoing dental care in the community.

SUMMARY

An area of correctional nursing practice not often part of nurses' practice in other settings is the assessment, triage, and referral of dental complaints. Nurses will often be the first health professional an inmate will see about a dental concern. The nurse's assessment and triage of the patient's health complaint is critical to ensuring timely and appropriate care. This chapter described key features in the assessment of dental conditions associated with trauma, infection, and pain. Guidelines for referral and timeframes to achieve definitive dental treatment were reviewed. There is growing evidence of the relationship between oral health and other medical conditions. The role of the nurse in oral cancer screening and addressing dental issues involved in the care of patients who are pregnant, diabetic, or immunosuppressed was reviewed. Finally, material for oral hygiene instruction and other dental health resources was provided for nurses' use in preventive care and health education.

DISCUSSION QUESTIONS

1. What are some of the reasons that inmates have poor oral health?
2. Which patients in the correctional setting are most at risk for dental problems and why?
3. What are the features of a good oral health education program?

REFERENCES

Adu-Tutu, M. (2009). Dental screening for nurses. *Building health care systems that work*. Orlando, FL: National Commission on Correctional Health Care.

American Correctional Association. (2002). *Performance based standards for correctional health care in adult correctional institutions*. Alexandria, VA: Author.

American Correctional Association. (2010). *2010 Standards supplement*. Alexandria, VA: Author.

American Dental Association. (n.d.). *Public resources, oral health topics, sensitive teeth*. Retrieved June 26, 2012, from ADA: American Dental Association: http://www.ada.org/3058.aspx?currentTab=1

American Nurses Association. (2007). *Corrections nursing: Scope & standards of practice*. Silver Spring, MD: Author.

Barak, S., Oettinger-Barak, O., Oettinger, M., Machtei, E., & Peled, M. O. (2003, September). Common oral manifestations during pregnancy: A review. *Obstetrical & Gynecological Survey, 58*(9), 624–628.

Barnett, M. (2006). The oral-systemic connection: An update for the practicing dentist. *Journal of the American Dental Association, 137*(2), 5S–6S.

Berman, A., Snyder, S., Kozier, B., & Erb, G. (2008). *Kozier & Erb's fundamentals of nursing: Concepts, process, and practice*. Upper Saddle River, NJ: Pearson Prentice Hall.

Bolin, K., & Jones, D. (2006). Oral health needs of adolescents in a juvenile detention facility. *Journal of Adolescent Health, 38*, 755–757.

Boyer, M. E., Nielsen-Thompson, N., & Hill, T. (2002). A comparison of dental caries and tooth loss for Iowa prisoners with other prison populations and dentate U.S. adults. *The Journal of Dental Hygiene, 76*(II), 141–150.

Brocklehurst, P. K. (2010). Screening programmes for the early detection and prevention of oral cancer (Review). *The Cochrane Library, (11)*, 1–28.

Centers for Disease Control and Prevention. (2006, November 21). *Oral health for adults*. Retrieved February 5, 2011, from Division of Oral Health: http://www.cdc.gov/oralhealth/publications/factsheets/adult.htm

Centers for Disease Control and Prevention. (2009). *Disparities in Oral Health*. Retrieved June 26, 2012, from Division of Oral Health: http://www.cdc.gov/oral health/oral_health_disparities.htm

Clare, J. (1998). Survey, comparison, and analysis of caries, periodontal pocket depth, and urgent treatment needs in a sample of adult felon admissions. *Journal of Correctional Health Care, 5*, 89–102.

Clare, J. (2002). Dental health status, unmet needs, and utilization of services in a cohort of adult felons at admission and after three years incarceration. *Journal of Correctional Health Care, 9*, 65–76.

Conklin, T., Lincoln, T., & Tuthill, R. (2000). Self-reported health and prior health behaviors of newly admitted correctional inmates. *The American Journal of Public Health, 90*(12), 1939–1941.

Cropsey, K. C. (2006, October). Relationship between smoking status and oral health in a prison poulation. *Journal of Correctional Health Care, 12*(4), 240–248.

Dasanayake, A., Gennaro, S., Hendricks-Munoz, K., & Chhun, N. (2008, January/February). Maternal periodontal disease, pregnancy, and neonatal outcomes. *The American Journal of Maternal/Child Nursing, 33*(1), 38–44.

Dean v. Coughlin, 623 F. Supp. 392 (S.D. N.Y. 1985).

Estelle v. Gamble, 429 U.S. 97 S. Ct. 285 (1976).

Forrester, D., Nash-Luchenbach, D., & Tistler, M. (2004). Help your patient manage dry mouth. *Nursing 2004, 34*(4).

Gilhooly, J., Simon, E. T., & Sells, C. (2001). A Look at the health of Oregon's adolescents in the adult correctional system. *Journal of Correctional Health Care, 8*, 55–65.

Makrides, N. (2009). *Oral health conditions for the non dentist. Building health care systems that work*. Orlando: National Commission on Correctional Health Care.

Makrides, N. C. (2006). Correctional dental services. In M. Puisis (ed.), *Clinical practice in correctional medicine* (pp. 559–561). Philadelphia: Mosby Elsevier.

Makrides, N., & Shulman, J. (2002). Dental health care of prison populations. *Journal of Correctional Health Care, 9*, 291–306.

May, J. (2006). Preventive health issues for individuals in jails and prisons. In M. Puisis (Ed.), *Clinical practice in correctional medicine* (pp. *357*, 367–370). Philadelphia, PA: Mosby Elsevier.

Metsch, L. C.-T. (2002, May). Met and unmet need for dental services among active drug users in Miami, Florida. *The Journal of Behavioral Health Services & Research, 29*(2), 176–188.

National Commission on Correctional Health Care (NCCHC). (2011). *Standards for health services in juvenile detention and confinement facilities*. Chicago, IL: Author.

National Commission on Correctional Health Care (NCCHC). (2008a). *Standards for health services in prisons*. Chicago, IL: Author.

National Commission on Correctional Health Care (NCCHC). (2008b). *Standards for health services in jails*. Chicago, IL: Author.

National Institute of Dental and Craniofacial Research. (2000). *Oral health in America: A report of the surgeon general*. Rockville, MD: Public Health Service, Centers for Disease Control and Prevention.

National Institute of Dental and Craniofacial Research. (2003). *A national call to action to promote oral health*. Public Health Service, Centers for Disease Control and Prevention, U.S. Department of Health and Human Services, Rockville, MD: NIH Publication No. 03-5303.

National Institute of Dental and Craniofacial Research. (2011). *Dry mouth*. National Institutes of Health. Bethesda, MD: NIH Publication No. 11-3174. Retrieved June 26, 2012, from http://www.nidcr.nih.gov/OralHealth/Topics/DryMouth/DryMouth.htm

New York State Department of Health. (2006). *Oral health care during pregnancy and early childhood: Practice guidelines (No. 0824)*. New York State Department of Health, Albany.

Registered Nurses Association of Ontario. (2008). *Oral health: Nursing assessment and interventions*. International Affairs and Nursing Best Practice Guidelines Program. Toronto: Registered Nurses Association of Ontario.

Treadwell, H., & Formicola, A. (2005). Improving the oral health of prisoners to improve overall health and well-being. *American Journal of Public Health, 95*(10), 1677–1678.

U.S. Bureau of Prisons. (2005, January 15). *Policy documents*. Retrieved January 28, 2011, from Federal Bureau of Prisons: http://www.bop.gov/policy/progstat/6400_002.pdf

Williams, N. (2007). Prison health and the health of the public: Ties that bind. *Journal of Correctional Health Care, 13*(2), 80–92.

EIGHT

End-of-Life Care

Catherine M. Knox

OVERVIEW OF END-OF-LIFE CARE IN CORRECTIONS

*T*erminal illness can be a time of great sorrow, loneliness, suspicion, pain, and suffering for prisoners. For many, their greatest fear is that they will die in prison alone, in pain, and without the support of family, friends, and spiritual advisors (Dubler & Heyman, 2006). Some correctional systems have established end-of-life care programs to cope with increasing numbers of inmates who die of natural causes while in prison or jail. The increase in numbers of inmate deaths is attributed to three trends:

1. Increasing numbers of people who are incarcerated.
2. Inmates who receive long sentences and then age while in prison.
3. Increasing numbers of persons who are middle aged or elderly at the time of sentencing and are admitted with chronic and life-limiting health problems (Dubler & Heyman, 2006; McAdoo, 2008; National Institute of Corrections Information Center, 1997).

The provision of end-of-life care to inmates with terminal illnesses is one of the distinguishing features of correctional nursing. Every correctional facility will inevitably have an inmate who is diagnosed with a terminal condition. Health care providers at the correctional facility will need to manage treatment, counseling, and initiate advance care planning for this inmate consistent with community standards. There are several reasons an inmate with terminal illness may remain at a correctional facility for end-of-life care:

■ The inmate may not be able to be released to the community for reasons of public safety.

■ The illness may be most appropriately cared for by the health care program at the facility.

■ The inmate may want to remain at the facility because he or she has a support system or family close by.

People with life-limiting or terminal illnesses suffer not only from the illness itself but from loss of function, diminished control of their body, and loneliness as others around them go on with life. A prisoner suffers these losses but also experiences the loss of family, the loss of freedom to determine their surroundings and schedule, as well as the loss of their individuality. The losses associated with incarceration magnify the suffering of an inmate with life-limiting illness (Maull, 2006).

The idea that people could have a "good death" has emerged over the last 15 years as clinicians focused on relief of their patients' pain and suffering, and curative treatment was no longer effective. When people with serious illness, their families, and health care providers were interviewed about what constituted a good death, the characteristics described as most important were symptom relief, communication, being prepared, spending time meaningfully, giving to others, and being understood as a whole person (Steinhauser, 2000).

There is no published research about what inmates with terminal illnesses would describe as a "good death," but anecdotal reports are consistent with these themes. In addition, prisoners often express the wish to die as a free person rather than in prison (Jervis, 2009; Leland, 2009; Linder & Meyers, 2007; Nelson, 1998; O'Conner, 2004; West, 2000). Stated in the negative, prisoners' fears or concerns about dying in prison are influenced by perceptions of inadequate health care and indifference of staff. These beliefs held true even though prisoners reported that they were satisfied or more than satisfied with health care provided by the correctional system (Aday, 2009; Levine, 2005). In a survey of older female inmates in five southern U.S. prisons, worries about experiencing pain and indignity while dying as well as concerns about substandard and indifferent care were more worrisome than the fear of death itself (Deaton, Aday, & Wahidin, 2009–2010).

As of 2008, hospice programs were in place in "75 prisons and jails in 41 states" according to a spokesperson at the National Hospice and Palliative Care Organization (Jervis, 2009; McAdoo, 2008). When the first programs started in prisons there were no standards for delivery of hospice services in correctional settings. Instead, the first programs sought and obtained licensure by the state licensing authority. This was important in assuring that services at the correctional facility met the community standard for hospice care (Bick, 2002). There were also many beliefs or myths about hospice care in correctional settings that were challenged by these first programs.

Eventually, the GRACE Project demonstrated that end-of-life care practices (listed in Exhibit 8.1) could be adapted to the correctional setting (Craig & Ratcliff, 2002; Price, 2008). Nurses are recognized as among those who can most effectively introduce and sustain changes in the delivery of end-of-life care in the correctional setting (Loeb et al., 2011b).

Both the American Correctional Association (ACA) and the National Commission on Correctional Health Care (NCCHC) have established accreditation standards

From the Experts . . .

"Harnassing nurses' expertise and applying their power of compassion may allow . . . prisoners to die with a modicum of dignity, respect, and humane care."

Loeb, Penrod, Hollenbeak, & Smith, 2011, p. 483

for end-of-life care. The four key aspects to end-of-life care covered in the NCCHC standard are:

- Hospice or palliative care is available if the inmate is not eligible or cannot be released to the community.
- Inmates have the opportunity to make informed decisions about the care they choose at the end of life.
- The program is effective in that it provides a supportive environment.
- The patient is treated with dignity, is without pain, and has the company of friends and family.
- Personnel (including inmate volunteers or workers) have been trained in hospice and palliative care (NCCHC 2008a, 2008b, 2011).

The ACA standards require a written treatment plan that provides direction to health care and other personnel about their respective roles in the care and supervision of a patient with terminal illness. The standards also explicitly allow offenders to

EXHIBIT 8.1
Practices From End-of-Life Care That Have Been Adapted
to the Correctional Environment

1. "Involvement of inmates as volunteers, serving as trusted peers, providing psychosocial support, and assistance with nonmedical care
2. Increased family involvement (including inmate family), made possible by modified visiting hours, locations, and protocols—including extended deathbed vigils
3. An interdisciplinary team of physicians, nurses, social workers, chaplains, and others, assigned to each patient
4. An individualized plan of care, including structured, documented discussions about treatment options with patient and family
5. Skilled pain and symptom management that includes access to analgesia, protocols for proper administration, and specialized palliative care training for clinical staff
6. Bereavement services for patients, family (including inmate family), volunteers, and staff, to cope with patient deaths
7. Adaptation of the environment to increase comfort and homelike quality, and the provision of comfort foods"

Source: Craig and Ratcliff (2002, p. 150).

provide hospice care as long as it is consistent with training received and within the requirements set forth in state law (2002).

Service Delivery Models

End-of-life care that combines outpatient, mainstreamed services with access to the services of highly specialized practitioners and programs is recommended by the National Consensus Project for Quality Palliative Care (2009). Early introduction to palliative care has been shown to reduce depression and increase quality of life. It has also been associated with less aggressive treatment at the end of life (Harvard Health Publications, 2011).

This combination of mainstreamed primary services with access to specialized consultation and clinical support has been adopted by correctional systems as well (Loeb et al., 2011a; Maull, 2006; Volunteers of America: GRACE Project (VOA), 2001). The advantages of making end-of-life care available to inmate patients wherever they are located include: the patient's family, social, and spiritual networks of support are maintained, and the patient is not isolated from other programs such as access to the chapel or yard (Anno, Graham, Lawrence, & Shansky, 2004; Maull, 2006). If patients have to leave a facility, family, or social supports in order to access end-of-life or palliative care, they may choose to forego services and suffer unnecessarily.

Inmate Hospice Workers

Half of the end-of-life programs in correctional facilities involve inmates as helpers and companions (McAdoo, 2008). The accreditation standards relating to inmate workers explicitly recognize the role of inmates in providing hospice care, which may include reading, playing cards or other games, writing letters, massage, holding hands, providing sips of water, helping the patient change position, or other activities of daily living when the patient is unable to do for themselves (ACA, 2002; NCCHC, 2008a, 2008b, 2011).

Inmates who provide hospice care must be trained and supervised appropriately. Typically, inmate hospice workers receive the same training as provided to volunteers in the community only supplemented with material specific to the facility and the scope of work the inmates will be assigned.

Expression of Grief and Loss

A framework suggested for understanding the normal process or tasks of grief is depicted in Exhibit 8.2. In addition to the losses experienced as a result of incarceration, prisoners often have experienced the loss of multiple family members, as well. This accumulation of losses accentuates the experience of grief (Taylor, n.d.). The process of mourning in correctional settings is often suspended or disrupted as a result of incarceration and the expression of grief or emotion, other than anger, is often not viewed as "safe" because it implies vulnerability and weakness (Ferszt, 2002; Hendry, 2009; Taylor, n.d.). The consequence of suspended or incomplete grief work includes numbness or detachment, sorrow, bitterness, depression, withdrawal, irritability or agitation, lack of trust in others, and difficulty carrying out normal routines (Howarth, 2011). Unresolved grief may manifest in altered relationships with others, agitated depression, and self-destructive behavior (Taylor, n.d.).

Until the establishment of hospice and palliative care programs in correctional settings, the opportunity for offenders to constructively grieve was very limited. Even

EXHIBIT 8.2
Worden's Tasks of Grieving

Accept the reality of the loss: talking about the death with supportive family and others, participating in vigil, viewing the body, attending the funeral or memorial service.

Experience the pain of grief: expression of emotion (anger, crying, sorrow, guilt, anxiety, loneliness, numbness, etc.), difficulty sleeping, pre-occupation with memories.

Adjust to the absence of the deceased: learning to cope without the presence of the deceased person, visitation, correspondence, financial or caretaking responsibilities.

Re-invest emotional energy: finding meaning in death and converting the relationship to memory, re-establish relationships without the deceased, and make new relationships.

Source: Taylor (n.d.) and Hendry (2009).

though provisions for grief and bereavement are now components of these programs, the setting and culture remain significant challenges (Loeb et al., 2011b; VOA, 2001; Zimmermann, 2006).

Expected Outcomes

The primary outcome of end-of-life care is to respect and carry out the wishes of the patient. If the patient wishes to spend one's remaining life in the care of family and friends in the community, and it is possible to release the inmate from incarceration, rigorous effort should be made to accomplish the inmate's release and transfer care to providers in the community.

Nearly all states as well as the federal government have a mechanism for early or compassionate release of prisoners with terminal illness. Although it is a time consuming and challenging process, nurses have a role in referring inmate-patients for compassionate or early release (Williams, Sudore, Griefinger, & Morrison, 2011). Nurses may also identify resources to continue the patient's care in the community and assist with transition.

For patients who are not able to be released, the primary outcome is that they not die alone. Other outcome measures are control of symptoms (Bick, 2002; Cahal, 2002; Tillman, 2000) and closure of family and other life issues (Cahal, 2002; Zimmerman, Wald, & Thompson, 2002).

NURSING CARE OF PATIENTS AT THE END OF LIFE

Assessment and then intervention to relieve distressful symptoms is the major role of nurses in end-of-life care. Regular, ongoing nursing assessment identifies changes in the patient's condition early so that symptoms can be addressed before the patient suffers. The use of a standardized approach to assessment ensures that information collected is consistent and objective (Soden et al., 2010). One tool that has been recommended is the Edmonton Symptom Assessment System-Revised, which may be obtained online at http://www.palliative.org/PC/ClinicalInfo/Assessment-Tools/ESAS%20ToolsIdx.html. It assesses the nine most common symptoms patients experience and has been validated in many different clinical settings (Institute for Clinical Systems Improvement, 2009).

In addition to report of symptoms, the nurse evaluates the patient for changes in cognition and functional ability by assessing mental status, degree of self-care, ambulation, activity level, and intake. The assessment also includes identification of any side effects the patient has as a result of treatment. New symptoms and worsening symptoms are communicated by the nurse to the treatment team (Soden et al., 2010). The use of order sets and treatment algorithms is recommended to facilitate quick response to symptoms that can be anticipated for each patient (National Consensus Project for Quality Palliative Care, 2009).

Pain

Pain is the predominant symptom for patients in end-of-life care; 70%–90% of patients with advanced disease will report pain and 72% of all dying patients report pain (Bass, 2010). This is why relief of pain and related suffering is a primary focus of palliative care. Aspects of pain management that are emphasized or unique in palliative care are that the pain will get worse, it is managed aggressively, and side effects must be anticipated.

Patients in end-of-life care will experience increasing pain. A stepped approach is used to control pain with analgesics and adjunctive medication methods (ICSI, 2009). Nonpharmacological measures are also very effective adjuncts in pain control (American Association of Critical-Care Nurses [AACCN], 2008; Bass, 2010; Registered Nurses Association of Ontario [RNAO], 2002, Supplement 2007). For more discussion of interventions to address pain, see Chapter 13, Pain Management, in this text. Two additional types of pain nurses providing end-of-life care should anticipate managing with as-needed medication (PRN) are breakthrough pain and incident pain.

Breakthrough pain is of greater intensity than the patient's normal or tolerated pain level. Breakthrough pain may be a result of the analgesic wearing off before the next dose and should be addressed with a supplemental dose of the same analgesic used for baseline pain. Repeated episodes of breakthrough pain in a 24-hour period may indicate the need to move up a step on the pain ladder (Soden et al., 2010).

Incident pain occurs when a particular action or movement takes place, such as walking or coughing. Nurses anticipate and treat incident pain so that the patient can carry out activities of daily living and participate in grief work. Treatment is an analgesic with fast onset of action to cover the pain while the activity takes place. This kind of analgesia may help a patient tolerate a dressing change, use the toilet, take a shower, or have a visit with family (Bass, 2010).

The nurse should put in place measures to prevent or mitigate common side effects of opioid analgesics. The nurse should also counsel the patient about constipation, nausea, respiratory depression, and sedation. If the patient is not tolerating measures to manage side effects, the nurse should obtain new or revised orders (Ferrell & Paice, 2008).

Skin Care

As a patient becomes less ambulatory skin care becomes more important. Any inmate admitted for inpatient care should have skin integrity assessed. Use of the Braden Scale for Predicting Pressure Sore Risk is recommended for the initial and periodic reassessment (ICSI, 2010, Second Edition; RNAO, 2005). The Braden Scale may be obtained at http://www.bradenscale.com/copyright.htm. A simple copyright permission form must be submitted in order to use the form, and it is provided at no charge to professionals who will not sell or profit from the use of the form.

Nursing actions to prevent skin breakdown are to use a positioning schedule, minimize friction and shear when turning or moving the patient, use of pressure-relieving material in bed and chair, encourage fluids and hydration, use pH-balanced cleansers and moisturizers, and use of protective barriers (films, padding, etc.) and absorbent material to wick moisture away from skin. Pruritus or dry itchy skin is treated with hydration, use of moisturizers, or emollients. Temporary relief may also be obtained from oatmeal bath products and over-the counter-topicals such as calamine lotion, antihistamine ointment, and anesthetic agents (Fauci et al., 2008; ICSI, 2010, Second Edition; VOA, 2001).

For patients who have skin breakdown, nursing actions anticipate and address pain in advance of wound care or dressing change; dressing products are used to manage exudate; odor is controlled by putting kitty litter, coffee grounds, or activated charcoal in tray under the bed; and foul orders are masked with peppermint oil or other aroma products (VOA, 2001).

Oral Hygiene

An oral health assessment should be included in the admission and periodic nursing assessment of inmates who are receiving end-of-life care in an inpatient setting. The results of the oral health assessment are used to develop a plan to maintain oral hygiene. The plan may include directions to staff about when and how to provide oral hygiene, to cue or remind the patient to attend to their oral hygiene, and what products to use to relieve symptoms of pain or other side effects. For patients who are unable to care for their own oral hygiene, nursing care should include scheduled

CASE EXAMPLE 8.1

Mr. George is a 56-year-old prisoner who has been incarcerated for the last 10 years within a state prison system. He has end-stage liver disease with severe ascites and Grade 3 esophageal varices. After an extensive workup at the regional medical center he is returned to the correctional facility for admission to the infirmary for end-of-life care. In addition to end-stage liver disease, Mr. George had been followed by mental health staff for major depression. He also is being treated for hypertension and gastroesophageal reflux disease (GERD). He has fallen twice while at the regional medical center and is considered a fall risk because of his ascites and general frailty. Medications on admission to the infirmary include lactulose, the antidepressant Remeron, propranolol, Lasix, and Colace. Orders for pain medication include a regular schedule for administration of intramuscular morphine. Breakthrough pain is managed with Norco, a combination of hydrocodone and acetaminophen, and Ativan. During the first 4 days on hospice, Mr. George refused his dose of regularly scheduled morphine on two occasions. The nurses document the patient's report of significant pain the following two shifts. Objective signs of pain that were also documented include clenching and grimacing. The PRN orders for Norco and Ativan were given after 8 hours of persistent reports of pain but did not significantly reduce symptoms. Create a plan of care for Mr. George, taking into consideration all available information.

oral care twice daily with specific instructions tailored to the patient's needs. Scheduling antimicrobial mouth rinse as a medication also can be a reminder for nursing staff to complete oral care (RNAO, 2008).

Dry mouth is addressed by increasing hydration, frequent rinsing of the mouth with water, and, if the patient does not have diminished swallowing, sugarless candy. The care plan may include use of mouth moisturizer or artificial saliva. For excessive secretions, have patient cough and deep breathe every hour while awake and encourage fluids for hydration. A room humidifier will help keep secretions fluid and less troublesome for respiration (National Consensus Project for Quality Palliative Care, 2009; Fauci et al., 2008).

Other Common Symptoms

A description of the other common symptoms patients experience along with recommended comfort care measures are listed alphabetically as a resource for care planning in Table 8.1 (AACCN, 2008; Fauci et al., 2008; ICSI, 2009; VOA, 2001). These measures are in addition to administering prescribed treatments that are ordered by the treating clinician to address symptoms as part of the patient's plan of care. Case Example 8.1 applies information from this section.

Recognizing Impending Death

There are a series of recognizable stages when death is imminent. The nurse in recognizing impending death can help the patient accomplish important tasks that remain undone, provide safety and reassurance as dependence increases, and communicate the patient's condition and wishes to the other members of the treatment team and to the family. Transition through each stage is highly variable; the entire process may take place in less than 24 hours or as long as 2 weeks or so (Weissman, 2009).

Early changes include decreased socialization; the patient is more lethargic, sleeping and resting. The patient may want to be alone or be with only one of a few people. Interest and/or ability to eat or drink is diminished; the patient may prefer liquid or soft foods. Be aware of diminished swallow reflex and position the patient with the head of the bed elevated slightly. The patient may verbalize that they are dying, may report visiting or seeing someone in their past who is dead, they may request a particular visit, or verbalize a task to finish. Cognitive changes include restlessness, confusion, and agitation. The patient may be frightened by the confusion and restlessness may be a manifestation of anxiety. Provide for the patient's safety but try not to interfere or restrain them; use quiet tones and reassuring phrases; explain what you are doing before you do it to reduce potential for alarm.

In the middle stage of dying, the patient's level of consciousness will decline further with only brief periods of wakefulness. The breathing pattern will be irregular and shallow, with periods of apnea. The patient should be prompted to deep breathe and cough every couple of hours. The swallowing reflex is diminished and secretions will collect in the throat (death rattle). This is managed by raising the head of the bed, turning the patient on their side, and reducing intake of fluid. Gentle suctioning of the mouth may be used, but is disturbing to the patient and ineffective in removing fluid beyond the mouth. Urine output will diminish and darkens in color. Both urinary and bowel incontinence take place. The patient should be kept clean and dry; linen changes can be avoided by using disposable pads. There may be periods of restlessness and agitation; the nursing action is to calm the patient and give reassurance. The patient may

TABLE 8.1 Common Symptoms With Nursing Actions for Comfort Care, Listed Alphabetically

SYMPTOM	SUGGESTIONS FOR COMFORT CARE
Anorexia & cachexia	Provide food and beverage pt. prefers Rest before and after eating Pleasant or diversionary activity while eating Frequent, small meals Frequent mouth care Minimize odors that suppress appetite
Belching	Keep mouth closed when chewing and swallowing Elevate head of bed Avoid foods that produce gas (beans, broccoli, cabbage, milk products) Avoid use of straws to drink fluid
Confusion & delirium	Explain what you are doing before providing care Reduce sensory stimulation Ensure pt. is using eyeglasses, hearing aids, etc. Establish or follow daily routine Avoid asking pt. questions Orient to time (morning, night) Offer reassurance Relaxation: massage, music
Constipation	Bowel regimen; use of stool softener & peristaltic stimulant Drink as much fluid as tolerated Physical activity as allowed by condition and energy Monitor bowel activity to intervene as early as necessary
Cough	Elevate the head of the bed Humidifier Sip warm H_2O with honey or lemon
Dyspnea	If on O_2, check for mechanical problems Positioning: sitting up, resting arms on a table Breathe through pursed lips Improve room air circulation: sit by window or a fan Cool room temperature Humidifier Relaxation: music, imagery, massage
Fatigue	Prioritize activity by pt. preference Schedule rest and activity periods Encourage mild exercise Assist with ADLs Improve sleep environment
Hiccups	Facilitate use of method patient reports worked before Hold breath Re-breathe into paper bag Bite a lemon Drink or gargle ice water Drink from opposite side of cup

(continued)

TABLE 8.1   *(continued)*

SYMPTOM	SUGGESTIONS FOR COMFORT CARE
	Spoonful of sugar or peanut butter If more than 48 hours, medical attention is required
Incontinence	Facilitate access to toilet: bedside commode, room with toilet Toilet regularly (every 2 hours) Avoid caffeine Provide skin care Change linen and clothing as needed Control odor Liquid stool may be due to impaction
Insomnia	Regular schedule for sleep and awake Avoid stimulants (caffeine, tobacco, etc.) Avoid napping: use television, radio, or other activity to prevent napping Encourage exercise Improve sleep environment Relaxation: breathing, imagery Explore possible underlying cause: fear of incontinence, nightmares, spiritual crisis
Nausea and/or vomiting	Wear loose clothing Elevate head of bed Avoid odors that trigger nausea Clear diet for 1 day; then bland, low-fat diet Avoid food that is difficult to digest Frequent, small meals Frequent mouth care Comfortable room temperature Good ventilation Relaxation techniques: breathing, imagery, music
Respiratory depression	Encourage deep breathing Monitor respiratory rate and depth for 1st 24 h after starting opioid medication Contact physician if rate less than 8 per minute
Restlessness & anxiety	Have someone remain with pt. Reduce sensory stimulation Restore routine Reorient to environment Ensure pt. is using eyeglasses, hearing aids, etc. Relaxation: massage, music, imagery Distracting activity: reading, television, cards Explore for possible spiritual concern or crisis Provide reassurance
Sedation	Monitor vital signs q 2 hours for first 12 h after starting opioid medication Encourage intake of caffeinated beverage Assess for fall risk and institute protective measures

Source: From Volunteers of America: GRACE Project (2001), Fauci et al. (2008), American Association of Critical-Care Nurses (2008), Institute for Clinical Systems Improvement (2009).

complain that they are cold or hot. Keep the patient warm with lightweight blankets; if hot, give lukewarm sponge bath. Vital signs are abnormal. Being with the patient is comforting, however, it is important that activities or loud conversation not contribute to fatigue. Use a normal tone of voice and speak directly to the patient; explain what is happening and be attentive to any response or participation on their part.

Near death the patient will be virtually unresponsive; their mouth and eyes partially or completely open or their jaw may drop to the side they are facing. The patient may hold a rigid position. The patient's vital signs are abnormal (respirations may be apneic, rapid, and cyclical; the pulse rapid, fever may be present, and the blood pressure low). The patient will have mottled extremities and the underside of the body will darken. Supportive care includes talking with the patient as described in the paragraph above, using gentle touch, providing for hygiene with as little disruption as possible, and moistening lips with lip balm or other emollient. The environment should be quiet, respectful, and private (Fauci et al., 2008; ICSI, 2009; VOA, 2001; Weissman, 2009).

Postmortem Care

The plan of care for the patient should specify actions to take place and responsibilities at the time of death and during the post-mortem period, including who pronounces that death has occurred, who is notified and by when, and preparation and disposition of the body following death. These arrangements should reflect the patient's cultural and spiritual practices as much as possible but still be consistent with facility policy and procedures regarding death of an inmate. Correctional facility policies concerning an inmate death may require that the patient and area be secured until released by the state police or another government agency. The body should be bathed, hair combed, and diapers or pads placed for incontinence. Once the body is placed in alignment, it should be covered with a sheet and the head of the bed elevated 20 degrees until it is to be removed. The nurse documents in the health record the time respirations and pulse ceased, general appearance of the body, who was present at the time of death, who was notified and when, and the time the body was removed and by whom. Other forms of documentation may be required as well.

The nurse should also be attentive to grief on the part of family, if present; inmate volunteers; and caregivers. A chaplain, if one is available at the facility, should be present to provide support. If one is not available, the nurse should provide support by active listening and expression of feelings about the patient and his or her death (Smith, 2010a; Sherman, Matzo, Pitorak, Ferrell, & Malloy, 2005).

COMMUNICATION IN END-OF-LIFE AND PALLIATIVE CARE
Interdisciplinary Plan of Care

Palliative and end-of-life care is distinguished from other types of health care by its focus on a comprehensive plan of care that is developed by an interdisciplinary team. Standards recommended by the GRACE Project are that the interdisciplinary team include at least a social worker or counselor and a chaplain, in addition to a physician and nurse (2001). Armed with a realistic understanding of the options available, the role of the patient is to make informed choices about care to be provided (ICSI, 2009). The patient also determines the level of family involvement, and their concerns should be addressed in the plan of care as well (VOA, 2001). There is growing recognition of the importance of incorporating any inmate who has become the patient's "family of choice" into the process of planning and providing end-of-life care (McAdoo, 2008). The term "family of choice" refers to inmates who have developed close and emotionally rich relationships with each other over the term of incarceration. An inmate with terminal illness may seek the participation and advice of these individuals when considering options for care, especially if biological family is distant or uninvolved.

Establishing a Therapeutic Relationship

A therapeutic nurse–patient relationship eases the suffering of patients receiving palliative care (Mok & Chiu, 2004). The features of a therapeutic nurse–patient relationship are respect, empathy, and validation or responsiveness to the patient (RNAO, 2002, Supplement 2006). Correctional nurses sometimes voice concern about whether the setting and patient population are conducive to the therapeutic relationship (LaMarre, 2006); however, the fundamentals are consistent with many of the provisos governing interaction in the correctional setting.

In a therapeutic relationship, communication with the patient always involves active listening, observation of nonverbal behavior, and respect. Respect is demonstrated by referring to the patient by proper name, introducing self by name, and explaining your role in the patient's care. Use of open-ended questions encourages the patient to voice concerns and allows the nurse to observe consistency of verbalization with nonverbal behavior (Smith, 2010b). Acknowledging the patient's situation validates the individual and can be an opportunity to demonstrate empathy. Empathy is not self-disclosure, the latter of which is discouraged in correctional settings, but instead is a nonjudgmental understanding of the subjective aspect of the patient's situation (RNAO, 2002, Supplement 2006). Finally, including the patient in choices or decision making about care supports the patient's autonomy and control, even in situations when the patient has little he or she can self-determine. Trust is established when the nurse explains or helps the patient understand a procedure or the next steps in care and is available to answer questions or address concerns. Providing privacy during care and honoring confidentiality convey respect and engender the patient's trust in the therapeutic relationship (Smith, 2010b). The result of a therapeutic nurse–patient relationship is simply effective communication of information important to the patient's well-being and provision of optimal care.

Emotional and Spiritual Preparation for End-of-Life

Many correctional facilities have chaplains and/or religious volunteers who are members of the interdisciplinary care team for patients receiving end-of-life care. The chaplain assesses needs, hopes, and resources and will identify spiritual concerns that either complicate or complement the plan of care. Spiritual and religious beliefs greatly influence the course of action taken by a patient and their family during end-of-life care (ICSI, 2009). Patients welcome inquiry into their spirituality especially as the severity of illness increases. Patients want health care providers to know how their beliefs influence how they deal with being sick, to understand them better as a person, and to understand how they make decisions (McCord et al., 2004).

Spirituality has long been a domain of nursing practice and the ethical principles used when addressing the spiritual concerns of patients include respecting the patient and their spiritual beliefs as integral to their person, acting in the best interests of the patient, maintaining personal integrity while not proselytizing, and being truthful (Hospice and Palliative Nursing Association, 2010; Puchalski et al., 2009; Ruder, 2008). The American Association of Colleges of Nursing (2004) has established competencies for nursing care of patients at the end of life that include assisting patients with emotional and spiritual issues, including distress. Nursing interventions to relieve symptoms of spiritual distress are listed in Table 8.2. The nurse who is attuned to these can help the patient identify and prioritize values in making decisions about treatment and comfort care (Browning, 2009; Callanan, 2008).

TABLE 8.2   Characteristics of Spiritual Distress and Related Nursing Interventions

CHARACTERISTICS OF SPIRITUAL DISTRESS	NURSING INTERVENTIONS
Change in behavior and mood (anger, crying, withdrawal, anxiety)	Assess spirituality, note participation in ritual and religious practices, impact of illness on spiritual outlook
Anger toward God or higher power	Use active listening to demonstrate focus on patient and to hear distress cues
Expressed desire for spiritual assistance	Approach patient in nonjudgmental way and keep conversation focused on the patient's spiritual values
Displaced anger toward religious representatives	Express willingness to discuss spirituality based upon patient wishes
Display of gallows humor	Assess desire for assistance coping with spiritual concerns
Expressed concern about meaning of life, belief systems, relationship with God or higher power	Provide information on grieving as well as the emotions and behaviors that accompany each stage to facilitate grief work
Expressed conflict about beliefs	Provide resources that address spiritual needs
Guilt	Acknowledge the patient's spiritual concerns and their validity
Inability to participate in religious practices	Make referral for spiritual assistance
Inability to express previous state of creativity	Provide privacy for chaplain visits
No interest in nature	Collaborate with clergy or spiritual healer in care of the patient
No interest in spiritual literature	Encourage patient to practice their religion or beliefs
Poor coping	Help patient define the problem causing conflict or distress
Questioning meaning of own existence and/or suffering	Encourage patient to have spiritual objects bedside or nearby
Questioning moral and ethical implications of treatment	Show willingness to pray with patient and provide spiritual support

Source: Taylor and Ralph (2010).

Patient Advocacy

Advocacy preserves the patient's autonomy, dignity, rights to privacy, confidentiality, and self-determination. Examples of advocacy for patients with terminal illness include achieving pain relief, limiting suffering, and resolving conflicts. Advocacy by nurses in the correctional setting is most certainly needed for the same purposes. It is also likely to involve changing or modifying institution rules, such as lifting limitations on visits to inmates in the infirmary for hospice or palliative care (ANA, 2007). Researchers with The Pennsylvania State University have partnered with the Pennsylvania Department of Corrections to support frontline workers, which include nurses, to adapt best practices for end-of-life care to correctional settings (Loeb et al., 2011b). Effective advocates are nurses who are experienced and confident in their practice, have an established therapeutic relationship with the patient, and have strong relationships with their colleagues (Taylor & Ferszt, 1998). Nurses who fail to advocate for patients are at risk of experiencing moral distress and professional burnout (AACCN, 2008; Pavlish, Brown-Saltzman, Hersh, Shirk, & Nudelman, 2011.

From the Experts ...

" ... it is up to you what kind of nurse you want to be. There is a whole lot of room to be innovative and an advocate. It is not always easy, but you are only limited by your imagination and how much advocacy you want to do."

Tanya Tillman, RN
Angola, LA
(Quinn, n.d.)

ETHICAL ISSUES

Ethical issues during end-of-life care concern decisions about treatment and care, including the person's capacity to decide from among treatment options, who is designated to make decisions in the event the patient is incapacitated and cannot decide for themselves, and whether a particular course of treatment is consistent

CASE EXAMPLE 8.2

The charge nurse for a 15-bed infirmary receives a phone call from the daughter of Mr. Arnold, a 56-year-old man who is recovering from surgery to remove a cancerous lesion in his left lung. She is calling to make arrangements to visit her father; she also wants to meet with the doctor and review his chart. She says that she has a power of attorney. The chart indicates a release of information from the patient, allowing discussion of his health information with the daughter. Mr. Arnold says that he has not given his daughter permission to make health care decisions for him, but she is handling some of his financial affairs while he is in prison. There is no indication that Mr. Arnold is incapacitated and unable to make decisions for himself, so even if the daughter had a health care power of attorney it does not apply at this point. What is the best response to the daughter?

with the patient's wishes. These same ethical issues are encountered in the care of inmates, but low levels of health literacy, separation from family and support systems, and limited decision-making authority while incarcerated add to the complexity of decision making for inmate-patients (Deaton, et al. 2009–2010; Enders, Paterniti, & Meyers, 2005; Levine, 2005). Case Example 8.2 can be used to apply information reviewed in this section.

Advance Care Planning

Advance care planning is a means to identify a person's preferences regarding treatment and care as they approach end of life. Ideally advance care planning prevents confusion and conflict among health care providers, the patient and family about the patient's treatment and care (Mohn-Brown, Burke, & Eby, 2010). Every state acknowledges the legality of written advance directives, but the forms and laws regarding their use vary (ICSI, 2009). Accreditation standards for correctional facilities also acknowledge the inmate's rights to make informed decisions about care and treatment (ACA, 2002; NCCHC, 2008a, 2008b, 2011). The NCCHC has a specific standard that recognizes an offender's ability to make end-of-life decisions but requires independent review before care and treatment may be withdrawn or withheld in the correctional setting (NCCHC, 2008a, 2008b, 2011). Patient safety standards proposed for correctional facilities include discussing advance directives with patients when admitted to inpatient settings and displaying those preferences prominently in the health record (Stern, Greifinger, & Mellow, 2010). Nurses need to be familiar with the terms and other characteristics defining advance care planning used in the correctional setting as well as in the local community.

Power of Attorney for Health Care

The term power of attorney for health care, or health care proxy, refers to the person who is designated by the patient to make decisions about their health care when the patient is unable to do so themselves. These individuals should be involved in discussions about care and treatment well in advance of the patient's incapacity so that they are fully informed (Fauci et al., 2008; ICSI, 2009).

Some correctional systems will not allow someone who is incarcerated to serve as a health care proxy for another incarcerated person to avoid potential for coercion and victimization (Federal Bureau of Prisons, 2005; Oklahoma Department of Corrections, 2011; Oregon Department of Corrections, 2008). Even if family members have been estranged from an inmate, often they are willing to serve as a designate when contacted. Care planning will be more satisfactory if a family member or other acceptable person is identified to serve as an inmate's health care designate early in the progression of a life-limiting illness. Identification of the health care proxy can be time consuming and is another reason to start this process sooner rather than later so that the patient is protected from unnecessary suffering or futile care.

Capacity to Make Health Care Decisions

The health care representative may make decisions regarding the patient only when the patient's health care provider or the court has determined the patient is incapable of making health care decisions. Nurses are often the providers who first identify concerns about diminished capacity to the other members of the treatment team

(Mohn-Brown et al., 2010; Taylor & Ferszt, 1998). Capacity to decide is demonstrated when the patient is able to perform all three of the actions listed here:

- Receive information about treatment and care options
- Evaluate or deliberate logically about the information received
- Communicate a treatment preference (ICSI, 2009; Mohn-Brown et al., 2010).

Living Will or Health Care Directive

The living will or health care directive documents the patient's preferences about life-prolonging intervention including resuscitation, use of antibiotics, nutritional support, and other medical interventions to be administered or withheld. It is used by the person designated as the health care proxy when the patient can no longer communicate his or her wishes (ICSI, 2009). Another form that assists in the enactment of advanced care decisions is the Physician's Order for Life-Sustaining Treatment (POLST), which consists of a written set of orders covering CPR, the degree of medical intervention, and nutritional support (Oregon POLST Task Force, 2011). The POLST Program is in place or being developed in states all across the United States (2008) and conveys information to health care providers from one setting to another about the care and treatment decisions at the end of life (ICSI, 2009).

Do Not Resuscitate Orders

Nurses still encounter orders to not resuscitate and/or take comfort measures only. The principle for obtaining the order is the same as other forms of advance care planning; that it expresses the patient's informed decision about medical intervention at the end of life. When used, these orders need to be clear and unambiguous so that there is no confusion about the patient's expectations for care. Nurses who are uncomfortable with the plan of care should bring those concerns forward to the provider or treatment team well in advance of a patient care crisis if at all possible. Nurses may also seek out a more experienced colleague or supervisor for advice and guidance (AACCN, 2008).

SUMMARY

The end of life is characterized as a time to review accomplishments, to resolve conflicts, to atone for wrongful acts, and to make peace with self and others who are important to the patient. Anger, sadness, despair, and anxiety are some of the emotions that patients experience as they prepare for death. Access to family, friends, and spiritual advisors are needed to reach a peaceful end to life.

Correctional nurses must be competent in the delivery of end-of-life care consistent with the standards for this type of care in the community. Correctional nurses use clinical knowledge, communication skill, ethical awareness, and organizational understanding to care for patients with terminal disease. Nursing care includes assisting the patient to make decisions about treatment, palliative care and life-sustaining measures, effectively addressing the concerns of the patient, coordinating care among multiple providers, and communicating with the patient's family and other members of the care team. Nurses actively support the diverse spiritual and cultural needs of patients and their families and advocate for modification of the correctional environment to ensure comfort, dignity, and respect in end-of-life care. The features of humane and compassionate end-of-life care enhance rather than challenge the safe and secure operation of correctional facilities.

DISCUSSION QUESTIONS

- What are some of the barriers to a patient experiencing a "good death" in your setting?
- What are the challenges in advance care planning with patients who are also incarcerated?
- How do you respond to a patient who asks you to pray with them?
- What are the support systems in place at your facility to support the expression of grief?

REFERENCES

Aday, R. (2009). The effect of health and penal harm on aging prisoner's views of dying in prison. *Omega: Journal of Death and Dying, 60*(1), 51–70.

American Association of Colleges of Nursing. (2004). *Peaceful death: Recommended competencies and curricular guidelines for end-of-life nursing care.* Retrieved May 16, 2011, from American Association of Colleges of Nursing: http://www.aacn.nche.edu/Publications/deathfin.htm

American Association of Critical-Care Nurses. (2008). *Palliative care and symptom management resource.* Retrieved September 3, 2011, from American Association of Critical-Care Nurses (AACN): http://www.aacn.org/WD/Palliative/Docs/Player/Topics/Topic01/Page01/Resources/Palliative%20Care%20and%20Symptom%20Management%20Resource.pdf

American Correctional Association. (2002). *Performance based standards for correctional health care in adult correctional institutions.* Alexandria, VA: Author.

American Nurses Association. (2007). *Corrections nursing: Scope & standards of practice.* Silver Spring, MD: Author.

Anno, B., Graham, C., Lawrence, J., & Shansky, R. (2004). *Correctional health care: Addressing the needs of elderly, chronically ill, and terminally ill inmates.* Washington, DC: U.S. Department of Justice, National Institute of Corrections.

Bass, M. (2010). Anatomy and physiology of pain and the management of breakthrough pain in palliative care. *International Journal of Palliative Nursing, 16*(10), 486–492.

Bick, J. (2002). Managing pain and end-of-life care for inmate patients: The California medical facility experience. *Journal of Correctional Health Care, 9,* 131–147.

Browning, A. (2009, January–March). Incorporating spiritual beliefs into end-of-life care. *Journal of Christian Nursing, 26*(1), 11–17.

Cahal, W. (2002). The birth of a Prison Hospice Program. *The Journal of Correctional Health Care, 9*(2), 125–129.

Callanan, M. (2008). *Final journeys: A practical guide for bringing care and comfort at the end of life.* New York, NY: Bantam Books.

Craig, E., & Ratcliff, M. (2002). Controversies in correctional end-of-life care. *Journal of Correctional Health Care, 9,* 149–157.

Deaton, D., Aday, R., & Wahidin, A. (2009–2010). The effect of health and penal harm on aging female prisoners' views of dying in prison. *Omega-Journal of Death and Dying, 60*(1), 51–70.

Dubler, N., & Heyman, B. (2006). End-of-life care in prisons and jails. In M. Puisis, *Clinical practice in correctional medicine* (2nd Ed., pp. 538–544). Philadelphia: Mosby Elsevier.

Enders, S., Paterniti, D., & Meyers, F. (2005). An approach to develop effective health care decision making for women in prison. *Journal of Palliative Medicine, 8*(2), 432–439.

Fauci, A., Braunwald, E., Kasper, D., Hauser, S., Longo, D., Jameson, J. et al. (2008). *Harrison's principles of internal medicine* (17th Ed.). New York: McGraw-Hill.

Federal Bureau of Prisons. (2005, January 15). *Program Statement 6031.01: Patient care.* Retrieved August 30, 2011, from Federal Bureau of Prisons Policy and Forms: http://www.bop.gov/policy/progstat/6031_001.pdf

Ferrell, B. L., & Paice, J. (2008). Managing pain from advanced cancer in the palliative care setting. *Clinical Journal of Oncology Nursing, 12*(4), 575–581.

Ferszt, G. (2002, July). Grief experiences of women in prison following the death of a loved one. *Illness, Crisis & Loss, 10*(3), 242–254.

Harvard Health Publications. (2011, February). Palliative care: Sooner may be better. *Harvard Health Letter*, 6–7.

Hendry, C. (2009). Incarceration and the tasks of grief: A narrative review. *Journal of Advanced Nursing, 65*(2), 270–278.

Hospice and Palliative Nursing Association. (2010, October). *HPNA Position Statement: Spiritual Care.* Retrieved May 17, 2011, from Hospice and Palliative Nursing Association: http://www.hpna.org/DisplayPage.aspx?Title=Position Statements

Howarth, R. (2011, January). Concepts and controversies in grief and loss. *Journal of Mental Health Counseling, 33*(1), 4–10.

Institute for Clinical Systems Improvement. (2009, November). *Health Care Guideline: Palliative Care.* Retrieved March 28, 2011, from Institute for Clinical Systems Improvement: http://www.icsi.org/guidelines_and_more/gl_os_prot/other_health_care_conditions/palliative_care/pallia-tive_care_11875.html

Institute for Clinical System Improvement. (2010, Second Edition, April). *Health care protocol: Pressure Ulcer Prevention and Treatment Protocol.* Retrieved March 31, 2011, from Institute for Clinical System Improvement: http://www.icsi.org/pressure_ulcer_treatment_ protocol__re-view_and_comment_/pressure_ulcer_treatment__protocol__.html

Jervis, R. (2009, November 30). *Inmates assist ill and dying fellow prisoners in hospices.* Retrieved April 3, 2011, from USA TODAY: http://www.usatoday.com/news/nation/2009-11-29-prison-hospices_N.htm

LaMarre, M. (2006). Nursing role and practice in correctional facilities. In M. Puisis, *Clinical practice in correctional medicine* (2nd Ed., pp. 417–425). Philadelphia, PA: Mosby/Elsevier.

Leland, J. (2009, October 17). *Fellow inmates ease pain of dying in jail.* Retrieved April 2, 2011, from *New York Times*: http://topics.nytimes.com/top/reference/timestopics/subjects/p/prisons_and_prisoners/index.html?query=DEATH%20AND%20DYING&field=des&match=exact

Levine, S. (2005). Improving end-of-life care of prisoners. *Journal of Correctional Health Care, 11,* 317–331.

Linder, J., & Meyers, F. (2007, August 22–29). Palliative care for prison inmates; "Don't Let Me Die in Prison." *Journal of the American Medical Association, 298*(8), 894–901.

Loeb, S., Penrod, J., Hollenbeak, C., & Smith, C. (2011a). End-of-life care and barriers for female inmates. *Journal of Obstetric, Gynecologic & Neonatal Nursing, 40,* 477–485.

Loeb, S., Penrod, J., Smith, C., Hollenbeak, C., & Kitt-Lewis, E. (2011b). Generalist strategies for enhancing end-of-life care. *National Commission on Correctional Health Care.* Phoenix: National Commission on Correctional Health Care.

Maull, F. (2006). Delivery of end-of-life care in the prison setting. In M. Puisis, *Clinical practice in corr-rectional medicine* (pp. 529–537). Mosby Elsevier, Philadelphia, PA.

McAdoo, C. (2008). Excellence in end of life care: New quality guidelines for hospice care. *National Commission on Correctional Health Care.* Chicago: NCCHC.

McCord, G., Gilchrist, V., Grossman, S., King, B., McCormick, K., Oprandi, A. et al. (2004, July/August). Discussing spirituality with patients: A reational and ethical approach. *Annals of Family Medicine, 2*(4), 356–361.

Mohn-Brown, E., Burke, K., & Eby, L. (Eds.). (2010, May 18). *Medical–Surgical Nursing Care - 3rd Ed., Chapter 13. Grief, Loss, and End-of-Life Care.* (I. Pearson Education, Producer) Retrieved May 9, 2011, from STAT!Ref Online Electronic Medical Library: http://online.statref.com.proxy.heal-wa.org/document.aspx?fxid=187&docid=95

Mok, E., & Chiu, P. (2004). Nurse–patient relationships in pallaitive care. *Journal of Advanced Nursing, 48*(5), 475–483.

National Commission on Correctional Health Care (NCCHC). (2008a). *Standards for health services in prisons.* Chicago, IL: Author.

National Commission on Correctional Health Care (NCCHC). (2008b). *Standards for health services in jails*. Chicago, IL: Author.

National Commission on Correctional Health Care (NCCHC). (2011). *Standards for health services in juvenile detention and confinement facilities*. Chicago, IL: Author.

National Consensus Project for Quality Palliative Care. (2009). *Clinical practice guidelines for quality palliative care* (2nd ed.). Retrieved March 29, 2011, from National Consensus Project for Quality Palliative Care: http://www.nationalconsensusproject.org

National Institute of Corrections Information Center. (1997, September). *Prison medical care: Special needs populations and cost control—Special issues in corrections*. Retrieved April 4, 2011, from National Institute of Corrections: http://nicic.gov/pubs/1997/013964.pdf

Nelson, L. (1998, January/February). Death among us. *The Angolite*, 18–27.

O'Conner, M. (2004). Finding boundaries inside prison walls: Case study of a terminally ill inmate. *Death Studies, 28*, 63–76.

Oklahoma Department of Corrections. (2011, February 17). *Offender living will/advance directive for health care and do not resuscitate (DNR) Consent*. Retrieved August 30, 2011, from Oklahoma DOC Policy and Procedure Manual - Health Services - 14: http://www.doc.state.ok.us/Offtech/op140138.pdf

Oregon Department of Corrections. (2008, October). *P-I-04 End-of-Life Decision Making*. Retrieved August 30, 2011, from DOC Health Services Policies and Procedures: http://www.oregon.gov/DOC/OPS/HESVC/docs/policies_procedures/Section_I/PI04.pdf

Oregon POLST Task Force. (2011, August). *POLST Physician Orders for Life-Sustaining Treatment paradigm guidance for oregon's health care professionals*. Retrieved August 30, 2011, from Oregon POLST Task Force, Center for Ethics in Health Care, Oregon Health Sciences University: http://www.ohsu.edu/polst/news/documents/Guidebook2011V2.pdf

Pavlish, C., Brown-Saltzman, K., Hersh, M., Shirk, M., & Nudelman, O. (2011). Early indicators and risk factors for ethical issues in clinical practice. *Journal of Nursing Scholarship, 43*(1), 13–21.

Price, C. (2008, November 11). *To adopt or adapt? Principles of hospice care in the correctional setting*. Retrieved April 4, 2011, from National Prison Hospice Association: http://www.npha.org/articles/6a.html

Puchalski, C., Ferrell, B., Virani, R., Otis-Green, S., Baird, P., Bull, J. et al. (2009). Improving the quality of spiritual care as a dimension of palliative care: The report of the consensus conference. *Journal of Palliative Medicine, 12*(9), 885–904.

Quinn, N. (n.d.). *A profile: Tanya Tillman, RN*. Retrieved November 5, 2011, from National Prison Hospice: http://www.npha.org/articles/Tillman7-1.html

Registered Nurse Association of Ontario. (2002, Supplement 2006). *Best practice guideline: Establishing therapeutic relationships*. Retrieved May 5, 2011, from Registered Nurse Association of Ontario: http://www.rnao.org/Page.asp?PageID=924&ContentID=801

Registered Nurse Association of Ontario. (2005, March). *Nursing best practice guideline: Risk assessment & prevention of pressure ulcers*. Retrieved March 31, 2011, from Registered Nurses Association of Ontario: http://www.rnao.org/Storage/12/638_BPG_Pressure_Ulcers_ v2.pdf

Registered Nurses Association of Ontario. (2002, Supplement 2007). *Assessment and management of pain*. International Affairs and Nursing Best Practice Guidelines Program. Toronto: Author.

Registered Nurses Association of Ontario. (2008). *Oral health: Nursing assessment and interventions*. Retrieved September 3, 2011, from International Affairs and Nursing Best Practices Guidelines Program: http://www.rnao.org/Page.asp?PageID=924&ContentID=1567

Ruder, S. (2008, March). Incorporating spirituality into home care at the end of life. *Home Healthcare Nurse, 26*(3), 158–163.

Sherman, D., Matzo, M., Pitorak, E., Ferrell, B., & Malloy, P. (2005, May/June). Preparation and care at the time of death: Content of the ELNEC curriculum and teaching strategies. *Journal for Nurses in Staff Development, 21*(3), 93–100.

Smith, N. (2010a, May 14). *Postmortem care*. Retrieved April 12, 2011, from Nursing Practice & Skill: http://web.ebscohost.com.proxy.heal-wa.org/nrc/detail?sid=d336a46e-5170-449b-a661-8009f8d41adc%40sessionmgr112&vid=1&hid=119&bdata=JnNpdGU9bnJjLWxpdmU%3d#db=nrc&AN= 5000011900

Smith, N. (2010 b, October 8). *Communication: Establishing nurse–patient relationships* (D. Pravikoff, Ed.) Retrieved May 5, 2011, from Nursing Practice & Skill: http://web.ebscohost.com.proxy.

heal-wa.org/nrc/detail?sid=545b7f66-a237-4306-8cad-5ff50445671e%40sessionmgr114&vid=5 &hid=127&bdata=JnNpdGU9bnJjLWxpdmU%3d#db=nrc&AN=5000011957

Soden, K., Ali, S., Alloway, L., Barclay, D., Perkins, P., & Barker, S. (2010). How do nurses assess and manage breakthrough pain in specialist palliative care units? A multicentre study. *Palliative Medicine, 24*(3), 294–298.

Steinhauser, K. C. (2000, May 16). The search of a good death: Observations of patients, families, and providers. *Annals of Internal Medicine, 132*(10), 825–832.

Stern, M., Greifinger, R., & Mellow, J. (2010, November). Patient safety: Moving the bar in prison health care standards. *American Journal of Public Health, 100*(11), 2103–2110.

Taylor, C., & Ralph, S. (2010). *Nursing diagnosis reference manual, Sparks & Taylor's* (8th ed.). USA: Lippincott Williams & Williams.

Taylor, P. (n.d.). *Healing after loss: Bereavement help for the correctional community.* Retrieved April 3, 2011, from National Prison Hospice Association: http://www.npha.org/articles/Taylor7-1. html

Taylor, P., & Ferszt, G. (1998, August). The nurse as patient advocate. *Nursing, 98*(8), 70–71.

Tillman, T. (2000, May). *Hospice in prison: The Louisianna State Penitentiary Hospice Program.* Retrieved April 3, 2011, from Innovations in End-of-Life Care: http://www2.edc.org/ lastacts/archives/archivesMay00/featureinn.asp

Volunteers of America: GRACE Project. (2001). *End-of-life care in correrctions: A handbook for caregivers and managers.* Volunteers of America: GRACE Project.

Weissman, D. (2009, March). *Syndrome of imminent death* (2nd ed.). Retrieved March 31, 2011, from Fast Facts and Concepts, End of Life/Palliative Education Resource Center: http://www.eperc. mcw.edu/fastfact/ff-003.htm

West, J. (2000). *Room number six.* Retrieved April 3, 2011, from Innovations in End-of-Life Care: www.edc.org/lastacts

Williams, B., Sudore, R., Griefinger, R., & Morrison, R. (2011). Balancing punishment and compassion for seriously ill prisoners. *Annals of Internal Medicine, 155,* 122–126.

Zimmermann, N. (2006). Bereavement care and services. *National Conference on Correctional Health Care.* Atlanta: National Commission on Correctional Health Care.

Zimmerman, N., Wald, F., & Thompson, A. (2002, July). The needs and resources for hospice care in the Conneticut prison system: A feasibility study. *Illness, Crisis & Loss, 10*(3), 204–232.

NINE

Women's Health Care

Lorry Schoenly

THE UNIQUE POPULATION OF FEMALE INMATES

The background, make-up, and health status of the population of women inmates differs greatly from that of men. This difference affects the type of conditions, frequency of interactions, and context of nursing care delivered to women in correctional settings. The population of incarcerated women is growing at an estimated rate of 5% per year (NCCHC, 2005). Although men still make up the majority of those behind bars, the increase in incarcerated female inmates has resulted in a greater focus on the unique needs of this population (Frost, Greene, & Paranis, 2006). There are seven female prisons in the federal prison system and 21 other facilities that house mixed populations (FBOP, n.d.) Every state has at least one designated women's prison. Larger states may have more. Nearly 200,000 women were incarcerated in prison or jail at year-end 2009 (Glaze, 2010).

Gender matters in the delivery of health care in the correctional setting. Nurses working with imprisoned women can improve health outcomes by understanding the socioeconomic background and unique health care needs of this patient population (Exhibit 9.1). Incarcerated women are likely to have a traumatic history including child abuse and domestic violence (Belknap, 2006; Kelly, Parlaz-Dieckmann, Chang, & Collins, 2010). Loss of contact with children, family, and other normal support systems that results from incarceration is a great stressor for women and can lead to depression and relational isolation. Female inmates have higher rates of mental illness and make greater use of medical services than their male counterparts (Binswanger et al., 2010). The majority of women enter the correctional system with substance abuse histories and many are sex workers (Clarke et al., 2006a; Frost et al., 2006).

EXHIBIT 9.1
National Profile of Female Inmate Population

- Disproportionately women of color
- In their early- to mid-30s
- Most likely to have been convicted of a drug or drug-related offense
- Fragmented family histories, with other family members also involved with the criminal justice system
- Survivors of physical and/or sexual abuse as children and adults
- Significant substance abuse problems
- Multiple physical and mental health problems
- Unmarried mothers of minor children
- High school degree/GED, but limited vocational training and sporadic work histories

Source: From Bloom, Owen, and Covington (2005), used with permission.

Women inmates report higher rates of most chronic conditions including cancer, asthma, diabetes, hypertension, and arthritis (Binswanger et al., 2010). All of these factors contribute to the health profile of the female inmate population.

From the Experts . . .

"Care of incarcerated women requires the nurse to be familiar with the unique characteristics of this population, including generally higher medical and mental health acuity and reproductive considerations. Nurses who integrate this knowledge into their practice are likely to be successful in caring for this underserved population."

Madeleine LaMarre, MN, FNP-BC
Atlanta, GA

Gender Responsive and Trauma Informed Care

The concept of gender responsiveness in correctional practice has gained traction as the female inmate population has spiraled upward. The prevailing demographic profile of women prisoners differs from that of men and must be considered in management and patient care perspectives. Six key principles (Exhibit 9.2) guide gender responsive programming starting with an acknowledgement of gender differences. Application of these principles to the provision of nursing care improves the patient's compliance and engagement in the plan of care.

Given the high degree of trauma women prisoners have experienced, a trauma-informed approach to interaction is recommended. Vivid memories of prior trauma can be triggered by a sight, sound, or smell and the flood of returning memory can overwhelm the patient. Self-protecting defenses such as screaming, violent outbursts,

EXHIBIT 9.2
Guiding Principles of Gender-Responsive Care

Principle 1: Gender. Acknowledge that gender makes a difference.
Principle 2: Environment. Create an environment based on safety, respect, and dignity.
Principle 3: Relationships. Develop policies, practices, and programs that are relational and promote healthy connections to children, family, significant others, and the community.
Principle 4: Services and supervision. Address substance abuse, trauma, and mental health issues through comprehensive, integrated, and culturally relevant services and appropriate supervision.
Principle 5: Socioeconomic status. Provide women with opportunities to improve their socioeconomic conditions.
Principle 6: Community. Establish a system of community supervision and reentry with comprehensive, collaborative services.

Source: McCampbell (2005), used with permission.

or withdrawal can occur at unlikely times. By understanding that these responses are self-protecting, the nurses can intervene to gain control using the recommendations in Exhibit 9.3 instead of escalating the situation further.

EXHIBIT 9.3
Measures to Regain Control in a Traumatized Inmate Situation

- Use a steady, slow, and modulated voice tone when giving instruction.
- Refocus the inmate on the present. Make statements about where they are.
- Confirm that the inmate is safe right now and should not fear harm.
- Ask simple questions about the present to refocus thoughts on the here and now.

Source: Adapted from S. S. Covington, personal communication, March 11, 2011.

COMMON MEDICAL CONDITIONS OF THE FEMALE INMATE

Women have many medical conditions that require care and treatment during incarceration. They have disproportionately high rates of medical and mental illness, which are discussed in other chapters. They also have health care needs specific to gender such as reproductive cancers, sexually transmitted infections, and pregnancy management.

Reproductive Cancers

From a public health perspective, incarceration is an opportunity to screen for high-risk conditions and provide patient education toward improving a women's health. Accreditation standards affirm that, depending on age and presentation, breast and pelvic exams, Pap smear, mammogram, and sexual history should be a part of intake

EXHIBIT 9.4
Standard Breast Cancer Screening Components

- Annual Mammogram starting at age 40 and continuing for as long as a woman is in good health.
- Clinical breast exam about every 3 years for women in their 20s and 30s and annually for women 40 and over.
- Breast self-exam is an option for women starting in their 20s. Women should know how their breasts normally look and feel. Instruct to report any breast change promptly.

Source: Adapted from American Cancer Society, 2010.

examination (NCCHC, 2005). Reproductive cancers are often silent killers that, without screening, only emerge after progressing to later stages.

Breast

Breast cancer is a leading killer of women and incarceration is an opportunity to screen for breast cancers and teach breast health skills. The rates of breast cancer and breast cancer deaths among young African American women are higher than those of White women (American Cancer Society, 2011). Correctional nurses have a great opportunity to affect general breast health of this vulnerable population by promoting breast cancer screening and providing education on the importance of screening and the benefits of early detection and treatment. Recommendations for initial and annual breast cancer screening are listed in Exhibit 9.4. The Centers for Disease Control provides excellent patient education resources (CDC, 2010a).

Cervical

Both African American and Hispanic minorities have greater incidence of cervical cancer than in the non-Hispanic White population (American Cancer Society, 2009, 2011). With greater proportions of both minorities among the incarcerated, increased attention to cervical cancer screening is warranted. Initial and periodic screening using accepted community standards is recommended (Exhibit 9.5).

Patients often refuse a pelvic exam because it is invasive. Patients with a history of emotional and physical abuse may be especially traumatized and vulnerable during the procedure. When nurses make the efforts to improve the patient's comfort and privacy (comfortable room temperature, draping, and limiting personnel in the area) refusal rates decrease. The Centers for Disease Control also provides excellent patient education resources regarding pelvic exams (CDC, 2010b).

Ovarian

Although characteristics of the female inmate population do not indicate an increased risk for ovarian cancer, the condition bears mention as a female-specific concern. In fact, ovarian cancer is of great concern to the health care providers and women in the general community due to a current lack of adequate screening mechanisms (CDC, 2010c). While the leading cause of death among gynecologic cancers, ovarian cancer eludes early detection. Fully 80% of ovarian cancers are diagnosed

EXHIBIT 9.5
Standard Cervical Cancer Screening Components

- Annual screening starting at 21 years or 3 years after beginning vaginal intercourse. Screening should be done every year with the regular Pap test or every 2 years using the newer liquid-based Pap test.
- Beginning at age 30, women who have had three normal Pap test results in a row may get screened every 2–3 years. Women older than 30 may also get screened every 3 years with either the conventional or liquid-based Pap test, plus the human papilloma virus test.
- Women 70 years of age or older who have had three or more normal Pap tests in a row and no abnormal Pap test results in the last 10 years may choose to stop having Pap tests.
- Women who have had a total hysterectomy (removal of the uterus and cervix) may also choose to stop having Pap tests, unless the surgery was done as a treatment for cervical cancer or pre-cancer.
- Women who have had a hysterectomy without removal of the cervix should continue to have Pap tests.

Source: Adapted from American Cancer Society (2010).

only after dissemination to other body organs (Ovarian Cancer Research Fund, n.d.). A consensus statement among leading gynecologic cancer entities suggest four early warning signs of ovarian cancers: bloating, pelvic or abdominal pain, difficulty eating or feeling full quickly, and the sudden urge to urinate or frequent urination (National Cancer Institute, 2007). Women identifying these conditions should be referred to a physician for a medical work-up for ovarian cancer.

Sexually Transmitted Infections

The majority of women were sexually active at the time of incarceration. A study of women in one large jail found 38% reported having more than two sexual partners in the last 90 days (Clarke et al., 2006a). Although almost 90% reported using condoms, most (66.7%) admitted inconsistency with birth control in general. These findings, along with the general lack of health care and high levels of substance use, indicate great need for screening and treatment of sexually transmitted infections (STIs). STI screening should consider the three primary infections—chlamydia, gonorrhea, and syphilis.

Early Detection and Treatment

Detection and treatment of STI is of primary importance during intake because it reduces transmission of infection in the community. Women are at high risk and have higher rates of chlamydia or gonorrhea than men (Table 9.1). One study of large jails found those with high rates of screening and treatment were motivated by state regulation and assisted by local public health services (CDC, 2011a). Early screening and treatment will prevent more complex disease since both chlamydia and gonorrhea infections are often asymptomatic until the woman presents with complications such as pelvic inflammatory disease (CDC, 2010d). In addition, stigmatization about these infections decreases understanding and perpetuates myths

TABLE 9.1   Rates of Sexually Transmitted Infections Among the Incarcerated by Gender

SEXUALLY TRANSMITTED INFECTIONS	FEMALE (%)	MALE (%)
Chlamydia	7.2	6.6
Gonorrhea	1.6	1.2
Syphilis	5	7

Source: Adapted from CDC (2009).

so that women are often ill-informed about STI detection and treatment (Friedman & Bloodgood, 2010). The correctional setting is an opportunity for the nurse to provide patient teaching about prevention and treatment.

Pelvic Inflammatory Disease (PID)

Pelvic inflammation can lead to chronic pelvic pain, ectopic pregnancies, and infertility (Friedman & Bloodgood, 2010). It is a common outcome of untreated STI in women, particularly chlamydia and gonorrhea. Pelvic inflammation should be considered whenever a patient presents with fever, nausea, vomiting, and severe pelvic and abdominal pain (Table 9.2).

Pregnancy Management

The majority (80%) of incarcerated women are of reproductive age and so pregnancy identification and management are fundamental components of the health care program (Richardson, 2006). Women entering the corrections environment should be routinely screened for pregnancy so that pregnancy status can be considered in all health decisions. Pregnancy should also be considered whenever women leave the facility, such as weekend leave, returning for a parole violation, or following conjugal visitation. Pregnancy testing should be offered on a regular basis.

Ectopic Pregnancy

Ectopic pregnancy occurs when a fertilized ovum implants somewhere outside the uterus and with fetal growth, rupture and hemorrhage can result (Ricci, 2009).

TABLE 9.2   Criteria to Establish the Diagnosis of PID

MINIMUM CRITERIA	ADDITIONAL SUPPORTIVE CRITERIA
• Presence of at least one of the following: Lower abdominal tenderness, adnexal tenderness (pain from the ovary and fallopian tube), cervical motion tenderness • STD risk profile • Signs of lower-genital-tract inflammation (predominance of leukocytes in vaginal secretions, cervical exudates, or cervical friability)	• Oral temperature >101° F (>38.3°C) • Abnormal cervical or vaginal mucopurulent discharge • Presence of abundant numbers of WBC on saline microscopy of vaginal fluid • Elevated erythrocyte sedimentation rate • Elevated C-reactive protein • Laboratory documentation of cervical infection with *N. gonorrhoeae* or *C. trachomatis.*

Source: From CDC (2010d), used with permission.

EXHIBIT 9.6
Common Causes of Acute Pelvic Pain*

- Appendicitis
- Ectopic pregnancy
- Endometriosis
- Ovarian cyst or torsion
- Pelvic inflammatory disease

*Alphabetic Order—Adapted from Kruszka and Kruszka (2010).

Women who smoke or with a history of genital infections or infertility are at increased risk of ectopic pregnancy (Lozeau & Potter, 2005).

Ectopic pregnancy should be suspected any time a woman of reproductive years experiences significant pelvic pain, which may be accompanied by vaginal bleeding (see Exhibit 9.6). If pregnancy status is unknown, the nurse should obtain a urine pregnancy test while making contact with a physician for an immediate medical evaluation. If a tubal rupture takes place, the pain will intensify and signs of shock such as low blood pressure and a rapid, thready pulse will be evident. Intra-peritoneal hemorrhage can cause referred pain to the shoulder area and a very tender abdomen. Emergency response protocols including establishment of intravenous access and fluid loading should be initiated with immediate transport to acute care. Case Example 9.1 applies information from this section.

CASE EXAMPLE 9.1

A 21-year-old female inmate is detained in an urban jail on charges of driving under the influence. At the intake medical assessment she is estimated to be 2 months pregnant. After 12 hours she complains of intensifying abdominal pain and is evaluated by the nurse 3 times over the next 14 hours. During the last visit the nurse notes the patient's pain is subsiding. One hour later the woman is found unconscious and is transported to the emergency room. What would have been the appropriate assessment and nursing actions in this situation?

High-Risk Pregnancy

High rates of STIs, drug and alcohol dependence, lack of prenatal care, and inadequate nutrition have caused many correctional health care programs to treat every pregnant woman as high risk (Richardson, 2006). Even with these considerable risk factors, each patient should be evaluated individually to determine her specific risk (NCCHC, 2005).

General Nursing Interventions

Improving maternal health and increasing the patient's knowledge and understanding of pregnancy needs are major goals during the prenatal period. Since the majority of women enter the correctional system without prenatal care, the initiation of routine prenatal visits is of primary importance (Exhibit 9.7). Small facilities may have a

EXHIBIT 9.7
Routine Prenatal Visit Schedule

- Every month to 28 weeks
- Biweekly during 28–30 weeks
- After 30 weeks: weekly until delivery

Source: Adapted from Richardson (2006).

relationship with a local obstetric provider and some larger women's prisons may have an obstetrician make onsite appointments. The facility and health care program should have procedures, equipment, and supplies to handle precipitous onset of labor.

General nursing care at each prenatal visit should include weight, blood pressure, and urine testing for protein, glucose, ketones, and nitrates. In addition, fundal height should be measured, fetal movement determined, if appropriate, and fetal heart rate measured and documented (Ricci, 2009). A program of patient education should be initiated to prepare the mother for childbirth and recognition of emergency conditions requiring attention.

Pregnancy care requires the engaged cooperation of security staff to ensure appropriate housing, transportation, and security (Richardson, 2006). Of note is the concern for injury or impeded labor and delivery through the use of custody restraint with pregnant inmates. The National Commission on Correctional Health Care (NCCHC) adopted a position statement that discourages use of restraints, especially in the third trimester (NCCHC, 2010). In addition, the American Corrections Association (ACA) adopted a similar accreditation standard in 2008 (ACA, 2010).

Substance Withdrawal During Pregnancy

Abrupt alcohol withdrawal is difficult to manage in the general inmate population and the addition of an unborn child complicates the process. Delirium tremens is an obstetric emergency and hospitalization is necessary if alcohol withdrawal could result in miscarriage (FBOP, 2009; Richardson, 2006). Frequent nursing assessment, vital signs, and fetal heart tones should be taken and documented while awaiting medical evaluation and transport.

From the Experts . . .

"Care of the pregnant inmate can often be complex due to the lack of prenatal care prior to incarceration. High-risk factors that can include drug abuse, alcohol abuse, and poor nutrition maximize the need to closely monitor the health status of these women and their unborn child. Besides regularly scheduled obstetric care, we also consider increased caloric intake, vitamin supplements, an extra mattress, and supportive footwear."

Maria C. Biuso, RN, BSN
Rochester, NY

One study indicated almost 90% of pregnant women entering a Midwest correctional facility reported drug dependence, the majority indicating multiple substances (Eliason & Arndt, 2004). Withdrawal is a concern when admitting any pregnant inmate and a thorough drug history with specific attention to amount, frequency, and last use needs to be obtained so that medical monitoring and treatment can be determined.

Heroin and other opioid analgesics, such as hydromorphone and oxycodone, are of greatest concern. Pregnant inmates should generally not be detoxified or should be moved to methadone maintenance. Detoxification increases the risk of miscarriage and premature labor (FBOP, 2009). Health care programs should have a relationship with an obstetric provider who can manage addiction.

Barbiturate and benzodiazepine withdrawal is less problematic but still a concern in pregnancy. If significant use is noted on history, monitor the withdrawing inmate closely and transport to a higher level of care with any indication of distress. Monitor fetal heart tones regularly.

Cocaine use has a major effect on the fetus and withdrawal must be managed carefully. Cocaine use in pregnancy has been associated with spontaneous abortion in early pregnancy and placental abruption and fetal demise in late pregnancy (Keegan, Parva, Finnegan, Gerson, & Belden, 2010). Cocaine withdrawal in the pregnant inmate should be managed in the inpatient setting.

Perinatal Loss

Pregnancy loss, whether unintentional or through pregnancy termination, can be emotionally and physically devastating. The grief of this loss is intensified by the incarcerated status of the mother and the lack of support systems. Correctional nurses can help grieving mothers cope with the overwhelming emotions brought on by this loss by referral for counseling and mental health services (Ricci, 2009). A grieving mother may lash out in anger at the correctional staff for the loss. Dispelling misconceptions about the causes of the perinatal loss and providing honest answers to the patient's questions can help resolve emotions and assist in resolution for the mother (Richardson, 2006).

REPRODUCTIVE HEALTH NEEDS

Taking a sexual history on intake is of particular importance for determining reproductive health needs. Although the majority of incarcerated women are heterosexual, some women are bisexual or lesbian, including women with children. Assumptions should not be made about the sexual preferences of a patient.

Contraception

A study of reproductive health in a large jail system found only 28% of women reporting consistent birth control at intake (Clarke et al., 2006b). Incarceration is an ideal opportunity for nurses to provide patient education about effective contraception. Women inmates hold many misconceptions about reproduction. Nurses can ask about current contraceptive practices during intake screening and provide counseling during the initial physical assessment. Nurses can also discuss and prepare women to use contraception during the prison discharge process. Women were more likely to start using birth control if it was offered in the correctional facility rather than through community health services after release (Clarke et al., 2006a).

Start discharge planning for contraception early by identifying options and assisting the patient in choosing the most appropriate method. Referrals to local public health departments or community-based organizations such as Planned Parenthood (2011) are also important.

Menopause and Osteoporosis

As the inmate population ages, there has been greater attention to menopause and its impact on women's health. The dramatic decline in estrogen experienced midlife affects almost every body system (Ricci, 2009). Menopausal women are at increased risk of cardiovascular disease, potential skin breakdown, and decreased bone density.

Long-term hormone replacement therapy is no longer the treatment of choice for menopausal conditions and so symptom management is accomplished through lifestyle adjustment and supplementation (Richardson, 2006). For example, dry eyes can be relieved by saline drops; lotion or creams for dry, fragile skin can be obtained from the commissary; and sleep hygiene principles can be applied for bouts of insomnia. Nurses can discuss with patients strategies to deal with body temperature fluctuation and support efforts to increase the clothing options so menopausal patients can layer clothing for increased comfort.

Osteoporosis is of great concern for aging women, especially those with years of poor nutrition, little exercise, and cigarette smoking. Bone loss accelerates after menopause with the greatest loss in the first 10–15 years without estrogen (Richardson, 2006). Other risk factors include history of steroid treatment, hyperthyroidism, anorexia, or bulimia. Nurses can educate older female patients to maximize calcium and Vitamin D intake, regularly engage in weight-bearing exercises such as walking, and protect against falls (Ricci, 2009). Healthy diet and exercise is often a challenge in the correctional setting. Nurses can also explore options with the patient for weight-bearing exercise and review high-calcium food options from the inmate cafeteria. Patients may be on vitamin supplements; if so, check the current medication profile for potential drug interactions (NIH, 2011a, b). Calcium can potentially interact with several significant medications and should be time-separated on the pill-pass schedule (NIH, 2011a).

MENTAL HEALTH CONDITIONS OF INCARCERATED WOMEN

Incarcerated women have significantly more mental health disease than their male counterparts. For example, women inmates have higher rates of depression, bipolar disorder, and post-traumatic stress which are discussed in Chapter 12, Mental Health (Binswanger et al., 2010). There are also some mental health conditions that are more specific to the female population, which are discussed here.

Psychogenic Seizures

Seizure activity is a common concern in the inmate population. Psychogenic nonepileptic seizures (PNES) are a particular type of seizure prevalent in greater degree in the female population (Famiglio, 2010). Psychogenic seizures do not have a physiologic cause but are a physiologic manifestation of psychologic distress (Alsaadi & Vinter, 2005).

PNES activity is involuntary and should not be confused with malingering. This condition is predominately experienced by women, not men, and peaks in the third decade of life (Famiglio, 2010). PNES is a coping mechanism for severe and deep-rooted stress and is related to post-traumatic stress disorder (PTSD), anxiety and depressive disorders, and personality pathology (Alsaadi & Vinter, 2005). History of significant physical and sexual abuse is at the core of 50%–60% of PNES cases.

PNES is often misdiagnosed as epilepsy and mistreated with ever stronger anti-epileptic medications. Correctional nurses play a major part in diagnosing this condition by observing and documenting the nature, timing, and context of seizure activity. As with other seizure activity, patient safety is of primary importance (Alsaadi & Vinter, 2005). Conventional treatment involves addressing the underlying psychologic causes such as depression, anxiety, and PTSD therapy, although there is little research to establish best practices or clinical guidelines (Alsaadi & Vinter, 2005). Case Example 9.2 applies information from this section.

CASE EXAMPLE 9.2

A 30-year-old female inmate with history of child sexual abuse is transferred to a medium security state facility. She has been taking Dilantin for seizure disorder for the last 10 years. The prison is 150 miles from her family and support system and she shows signs of increased anxiety and erratic behavior. The nurse is called to her dorm room and witnesses a seizure in progress. The patient is rocking back and forth while moving her legs in a bicycle motion. She is unresponsive to voice command or touch. She does not lose bowel or bladder control and does not injure herself. Which elements of this case suggest psychogenic seizure activity?

Deliberate Self-Harm

Self-harm is another mental health condition of greater concern when caring for women prisoners. Although the size of this segment of the population is unclear, a small study (Gorsuch, 1998) found 54% of incarcerated women engaged in deliberate self-harm (DSH) and a more recent study found 30% participated in the behavior (Chapman & Dixon-Gordon, 2007). DSH is distinguished from suicide attempt in that the individual most often engages in self-harm activity as an active coping mechanism rather than an attempt to die. However, some overlap exists between DSH and suicide, so the intent is not always clear (Mangnall & Yurkovich, 2008).

The majority of self-injury behavior is cutting or scratching with an object. Other injuries are head banging, opening old wounds, inserting objects into the body, burning, pulling hair, and bone breaking (Kaminski, Smith, & DeHart, 2009). Women found performing any of these activities should be referred to mental health, evaluated for DSH, and started in a treatment program.

Physical, emotional, and sexual child abuse, psychiatric co-morbidity, and drug abuse are risk factors for DSH among women inmates (Mangnall & Yurkovich, 2010). Situational conditions such as poor adaption to incarceration have also been suggested as risk factors (Thomas, Leaf, Kazmierczak, & Stone, 2006).

Correctional nurses can assist self-harming patients by showing understanding and "hearing" the patient's expression of and efforts to cope with distress. Avoid labeling self-harm as manipulative, focus on developing a therapeutic relationship

EXHIBIT 9.8
SCOFF Eating Disorder Questionnaire

S Do you make yourself SICK (vomit) because you feel uncomfortably full?
C Do you worry that you have lost CONTROL over how much you eat?
O Have you recently lost more than ONE stone (15 pounds) in a 3-month period?
F Do you believe yourself to be FAT when others say you are thin?
F Would you say that FOOD dominates your life?

Source: Hill et al. (2010), used with permission.

with the patient, and assist her to use alternative methods to relieve psychologic stress (Mangnall & Yurkovich, 2008).

Postpartum Depression

Postpartum depression (PPD) should be considered for all female inmates after delivery. Factors associated with PPD include prior depression or anxiety, recent life stresses, and poor social support (Stewart, Robertson, Dennis, Grace, & Wallington, 2003). These are prevalent in the women's prison population and are cause for greater concern.

PPD occurs most frequently within the first 4 weeks after birth but can occur up to a year later (Mayo Clinic, 2010). Women who have recently delivered and have significant changes in appetite, unintended weight change, insomnia, hypersomnia, or severe restlessness should be referred for evaluation.

Eating Disorders

The eating disorders anorexia nervosa (AN) and bulimia nervosa (BN) are more common among White women and stem from fear of gaining weight, desire to lose weight, and unhappiness with body size and shape (National Women's Health Information Center, 2009). One study found 25% of female inmates in a British prison to be at risk for an eating disorder (Milligan, Waller, & Andrews, 2002). This is much higher than the reported prevalence in the general population of less than 1% (Gentile, 2010).

Eating disorders may manifest in women who feel powerless and out of control as a result of incarceration. Correctional nurses can assist women with these disorders by being alert and attentive to signs and symptoms of disordered eating. The SCOFF questionnaire (Exhibit 9.8) is an effective screening tool for eating disorders (Hill, Reid, Morgan, & Lacey, 2010). These five short questions, if answered honestly, reveal a majority of eating disorders among women. Questions can be incorporated into the intake process for women or used at any point that anorexia or bulimia is suspected. Should the patient score high on the questionnaire, referral for medical and mental health evaluation is warranted.

Anorexia (AN) manifests during adolescence, although the number of cases diagnosed under age 14 is growing. These patients have an irrational fear of body fat and it is one of the most medically serious mental health conditions. Women with AN are at high risk for suicide, osteoporosis, and electrolyte imbalances. All of these conditions should be closely monitored in any patients who are diagnosed with AN. Women with BN are more common but less identifiable than those with AN. One to 1.5% of women in the general population have characteristics of this condition. Prevalence among incarcerated women is unknown. Patients with BN often maintain a normal weight with regular episodes of binge eating followed by purging or excessive exercise, fasting, and other diet restriction (Sim et al., 2010). Medical outcomes of BN are less severe as there is less significant prolonged starvation (Sim et al., 2010).

SPECIAL ISSUES WITH FEMALE INMATES

Women are often the primary care providers for children and other family members in modern western society. During incarceration, correctional nurses have an opportunity to encourage healthy living habits and improve women's knowledge and understanding as caregivers.

Health Education

Contact with nursing services, may be relatively unavailable to individuals in an underserved community setting, but is increased to those who may be incarcerated for a period of time. Therefore every health care encounter during incarceration or detention is an opportunity to improve the woman's health, as well as the health of her children and family. Low literacy is a concern and many people understand spoken much better than written words (Easton, Entwistle, & Williams, 2010). Nurses should assure that any written material is offered at a low literacy level with a lot of graphics and only to supplement verbal explanations. General health information for these patient encounters can be found at the Centers for Disease Control's Division of Nutrition, Physical Activity, and Obesity website (CDC, 2011b).

Parenting Issues

The majority of women prisoners have minor children (62% of state and 56% of federal) and more than half are the primary financial support for their children (Glaze & Maruschak, 2008). While incarcerated, mothers depend on others to care for their children, which is an additional life stress (Table 9.3). Correctional nurses may assist mothers in developing additional knowledge and skills related to healthy living and disease prevention. Suggested topics are listed in Exhibit 9.9.

Sexual Assault Vulnerability

The true extent of custodial sexual misconduct in women's prisons is unknown (U.S. Department of Justice, 2005). Although reported cases are relatively small, it is widely held that sexual abuse of women prisoners by custody staff is greatly underreported. The power-over structure and authority position of correctional staff combined with the high level of abuse history in the inmate population increase vulnerability for sexual assault.

Female inmates are also twice as likely to have been sexually coerced by another inmate (Beck, Harrison, Berzofsky, Caspar, & Krebs, 2010). Inmate-on-inmate sexual misconduct is difficult to distinguish. Inmate relationships can begin as consensual and turn coercive later (Moss, 2007). For this and other reasons, most facilities prohibit inmate–inmate sexual conduct.

TABLE 9.3   Current Caregivers of Minor Children of Women in State Prison

CAREGIVER	PERCENTAGE (%)
Father	37
Grandparent	45
Other relative	23
Other: Foster home, agency, friend	19

Source: Adapted from Glaze and Maruschak (2008).

The Prison Rape Elimination Act of 2003 makes all forms of inmate–staff contact illegal, even if voluntary by the inmate. Health care staff must understand that this law is intended for all staff members, including health care staff. Correctional nurses working in women's prisons should be especially vigilant in identification of potential for and alert to signs of sexual assault in the patient community. Nurses play an important part in helping to shape a culture of sexual safety in correctional facilities.

Development of Inmate Family Groups

The specialized needs of female prisoners along with the small numbers relative to the size of the male inmate population means there are often only one or two locations for female prisoners in a large geographic area. Women in prison, therefore, can be kept a great distance from their family and friends, making visitation difficult. The isolation created by geographic distance can be intense. Female inmates received fewer visitors than their male counterparts (Bedard, 2009). Add to this the relational nature of this gender and a great desire for belonging and group identity emerges. Pseudo-family units provide financial, psychological, and safety benefits to inmates and can be, but are not always, sexual in nature. These factors contribute toward a pseudo-family subculture in long-term women's correctional facilities (Collica, 2010).

The interaction within female family groups can impact care and communication with the nursing staff. Patients may seek the input and approval of pseudo-family members before agreeing to critical treatments or procedures. Family member input may be a factor in folk remedies tried by the patient. Correctional nursing practice is improved through an understanding of this dynamic within the women's prison system.

EXHIBIT 9.9
Healthy Living and Disease Prevention Topics for Mothers

- Basic child safety
- Nutrition and family meals
- Preventing the spread of infection
- Dangers of smoking and heavy drinking
- Encouraging physical activity
- Preventing dental caries
- Sun safety
- Basic first aid

Source: Adapted from CDC (2011c).

SUMMARY

Gender matters in the nursing care of women in jails and prisons. Nurses working in women's facilities need a thorough understanding of medical conditions prevalent in the female population. In addition, a contextual understanding of the nature of the prison culture in which patients live and their dominant past history of high levels of trauma, abuse, and victimization assist in establishing professional boundaries and therapeutic communication in the nurse-patient relationship. Correctional nurses must work within the custody community, collaborating with corrections peers while advocating for the health needs of their patients. Incarceration is an opportune time for disadvantaged and marginalized women to gain a better understanding of healthy living and disease prevention strategies with the help of patient teaching from facility nursing staff.

DISCUSSION QUESTIONS

1. Name at least three conditions more prevalent among incarcerated women than men and discuss the reasons.
2. How would you describe the difference in nursing practice with incarcerated women to a nurse working in a male prison?
3. What traumatic history is most prevalent in the female inmate population and how does this affect nursing practice?

REFERENCES

Alsaadi, T. M., & Vinter, A. (2005). Psychogenic nonepileptic seizures. *American Family Physician*, 72(5), 849–856. Retrieved from http://www.aafp.org/afp/2005/0901/p849.pdf

American Cancer Society. (2009). *Cancer facts and figures for Hispanic/Latino Americans 2009–2011*. Retrieved from http://www.cancer.org/acs/groups/content/@nho/documents/document/ffhispanicslatinos20092011.pdf

American Cancer Society. (2010). *Guidelines for the early detection of cancer*. Retrieved from http://www.cancer.org/Healthy/FindCancerEarly/CancerScreeningGuidelines/american-cancer-society-guidelines-for-the-early-detection-of-cancer

American Cancer Society. (2011). *Cancer facts and figures for African Americans 2011–2012*. Retrieved from http://www.cancer.org/acs/groups/content/@epidemiologysurveilance/documents/document/acspc-027765.pdf

American Corrections Association. (2010). *2010 standards supplement*. Alexandria, VA: Author.

Beck, A. K., Harrison, P. M., Berzofsky, M., Caspar, R., & Krebs, C. (2010). *Sexual victimization in prisons and jails reported by inmates, 2008–09*. NCJ 231169 http://bjs.ojp.usdoj.gov/content/pub/pdf/svpjri0809.pdf

Bedard, L. (2009). The pseudo-family phenomenon in women's prisons. Women in corrections. Correctionsone. Retrieved from http://www.correctionsone.com/jail-management/articles/1956587-The-pseudo-family-phenomenon-in-womens-prisons/

Belknap, J. (2006). *The invisible woman: Gender, crime, and justice*. Belmont, CA: Wadsworth/Thompson Learning.

Binswanger, I. A., Merrill, J. O., Krueger, P. M., White, M. C., Booth, R. E., & Elmore, J. G. (2010). Gender differences in chronic medical, psychiatric, and substance-dependence disorders among jail inmates. *American Journal of Public Health*, 100(3), 476–482.

Bloom, B., Owen, B., & Covington, S. (2005). *Gender-responsive strategies: A summary of research, practice, and guiding principles for women offenders*. National Institute of Corrections. Retrieved from http://www.idoc.idaho.gov/sites/default/files/webfm/documents/education_and_treatment/program_services/Gender%20responsivity.pdf

CDC. (2009). *Centers for disease control: STDs in persons entering corrections facilities.* Retrieved from http://www.cdc.gov/std/stats09/corrections.htm

CDC. (2010a). *Centers for disease control: Breast cancer and you–what you need to know.* Retrieved from http://www.cdc.gov/cancer/breast/pdf/BreastCancerFS_Dec2010.pdf

CDC. (2010b). *Centers for disease control: Cervical cancer.* Retrieved from http://www.cdc.gov/cancer/cervical/pdf/Cervical_FS_0510.pdf

CDC. (2010c). *Centers for disease control: Cervical ovarian cancer.* Retrieved from http://www.cdc.gov/Features/dsOvarianCancer/

CDC. (2010d). *Centers for disease control: Sexually transmitted diseases treatment guidelines.* Retrieved from http://www.cdc.gov/std/treatment/2010/pid.htm

CDC. (2011a). *Centers for disease control: Evaluation of large jail STD screening programs, 2008–2009.* Retrieved from http://www.cdc.gov/std/publications/JailScreening2011.pdf

CDC. (2011b). *Centers for disease control: Division of nutrition, physical activity, and obesity.* Retrieved from http://www.cdc.gov/nccdphp/dnpao/index.html

CDC. (2011c). *Centers for disease control: Family health.* Retrieved June 22, 2011, at http://www.cdc.gov/family/index.htm

Chapman, A., & Dixon-Gordon, K. (2007). Emotional antecedents and consequences of deliberate self-harm and suicide attempts. *Suicide and Life-Threatening Behavior, 37*(5), 543–552.

Clarke, J. E., Herbert, M. R., Rosengard, C., Rose, J. S., DaSilva, K. M., & Stein, M. D. (2006a). Reproductive health care and family planning needs among incarcerated women. *American Journal of Public Health, 96*(5), 834–839.

Clarke, J. G., Rosengard, C., Rose, J. S., Hebert, M. R., Peipert, J., & Stein, M. D. (2006b). Improving birth control service utilization by offering services prerelease vs postincarceration. *American Journal of Public Health, 96*(5), 840–845.

Collica, K. (2010). Surviving incarceration: Two prison-based peer programs build communities of support for female offenders. *Deviant Behavior, 31*(4), 314–347.

Easton, P., Entwistle, V. A., & Williams, B. (2010). Health in the "hidden population" of people with low literacy. A systematic review of the literature. *BMC Public Health, 10,* 459. Retrieved from http://www.ncbi.nlm.nih.gov/pmc/articles/PMC2923110/pdf/1471-2458-10-459.pdf

Eliason, M. J., & Arndt, S. (2004). Pregnant inmates: A growing concern. *Journal of Addicitons Nursing, 15,* 163–170.

Famiglio, G. (2010). Psychogenic nonepileptic seizure activity in corrections. *CorrDocs: The Newsletter of the Society of Correctional Physicians, 13*(2). Retrieved from http://www.corrdocs.org/framework.php?pagetype=newsstory&newsid=12185&bgn=1

FBOP. (2009). *Detoxification of chemically dependent inmates federal bureau of prisons clinical practice guidelines.* Retrieved from http://www.bop.gov/news/PDFs/detoxification.pdf

FBOP. (n.d.). *Federal bureau of prisons: Institutions housing female offenders.* Retrieved from http://www.bop.gov/locations/female_facilities.jsp

Friedman, A. L., & Bloodgood, B. (2010). "Something we'd rather not talk about": Findings from CDC exploratory research on sexually transmitted disease communication with girls and women. *Journal of Women's Health, 19*(10), 1823–1831. DOI: 10.1089/jwh.2010.1961

Frost, N., Greene, K., & Paranis, K. (2006). *Hard hit: The growth in the imprisonment of women, 1977–2006.* Women's Prison Association. Retrieved from http://www.wpaonline.org/pdf/HARD%20HIT%20Full%20Report.pdf

Gentile, M. G. (2010). Anorexia nervosa: Identification, main characteristics and treatment. *Nutritional therapy & Metabolism, 28*(4), 185–192.

Glaze, L. E. (2010). *Bureau of justice statistics: Correctional populations in the United States, 2009.* NCJ 231681. Retrieved from http://bjs.ojp.usdoj.gov/content/pub/pdf/cpus09.pdf

Glaze, L. E., & Maruschak, L. M. (2008). *Bureau of justice statistics special report: Parents in prison and their minor children.* Retrieved from http://bjs.ojp.usdoj.gov/content/pub/pdf/pptmc.pdf

Gorsuch, N. (1998). Unmet needs among disturbed female offenders. *The Journal of Forensic Psychiatry, 9*(3), 556–570.

Hill, L. S., Reid, F., Morgan, J. F., & Lacey, J. H. (2010). SCOFF, the development of an eating disorder screening questionnaire. *International Journal of Eating Disorders, 43*(4), 344–351.

Kaminski, R. J., Smith, H. P., & DeHart, D. D. (2009). *National survey of self-injurious behaviors in prison, 2008.* Department of Criminology and Criminal Justice, University of South Carolina. Retrieved from http://www.cas.sc.edu/crju/research/self_injurious_behavior_final2008.pdf

Keegan, J., Parva, M., Finnegan, M., Gerson, A., & Belden, M. (2010). Addiction in pregnancy. *Journal of Addictive Diseases, 29*, 175–191.

Kelly, P. J., Parlaz-Dieckmann, E., Chang, A. L., & Collins, C. (2010). Profile of women in a county jail. *Journal of Psychosocial Nursing, 48*(4), 38–45.

Kruszka, P. S., & Kruszka, S. J. (2010). Evaluation of acute pelvic pain in women. *American Family Physician, 82*(2), 141–147. Retrieved from http://xa.yimg.com/kq/groups/17358357/514409291/name/Acute%20Pelvic%20Pain%20in%20Women.pdf

Lozeau, A. M., & Potter, B. (2005). Diagnosis and management of ectopic pregnancy. *American Family Physician, 72*(9), 1707–1714. Retrieved from http://www.aafp.org/afp/2005/1101/p1707.pdf

McCampbell, S. W. (2005). *Gender responsive strategies for women offenders.* Retrieved from http://www.urban.org/reentryroundtable/mccampbell_paper.pdf

Mangnall, J., & Yurkovich, E. (2008). A literature review of deliberate self-harm. *Perspectives in Psychiatric Care, 44*(30), 175–184.

Mangnall, J., & Yurkovich, E. (2010). A grounded theory exploration of deliberate self-harm in incarcerated women. *Journal of Forensic Nursing, 6*, 88–95.

Mayo Clinic. (2010). *Postpartum depression: Tests and diagnosis.* Retrieved from http://www.mayoclinic.com/health/postpartum-depression/DS00546/DSECTION=tests-and-diagnosis

Milligan, R. J., Waller, G., & Andrews, B. (2002). Eating disturbances in female prisoners: The role of anger. *Eating Behaviors, 3*(2), 123–132.

Moss, A. (2007). *The prison rape elimination act: Implications for women and girls.* Retrieved from http://www.aca.org/publications/pdf/Moss_Aug07.pdf

National Cancer Institute. (2007). Groups say common symptoms may indicate ovarian cancer. *NCI Cancer Bulletin, 4*(20). Retrieved from http://www.cancer.gov/aboutnci/ncicancerbulletin/archive/2007/062607/page4

National Women's Health Information Center. (2009). *Eating disorders.* Retrieved from http://womenshealth.gov/bodyimage/eatingdisorders/

National Commission on Correctional Health Care (NCCHC). (2005). *Position statement: Women's health care in correctional settings. National commission on correctional health care.* Retrieved from http://ncchc.org/resources/statements/womenshealth2005.html

National Commission on Correctional Health Care. (2010). *Position statements: Restraint of pregnant inmates.* Retrieved August 18, 2011, from National Commission on Correctional Health Care: http://www.ncchc.org/resources/statements/restraint_pregnant_inmates.html

NIH. (2011a). *National Institutes of Health: Daily supplement fact sheet-calcium.* Retrieved from http://ods.od.nih.gov/factsheets/calcium/

NIH. (2011b). *National Institutes of Health: Daily supplement fact sheet-vitamin D.* Retrieved from http://ods.od.nih.gov/factsheets/vitamind/

Ovarian Cancer Research Fund. (n.d.). *About ovarian cancer.* Retrieved November 21, 2011, from http://www.ocrf.org/indexphp?option=com_content&view=category&layout=blog&id=36&Itemid=293&gclid=CKKPjp7AyqwCFQ1x5QodszUEpw

Planned Parenthood. (2011). *What to do if you forget to take the pill.* Retrieved from http://www.plannedparenthood.org/health-topics/birth-control/if-forget-take-pill-19269.htm

Ricci, S. S. (2009). *Essentials of maternity, newborn, & women's health nursing.* Philadelphia: Wolters Kluwer/Lippincott Williams & Wilkins.

Richardson, S. (2006). Women's health care in the incarcerated setting. In M. Puisus (Ed.), *Clinical practice in correctional medicine* (2nd ed.). Philadelphia: Mosby Elsevier.

Sim, L. A., McAlpine, D. E., Grothe, K. B., Himes, S. M., Cockerill, R. G., & Clark, M. M. (2010). Identification and treatment of eating disorders in the primary care setting. *Mayo Clinic Proceedings, 85*(8), 746–751.

Stewart, D. E., Robertson, E., Dennis, C. L., Grace, S. K., & Wallington, T. (2003). *Postpartum depression: Literature review of risk factors and interventions.* University Health Network Women's Health Program. Retrieved from http://www.who.int/mental_health/prevention/suicide/lit_review_postpartum_depression.pdf

Thomas, J., Leaf, M., Kazmierczak, S., & Stone, J. (2006). Self-injury in correctional settings: "Pathology" of prisons or of prisoners? *Criminology and Public Policy, 5*(1), 193–202.

U.S. Department of Justice. (2005). *Deterring staff sexual abuse of federal inmates.* Retrieved from http://www.justice.gov/oig/special/0504/final.pdf

TEN

Infectious Diseases

Sue Smith

Nurses have a key role in the identification, treatment, and control of the transmission of infection within the correctional setting. Correctional facilities have been termed "reservoirs" and even "breeding grounds" for communicable and infectious diseases (Hammett, Harmon, & Rhodes, 2002; Restrum, 2005). A study conducted in 1995 estimated that 12%–35% of the burden of key infections were found in incarcerated populations (Hammett et al., 2002). The prevalence of infectious disease among the incarcerated has great impact on the safety and security of correctional facilities and on the public health. Nursing interventions that prevent communicable disease include screening, patient education and counseling, immunization, monitoring treatment compliance, and symptom management.

INFECTION CONTROL BASICS

An important concept to understand in managing communicable disease is the *chain of infection*; a series of events that includes:

- The organism—the bacteria, virus, or parasite that causes the infection,
- The reservoir—the continual source of the organism; where it is found between outbreaks,
- Portal of exit—how the organism leaves the reservoir (i.e., feces, blood, mucus, etc.),
- Transmission—how the organism gets from one host to another,
- Portal of entry—how the organism enters a vulnerable host,
- Vulnerable host—persons who are most vulnerable to the organism (Zeigler, 2010).

TABLE 10.1 Transmission of Communicable Disease

TYPE OF TRANSMISSION	DESCRIPTION
Airborne	Very small droplets that are aerosolized when sneezing or coughing and then inhaled by another through the respiratory system or absorbed through mucus membrane.
Droplet	Larger droplets created when talking, coughing, or sneezing and then inhaled or absorbed. May also be transmitted during procedures such as suctioning.
Bloodborne	Infected blood or blood-containing body fluid is introduced into the blood of another person; typical ways in which this occurs are needlesticks, splashes to mucous membranes, and blood contacting open areas of the skin.
Vector-borne	An organism is transmitted through another source like ticks, fleas, or mosquitoes.
Sexual transmission	Sexual contact with an infected person.
Casual or household contact	Close body-to-body contact; contact with linens or other items in the environment.

Source: Bick (2006a) and Kennamer (2007).

All links of the chain of infection must be present for the infection to be transmitted; if any part is missing, the infection cannot be transmitted. Infection control procedures are based on the concept that if any part of the chain of infection can be removed, transmission of the infection can be controlled. Transmission of communicable disease takes place in several ways; these are listed in Table 10.1.

ESSENTIAL ELEMENTS OF INFECTION CONTROL
Prevention and Control Procedures

Handwashing, or hand hygiene, is arguably the best overall workplace practice for preventing spread of infection. The use of plain soap and water will facilitate removal of soil from hands; use of antibacterial soaps has the additional benefit of killing bacteria (Bick, 2006a). Hand hygiene needs to be performed:

- Before and after patient contact,
- After contact with blood, body fluids, or potentially contaminated surfaces,
- Before and after invasive procedures,
- After removing gloves (wearing gloves is *not* enough to prevent transmission of pathogens in health care settings), and
- Whenever there is the potential of pathogen transmission—when in doubt, wash your hands (CDC, 2011a; Kennamer, 2007).

When handwashing with soap and water is not possible or is inconvenient, alcohol-based hand sanitizers are effective substitutes as long as they contain 60%–95% alcohol (Bick, 2006a).

Biohazard containers, or sharps containers, are closable, puncture-resistant containers that are leak proof and color coded (red), used for the disposal of contaminated needles and other disposable sharps.

Medical devices, such as injection needles and intravenous needle sets, are manufactured with protective sheaths or allow push-button retraction of the needle following use to prevent needle stick injury (Kennamer, 2007).

Personal Protective Equipment (PPE) consists of clothing and equipment made to protect its wearers from contaminated air, body fluids, or blood and consists of: respirators, gloves, eye goggles, face shields, gowns, and foot coverings. PPE needs to be maintained in appropriate sizes and quantities, be easily accessible, and available to employees at no charge (Bick, 2005; OSHA, 2007).

Engineering Controls place a barrier between the worker and the hazard or will completely remove the hazard (OSHA, 2007). An example of an engineering control is air cleaning or filtration systems to dilute and remove contaminated air, control the direction of the airflow, and control airflow patterns within a room such as an airborne infection isolation (AII) or negative pressure room.

Correctional Standard Precautions and Isolation Procedures

Standard precautions incorporate the use of PPE, components of universal precautions, and body substance isolation; they are used with all patients and apply to nonintact skin, mucous membranes, and all body secretions except sweat (Bick, 2004, 2006a; Kennamer, 2007). The Federal Bureau of Prisons (FBOP) developed directions for standard precautions in the correctional setting, which refine standard precautions to apply more directly to correctional settings. The correctional standard precautions require correctional staff to assume that all inmates are potentially infectious and to take precautions whenever contact with blood or bodily fluids is even possible. This material is available within guidelines for managing HIV, MRSA, and in the Pandemic Influenza Plan at the FBOP website, http://www.bop.gov, by typing the words "correctional standard precautions" into the search field. Isolation procedures used to control transmission of disease when treating patients with known or suspected transmissible infections are described in Table 10.2.

Nursing Procedures

Nursing procedures involved in prevention and control of communicable diseases include medication administration, monitoring inmate adherence to the treatment plan, education, counseling to reduce risk of disease transmission, collaboration with public health organizations, and discharge planning.

Medication Administration

Many public health and correctional experts advocate strongly for the use of directly observed therapy (DOT) when administering certain treatments to inmates, particularly for tuberculosis and HIV disease (Altice & Springer, 2006; CDC, 2006; Lobato & Goldenson, 2006). It is well known that DOT increases adherence to treatment regimens and can greatly improve treatment outcomes. DOT also allows nurses to monitor adherence so that they can contact inmates who have missed doses to determine the possible reasons for the missed doses and provide education about the need of strict adherence. Disadvantages to DOT include long medication lines that may discourage inmates, increased expense because DOT requires intensive nursing time, potential loss of confidentiality if other inmates can view the medications being dispensed, and logistical obstacles presented by secure environments (Altice & Springer, 2006). Accordingly, DOT is primarily employed when the need

TABLE 10.2   Isolation Procedures

TYPE OF ISOLATION	DESCRIPTION	REQUIREMENTS
Airborne	Reduces risk of transmission of airborne organisms less than 5 μm. Examples: tuberculosis, measles, chickenpox, and disseminated shingles.	1. Isolation in an Airborne Infection Isolation (AII) room. If an AII room is not available, patients may be housed in a private room or groups of patients may be cohorted in a designated multi-bed room or ward. 2. Only those persons needed for patient care enter the isolation room wearing an N-95 respirator mask. 3. The door to the room is kept closed when not being used.
Droplet	Reduces transmission of droplets greater than 5 μm in size. Examples: seasonal flu and invasive *Neisseria meningitis*.	1. The patient is in a private room or may be cohorted with other patients with the same illness. 2. Staff wear an N-95 respirator when within 3 feet of the patient. 3. The patient wears a surgical mask when out of room.
Contact	Reduces transmission spread by direct contact with infected patients, their linens, or other items in their environment. Examples: *Clostridium difficile*, Herpes simplex virus, Hepatitis A virus, varicella zoster virus (VZV), methicillin-resistant *Staphylococcus aureus* (MRSA), scabies, and lice.	1. House patient in a private room or cohort multiple patients with the same infection in a multi-bed room. 2. Gloves and gowns worn when entering the patient(s) room and removed when leaving. 3. Hands are washed after removing gowns and gloves. 4. Whenever possible, patient care equipment is dedicated to use by the infected patient(s) only. 5. Movement of infected patients is limited.

Source: Kennamer (2007), OSHA (2007), and Bick (2006a).

for strict adherence to therapeutic regimens is most strong; for instance, for airborne illnesses like active tuberculosis disease.

Education

Training about infectious diseases for correctional staff and inmates is critical. Education specific to infectious diseases needs to include information about the infection control program, the exposure control program, correctional standard precautions, handwashing, proper use of PPE, recognition of the symptoms of infectious diseases, and the importance of reporting them and following up on treatment regimens (Schoenly, 2008). Correctional nurses are particularly well positioned to offer targeted education to correctional staff and inmates especially when interest in personal protection is heightened because of potential exposure to communicable disease (P. Voermans, personal communication, Nov. 5, 2011).

Risk Reduction Techniques

The goal of the risk reduction model of education and counseling is to reduce the harmful effects of substance abuse and any other behaviors that increase risk of infection. Some of the techniques use education and counseling to inform patients of the possibility of disease transmission, how those diseases are transmitted, and ways to avoid becoming infected or transmitting the disease. Risk reduction also advocates making condoms and clean needle exchange programs readily available to inmates (Hammett, 2006; Hogben & St. Lawrence, 2000; Johnson-Mallard et al., 2007).

Public Health Outreach

Cooperation and collaboration between correctional facilities and public health agencies is vital. Correctional facilities, public health, and community health agencies can form a collaborative triad to address gaps in knowledge and resources so that the burden of infection is decreased. (Lincoln & Miles, 2006). Public health and community health agencies have significant expertise in surveillance and contact investigation activities, educational materials, and case management capabilities that are of tremendous value to correctional facilities. Correctional facilities have a significant number of persons with various infectious diseases in one place that will eventually be returning to their communities; in this way, correctional facilities may serve as "sentinels" for monitoring the level of disease in communities (CDC, 2006; Conklin et al., 1998; Lincoln & Miles, 2006; Spaulding et al., 2006). In order to avoid duplication of services, confusion, costs, and missed opportunities, correctional facilities and public health agencies need to work together to establish clear roles and responsibilities.

(*continued*)

From the Experts ... (*continued*)

source of information on many of the infectious diseases we encounter in corrections. Forge a relationship with them, and you'll find their guidance and counsel to be invaluable time and again."

Kevin Connor, RN, BSN, CCHP
Rancho Cucamonga, CA

Inmate Discharge Planning

Effective discharge planning and post-release follow-up services require cooperation between correctional facilities and public health agencies. Discharge planning needs to begin as soon as possible after diagnosis of an infectious disease, particularly if the inmate will return to the community before the treatment regimen is completed. Correctional nurses must collaborate with other correctional case management staff to coordinate referrals and post-release follow-up care with community health agencies. There are several models of effective collaboration between correctional systems and public health, including the Hampden County Correctional Center public health model, pre-release programs supported by Ryan White funding like those developed in Ohio and many other states, AIDS Drug Assistance Programs (ADAP), and the CDC/HRSA Corrections Demonstration Project (CDC, 2006; Conklin et al., 1998; Lane, 2006; Parvez, Lobato, & Greifinger, 2010).

IDENTIFICATION, MANAGEMENT, AND PREVENTION OF COMMON COMMUNICABLE DISEASES

As it is well-established that inmates have a remarkably high prevalence of contagious diseases (Bick, 2006a; CDC, 2006; Hammett, 2006; Lane, 2006), it is important to identify those diseases that are most likely to flourish in the closed confines of correctional facilities.

Ectoparasites

Prevalence: Within the congregate setting of correctional facilities, ectoparasite cases (lice and scabies) tend to appear sporadically with episodic outbreaks. There are three types of lice—head lice (pediculus humanus capitus), body lice (pediculus humanus corporis), and pubic lice (pthiris pubis). The parasite responsible for scabies is a mite called *Sarcoptes scarpiei* (Bick, 2006a; CDC, 2010a, 2010b; FBOP, 2011a).

Transmission and susceptibility: Transmission generally requires close skin-to-skin contact; lice can live in the seams and inner surfaces of clothing, linen, and on personal care items. Susceptibility is general. Risk factors include poor hygiene and being unable to change clothing regularly. Persons with mental illnesses and immune deficiency are at risk for a severe form of scabies called crusted scabies (Bick, 2006a; CDC, 2010a, 2010b; FBOP, 2011a).

Signs and symptoms: The primary symptoms are itching at the affected area. Head lice typically infest head and facial hair, body lice typically infest the inner seams of clothing, and pubic lice typically infest pubic hair. Scabies rashes often present as linear, papular lesions that are most commonly found in the webs between fingers and toes, axillae, under female breasts, and in male pubic areas (CDC, 2010a, 2010b).

Patient treatment: Scabies usually can be successfully treated with a 5% preparation of permethrin that is applied after bathing and left on overnight. All clothing and linens used by the patient must be washed separately from other laundry. Permethrin can also be used for treatment of lice, but is often unsuccessful. Malathion has also been approved for treatment of lice. As with scabies, the antiparasitic medication of choice is applied after the person showers and washes his or her hair and all clothing and linens are washed separately from other laundry. Combs and personal care items should be washed and soaked in hot (130°) water (Bick, 2006a; CDC, 2010a, 2010b; FBOP, 2011a).

Prevention and control: Transmission is prevented by avoiding skin-to-skin contact with infested persons or sharing personal items like bedding, clothing, combs, or brushes. Persons with itching or skin rashes should be reported promptly to health care staff for evaluation. Persons with confirmed scabies or lice should be isolated with contact precautions (Bick, 2006a; CDC, 2010a, 2010b; FBOP, 2011a).

Contact investigations: Outbreaks of scabies or lice are reportable to local public health authorities. Outbreak investigations begin with confirming the diagnosis of scabies or lice by examining skin scrapings under a microscope, if possible. When the index case is confirmed, staff should develop a list of all persons with whom the patient has had direct, physical contact. Treatment should be coordinated so that all cases and contacts are treated at the same time (Bick, 2006a; CDC, 2010a, 2010b; FBOP, 2011a). Case Example 10.1 applies information from this section.

CASE EXAMPLE 10.1

The institution physician has just diagnosed scabies in a patient you saw on sick call earlier today. What actions are you going to advise the inmate and the housing officer to take?

Hepatitis A

Prevalence: Hepatitis A is caused by the Hepatitis A virus (HAV) and results in swelling and inflammation of the liver. Approximately 22%–39% of inmates show evidence of previous infection with HAV; however, incidence of new infections in correctional facilities is generally very low (FBOP, 2008).

Transmission and susceptibility: HAV is transmitted through contaminated food or water and direct contact with infected persons through the fecal–oral route. HAV can live on unwashed hands for up to 4 hours, so good handwashing is highly important to prevent spread of HAV. Susceptibility is general, but risk factors for HAV infection include men who have sex with men (MSM), persons who inject illegal drugs, persons who are on medications to treat a clotting disorder, and those who are close contacts of infected persons (FBOP, 2008; Kennamer, 2007).

Signs and symptoms: Many patients have no symptoms. When symptoms occur they are usually mild and include right upper quadrant abdominal pain, nausea, anorexia, fever, weakness, and jaundice.

Patient treatment: Treatment is generally supportive with an emphasis on managing symptoms.

Prevention and control: All persons caring for a patient with HAV need to follow standard precautions with an emphasis on good handwashing. Contact precautions, particularly with fecal material, must be taken. An inactivated Hepatitis A vaccine is available and is recommended by the CDC for all health care workers and may be used for postexposure prophylaxis (FBOP, 2008; Kennamer, 2007). Immunization for HAV is not generally recommended for inmates unless there is a significant exposure or significant risk factors (Lincoln et al., 2006).

Contact investigations: Hepatitis A reporting is required by all state health departments. Correctional facilities may consult with local or state public health authorities to identify close contacts of the source patient during the infectious period, which extends from 2 weeks before and after symptom onset. Close contacts include cellmate(s), sexual contacts, contacts sharing toilet facilities, persons sharing injection drug supplies, and persons sharing eating utensils.

Hepatitis B

Prevalence: Hepatitis B is transmitted by the Hepatitis B virus (HBV) primarily by direct contact with blood and body fluids. The incidence of HBV infection in correctional facilities ranges from 3.6% to 19% in juvenile facilities and from 13% to 47% in adult facilities and varies by region of the country. This incidence is 2–6 times greater than the general population, making the burden of infection much higher in correctional facilities (CDC, 2003a). Risk factors include unprotected sex with multiple partners, injection drug use, and occupational exposures from percutaneous and mucous membrane exposures. Potential, but less certain, risk factors include unsafe tattooing practices and bites (Bick, 2004; CDC, 2003a).

Transmission and susceptibility: Transmission is through exposure to blood and body fluids containing blood, most often through contact with contaminated needles or other sharps, sexual contact, and occupational exposures (Bick, 2004; Kennamer, 2007). Risk from percutaneous needlesticks if the blood contains Hepatitis B surface antigen and Hepatitis B antigen is 22%–31%. However, there have been reports of transmission without known percutaneous injury. HBV can survive in dried blood for up to 1 week (CDC, 2003a).

Signs and symptoms: Infected patients usually report flu-like symptoms including fever, joint pain, weakness, fatigue, anorexia, nausea, and vomiting; jaundice is often present. Symptoms are usually mild–moderate in intensity; fulminant hepatitis is rare (Bick, 2004; Kennamer, 2007).

Patient treatment: Treatment is generally supportive. Hepatitis B is self-limiting in the vast majority of patients; only 1%–2% of patients with HBV develop sustained chronic HBV infection. Recent developments in antiviral drug therapies have yielded a number of antiviral medications that may be useful in treating patients with chronic hepatitis B (FBOP, 2011b).

Prevention and control: Standard precautions are necessary, with emphasis on good handwashing. A recombinant vaccine is available and is administered as a series of three injections. The CDC recommends vaccination for all children, all health care workers, and adult inmates in correctional facilities (Bick, 2004; Buck et al., 2006; CDC, 2003a; NCCHC, 1997). The vaccine may also be used for postexposure prophylaxis.

Contact investigations: Like Hepatitis A, Hepatitis B is reportable to state public health authorities. Correctional facilities may consult with local or state public health authorities to identify close contacts of the source patient, which may include sexual contacts, persons sharing injection drug supplies, and persons who come into contact with the source patient's blood or body fluids that contain blood. All exposures to blood or bodily fluids that may contain blood need to be investigated for the potential to transmit HBV based on the type of bodily substance involved, the route, and severity of the exposure (CDC, 2003a).

Hepatitis C

Prevalence: The incidence of HCV infection in the United States is about 1.8%; however, incidence among incarcerated juveniles is estimated at 2%–3.5%, and among incarcerated adults is 16%–41%. The vast majority of inmates with evidence of HCV infection report a history of injection drug use; sexual transmission is rare, but possible. Incidence among corrections staff is estimated to be similar to that of the general population (CDC, 2003a).

Transmission and susceptibility: Hepatitis C virus is a bloodborne pathogen that is most efficiently transmitted by direct percutaneous exposure to infected blood. Risk of infection when exposed to blood infected with HCV is estimated to be 1.8% (CDC, 2003a; FBOP, 2011c).

Signs and symptoms: Most persons infected with HCV are asymptomatic; only about 20% of patients will exhibit symptoms. When symptoms are present, they typically present as flu-like symptoms including fever, joint pain, weakness, fatigue, anorexia, nausea, and vomiting; jaundice is often present as well. Chronic HCV infection occurs in 60%–70% of infected persons, but most do not develop long-term complications due to this infection. Approximately 10%–20% of persons with chronic HCV infection will develop liver cirrhosis and 1%–5% may develop hepatocellular cancer.

Patient treatment: Patients who present with symptoms of acute HCV infection are treated symptomatically, as with other forms of acute hepatitis. Patients with evidence of chronic HCV infection should receive detailed screening that consists of assessment for risk factors; a targeted history and physical examination; and lab evaluation including HIV and HBV screening, CBC with differential and platelet count, liver panel, and ferritin levels. It is recommended that patients with chronic HCV infection receive HBV immunization; HAV immunization may additionally be needed. If patients exhibit signs of progressive liver disease, additional lab evaluation that includes a liver biopsy may be needed (FBOP, 2011c). Treatment with antiviral therapy that includes Ribavirin and pegInterferon is considered based on the likelihood of disease progression and whether the treatment will be effective (FBOP, 2011c; Spaulding et al., 2006). Recent developments in the treatment of HCV include HCV specific protease inhibitors. These new medications are presently only used in combination with standard therapy and under very specific conditions, so it is advisable to work closely with a medical practitioner specializing in HCV care when considering this new treatment regimen (Fisher, 2011).

Prevention and control: Standard precautions are necessary, with emphasis on good handwashing (Kennamer, 2007). There is no vaccine available to prevent HCV infection and treatment with immunoglobin and antiviral agents is not recommended (CDC, 2003a; FBOP, 2011c).

Contact investigations: As with HAV and HBV infections, HCV infection is reportable to state public health authorities; both organizations should work together to identify possible contacts of the source patient. In the event of occupational blood exposure, every attempt should be made to identify the source patient and assess HCV serologic status (CDC, 2003a; FBOP, 2011c).

Human Immunodeficiency Virus

Prevalence: In 2008, the Bureau of Justice Statistics (BJS) reported that 21,987 inmates (1.5%) held in state or federal prisons were HIV positive or had confirmed AIDS (BJS, 2009).

Transmission and susceptibility: HIV is a bloodborne pathogen and is primarily transmitted through direct contact with infected blood and body fluids containing blood and sexual contact. Risk factors include preexisting sexually transmitted infections (STIs), intravenous drug use with shared needles, and unprotected vaginal or anal sex with multiple partners (FBOP, 2011d; Kennamer, 2007).

Signs and symptoms: HIV infection may take many years to manifest. Symptoms may vary, but many HIV-infected patients complain of fatigue, night sweats, fever, diarrhea, swollen lymph nodes, skin lesions, and unexplained weight loss. Because HIV infection weakens the immune system, opportunistic infections are common (Kennamer, 2007).

Patient treatment: Patient treatment for HIV infection and AIDS is complex and treatment guidelines change rapidly; it is recommended that HIV treatment be managed by a medical practitioner skilled and up-to-date in treatment of HIV/AIDS. Generally, it is recommended that antiretroviral treatment (ART) be initiated for patients who are diagnosed with an opportunistic infection, patients with CD4 levels of 350–500, or patients who are diagnosed with HIV neuropathy or co-infection with HBV.

Prevention and control: Use correctional standard precautions when contact with an infected patient's blood or body fluids is possible. If a blood or body fluid exposure is reported, it is important to immediately implement the facility's exposure control plan (Bick, 2006a).

Contact investigations: HIV infection is reportable to the state public health authority; both organizations should work together to identify possible contacts of the source patient. In the event of occupational blood exposure, every attempt should be made to identify the source patient and assess HIV serologic status (CDC, 2005; FBOP, 2011d).

Influenza (Flu)

Epidemiology: *Influenza* has caused outbreaks of respiratory illness for centuries, including three pandemics, or worldwide outbreaks, in the 20th century. There are three types of human influenza—types A, B, and C. Health care staff and the public are most familiar with *Seasonal flu*, which is caused by strains of influenza types A and B. *Pandemic influenza* is caused by a new influenza type A virus, against which most people have little or no immunity (OSHA, 2007).

Transmission and susceptibility: Persons infected with influenza are typically contagious for about 6 days, from 1 day before symptoms appear until about 4 days following appearance of symptoms. Transmission can be airborne via aerosolized droplet nuclei or by contact with surfaces contaminated with droplets. Susceptibility is general, although medical conditions that can lead to immune deficiency may increase risk of infection (OSHA, 2007).

Signs and symptoms: Influenza generally has an abrupt onset. Symptoms usually include fever, chills, fatigue, muscle aches, headache, dry cough, upper respiratory congestion, and sore throat (OSHA, 2007).

Patient treatment: Health care is usually supportive and focused on making symptoms more tolerable. Antiviral medications like amantadine, rimantadine, and neuraminidase inhibitors are available for treatment and prophylaxis and could reduce the morbidity and mortality associated with pandemic influenza, but are generally not used for seasonal influenza (Kennamer, 2007; OSHA, 2007).

Prevention and control: Primary prevention measures include standard and droplet or correctional standard precautions. Inmates suspected of having influenza may be isolated in single cells; if multiple inmates are diagnosed, they may be cohorted in a multi-bed cell (CDC, 2009). Identified close contact of infected inmates may be quarantined, or cohorted, as well (FBOP, 2009a). Vaccines are available for seasonal influenza and the CDC strongly recommends annual flu vaccination for all health care workers. As pandemic influenza will likely be a novel virus, a vaccine would probably not be available until after the pandemic begins. Antiviral medications may be used for prophylaxis and treatment of influenza.

Contact investigations: It is generally not required for individual cases of seasonal influenza to be reported to public health authorities; however, suspected or confirmed outbreaks of disease, as well as all hospitalization and deaths due to influenza are to be reported to local or state public health authorities as required by state law (CDC, 2010c). If public health authorities suspect a novel influenza virus is circulating and that a pandemic has developed, reporting of all cases of the novel influenza will be required.

Methicillin-Resistant *Staphylococcus aureus* (MRSA)

Prevalence: There are no incidence or prevalence figures available for MRSA infections; the skin and soft-tissue infections (SSTIs) that MRSA causes tend to appear sporadically, with episodic outbreaks. Many cases of MRSA infection are missed because wounds were not cultured and because they were misdiagnosed as "spider bites." It is estimated that 30%–50% of the general population of the United States is colonized with *Staphylococcus aureus* on the skin or in the nares; however, most of these people are asymptomatic (Bick, 2007; FBOP, 2011e). Risk factors identified in correctional settings include: sharing towels or soap, poor sanitation of exercise equipment, poor hygiene practices, self-care of SSTIs, and poor access to medical care (CDC, 2003b; Deger & Quick, 2009; FBOP, 2011e; Webb & Czachor, 2009; Romero, Treston, & O'Sullivan, 2006).

Transmission and susceptibility: Transmission is via person-to-person contact, sharing of personal items, close contact sports, sharing sports equipment, sharing injection drugs, or tattooing equipment. Persons who carry MRSA in their nares can transmit it during a viral upper respiratory infection and it can be transmitted via food, causing gastroenteritis (FBOP, 2011e). Susceptibility is general, but persons with chronic health conditions like diabetes and immune deficiency, recent surgical procedures, indwelling medical devices such as catheters, implanted medical devices, and open and chronic wounds are at greatest risk (FBOP, 2011e).

Signs and symptoms: Most MRSA infections present as SSTIs, often appearing as raised, red lesions with a necrotic center that may be accompanied by fever, swelling, severe pain, purulent drainage, and warmth (FBOP, 2011e; Romero et al., 2006). Because the lesions often appear suddenly and are very painful, many persons misidentify these infections as "spider bites."

Patient treatment: Conservative treatment using warm, moist compresses may be sufficient for early or small lesions; incision and drainage of wounds may be needed if more conservative treatment is not effective. If antibiotic therapy is indicated, the most effective medications include trimethoprim-sulfamethoxazole

(TMP-SMX), clindamycin, gentamycin, vancomycin, and tetracycline with or without Rifampin. MRSA infections are not susceptible to beta-lactam antibiotics such as cephalexin, methacillin, or penicillin (FBOP, 2011e; Romero et al., 2006).

Prevention and control: Correctional contact precautions should always be used, with emphasis on meticulous hand hygiene, using gloves and, decontaminating linens and "high contact" surfaces (FBOP, 2011e; Romero et al., 2006). All inmates should be screened for skin lesions or risk factors at the time of admission to correctional facilities (Bick, 2007). Additionally, correctional facilities have reported that success in controlling and preventing MRSA outbreaks by dispensing antibacterial soaps at all handwashing facilities, educational programs about handwashing and wound care, isolation of inmates with draining wounds, daily showering for inmates, and issuance of alcohol-based hand sanitizers to correctional staff (Deger & Quick, 2009; FBOP, 2011e; Romero et al., 2006; Webb & Czachor, 2009).

Contact investigations: MRSA infections are reportable, but the conditions for reporting and reporting area vary by state. Lesions with purulent drainage should be cultured to determine if there are epidemiological links between multiple patients with lesions. However, clinicians should not try to drain lesions that do not contain purulent material. If epidemiological links are found between two or more cases, an investigation should be initiated to look for more cases (FBOP, 2011e).

Norovirus

Prevalence: Noroviruses are the most common cause of widespread gastroenteritis, a major cause of foodborne illnesses, and are responsible for about 50% of all cases of gastroenteritis worldwide (CDC, 2011a).

Transmission and susceptibility: Norovirus is extremely contagious. Humans are the only known reservoir for human norovirus. It is transmitted in three ways; person-to-person, foodborne, and waterborne. Person-to-person contact is the fecal–oral route via contaminated, unwashed hands, exposure to aerosolized vomit, or by indirect exposure to contaminated surfaces. Foodborne transmission occurs by contamination of food by infected food handler or by contamination of food by human wastes. Waterborne transmission usually involves contamination of water sources by septic tank leakage or sewage. Susceptibility is general, but persons with weakened immune systems are at greater risk (CDC, 2011a).

Signs and symptoms: Norovirus infections are often called "stomach flu," although the virus has no association with influenza. Onset is usually abrupt; signs and symptoms include nonbloody diarrhea, vomiting, nausea, and abdominal cramps.

Patient treatment: Treatment is usually supportive and aimed at making symptoms more tolerable. Occasionally, infected persons develop more serious symptoms including dehydration, chronic diarrhea, and necrotizing enterocolitis and require more intense medical attention (CDC, 2011a).

Prevention and control: Meticulous handwashing is the single most important means of preventing transmission of norovirus; even alcohol-based hand sanitizers are not as effective in reducing norovirus. Isolation should be considered for infected persons in congregate settings, like correctional facilities. Quarantining close contacts of infected persons may also be needed. Surfaces that may be contaminated with noroviruses should be frequently cleaned with chemical disinfectants (CDC, 2011a).

Contact investigations: As with influenza, reporting of individual cases of norovirus is not required. However, all suspected outbreaks need to be reported as required by state or local regulations.

Sexually Transmitted Infections (STIs)

Prevalence: There are several infections that can be transmitted sexually. Information included in this section will be related to syphilis, gonorrhea, and chlamydia. In 2009, nationwide syphilis cases were reported to be 4.6/100,000, gonorrhea is reported at 99.1/100,000 and Chlamydia is reported at 409.2/100,000 (CDC, 2011b). Prevalence in correctional facilities is difficult to estimate because (1) most state jurisdictions do not separate reported correctional cases from general population reports, (2) there is great variability in reporting from correctional facilities, and (3) not all correctional facilities conduct routine screening for sexually transmitted infections, so information is not available. Multiple studies conducted in different states indicate that prevalence among inmates and detainees is significantly higher than the general population (Conklin, Lincoln, & Flanigan, 1998; Hammett, 2006; Hammett et al., 2002; Kahn et al., 2006).

Transmission and susceptibility: STIs are primarily transmitted through sexual contact with infected ulcers or drainage in sexual organs. Susceptibility is general, but risk factors include substance abuse, risky sexual behaviors like unprotected sex with multiple partners, and sharing injection drug supplies (Hammett, 2006; Kahn et al., 2006; Kennamer, 2007).

Signs and symptoms: Signs and symptoms vary according to the type of infection, but generally include dysuria, or purulent vaginal or urethral drainage. Symptoms of syphilis may also include development of a chancre ulcer, skin rash, or, in late stages, central nervous system problems. If untreated, gonorrhea and clamydia can lead to pelvic inflammatory disease or sterility (Kennamer, 2007).

Patient treatment: Treatment for STIs is specific to the type of infection and generally consists of antibiotic therapy and supportive care (Kahn et al., 2006; Kennamer, 2007). Correctional facilities should collaborate with local or state public health authorities to determine the best therapies and dosages to prescribe for infected inmates.

Prevention and control: Contact and correctional standard precautions are indicated for all STI cases. Caution needs to be taken with patient linens and strict handwashing procedures should be followed (Kahn et al., 2006; Kennamer, 2007).

Contact investigations: STIs are reportable, by law, to local or state public health departments; care must be taken to determine local reporting requirements (Kahn et al., 2006). Correctional facilities should collaborate with the local or state public health department to identify potential sexual contacts; public health departments have specific resources to provide confidential contact notification procedures (Kahn et al., 2006).

Tuberculosis

Incidence: The rate of tuberculosis (TB) infections in federal prisons is 29.4/100,000 and state prisons is 24.2/100,000; this is remarkably higher than the general population rate, which is 6.7/100,000 (Bick, 2006b). Tuberculosis is caused by the *Mycobacterium tuberculosis bacillus* (MTB); it is an ancient disease that remains a significant public health concern (CDC, 2006).

Screening procedures: The CDC recommends careful and systematic screening for tuberculosis in prisons and jails, especially at intake, to detect disease (CDC,

2006). Screening forms must contain questions specific to signs and symptoms of tuberculosis and should solicit information about health conditions that increase risk for infection.

Inmates who report symptoms or risk factors for tuberculosis are then screened for active TB with a tuberculin skin test (TST), a QuantiFERONw-Gold blood test, or chest x-ray. Tuberculin skin tests are most commonly used because they are cost-effective and have good specificity for TB (CDC, 2006). While the TST procedure is fairly simple, it is very important that the test be planted properly and evaluated precisely. Unfortunately, improper TST administration and evaluation is commonplace. Proper TST administration technique and evaluation process is outlined in Table 10.3.

TABLE 10.3   Placing and Reading Mantoux Skin Tests

Planting a TST

1. Draw 0.1 mL of purified protein derivative (ppd) into a ppd syringe (1 mL syringe calibrated in 0.01 mL with a 25g needle). DO NOT use an insulin syringe, the calibrations are different.
2. Clean an area in the middle section of the inner surface of the forearm with alcohol— allow to dry completely.
3. Insert needle at a 15° angle, bevel side up. Insert until *just the bevel* is under the skin. This is an intradermal injection—DO NOT insert entire needle into the skin. Inject ppd solution into the dermis of the skin (you should feel a slight resistance as the solution enters the skin surface).
4. Remove needle. Dab area with a dry cotton ball to absorb any bleeding.
5. Inform the patient that the test will be read in 48–72 h.

Reading a TST

1. Test must be read in 48–72 h. If the test is not read within 72 h, it must be repeated.
2. Palpate the area of the TST with pads of fingers—feel for induration—a palpable raised, hardened swelling. The reader should *not* measure erythema or bruising.
3. Measure any induration by palpating the lateral boundaries (transversely across the arm) and making a small mark. Measure only the induration and record in mm. TSTs are not recorded as positive or negative.

Classification of the Reaction

Induration of ≥5 mm is **positive** if:

- Pt is HIV +
- Pt has had recent contact of someone with TB disease
- Pt has fibrotic changes on a chest x-ray consistent with TB disease
- Pt is immunosuppressed for any reason.

Induration of ≥10 mm is **positive** if:

- Pt is a recent immigrant
- Pt is an injection drug user
- Pt is a inmate
- Pt has a high risk clinical condition
- Pt is under 4 years of age.

Induration of ≥15 mm is **positive** if:

- Pt has no other known risk factors for TB.

Source: Adapted from TB Elimination: Tuberculin Skin Testing (CDC, 2010d).

Transmission and susceptibility: MTB is an airborne pathogen that can be transmitted via inhalation of droplets from a cough or sneeze. Persons can become exposed to MTB when in prolonged, close contact with a patient with active tuberculosis disease. Persons at greatest risk of exposure include those with compromised immune systems, the very old, and the very young (Kennamer, 2007).

Signs and symptoms: Tuberculosis can remain in a dormant state in the body for many years; this is known as latent TB infection (LTBI). Persons with LTBI are not contagious and may never develop active TB disease. Active TB disease can affect any part of the body, but most commonly affect the lungs. Symptoms include persistent cough, sputum production (which may be blood-stained), fever, unexpected weight loss, night sweats, and fatigue.

Patient treatment: LTBI can be treated with isoniazid or rifampin to reduce the chance that active TB disease will develop. Active TB disease requires much more aggressive treatment with a multi-drug regimen that includes isoniazid, rifampin, pyrazinamide, and ethambutol (CDC, 2006). The CDC recommends that all treatment for LTBI and active TB disease be administered via directly observed therapy (DOT), as this has been found to significantly increase adherence to the treatment regimen (CDC, 2006).

Prevention and control: If the person has LTBI only, the patient is not contagious; no particular precautions are needed. If the patient has active TB disease, airborne and standard precautions must be observed. Environmental controls consist of use of an AII negative-pressure isolation room and use of N-95 respirator masks whenever close contact with the patient is anticipated.

Contact investigations: Tuberculosis must be reported to local or state public health authorities as required by state law. Correctional and public health staff need to work together to identify, isolate, and treat any person(s) diagnosed with active TB disease, and to identify potential contacts of the source patient(s). Identified contacts need to be stratified by the duration and intensity of exposure to the source patient(s) and by any medical conditions that may increase the risk of infection. All contacts should be screened for symptoms of TB. The primary diagnostic tests for LTBI and active TB disease include the tuberculin skin test (TST), the QuantiFERON®-Gold blood test, and the chest x-ray. Case Example 10.2 applies information from this section.

CASE EXAMPLE 10.2

A 28-year-old male has just arrived at intake and during initial health screening is found to have a productive cough and a fever. He gives a history of having been treated with cough syrup for persistent cough and upper respiratory infection while at another correctional facility the past 5 months. His past medical history was otherwise unremarkable. What diagnosis do you suspect? What are your first actions?

Varicella

Prevalence: Varicella Zoster virus (VZV) is the cause of varicella (chickenpox) and varicella zoster (shingles). Greater than 90% of persons in the United States develop VZV infection in the form of chickenpox before age 15. It is estimated that 97% of U.S.-born persons are immune (FBOP, 2009b). Herpes Zoster or shingles is a reactivation of the VZV infection and is usually found in persons over 50 and persons with immune deficiency disorders. Approximately 50% of persons aged between 50 and 85 will develop shingles (Bick, 2006a; FBOP, 2009b).

Transmission and susceptibility: VZV is an airborne infection that is spread via air droplets from nasopharyngeal secretions. Patients with chickenpox are contagious from 48 hours before lesions appear on the body until all lesions are crusted and no longer draining. VZV can also be transmitted to nonimmune persons via direct contact with zoster lesions or exposure to aerosolized virus from contaminated linen or clothing (Bick, 2005, 2006a). Exposure to uncomplicated shingles is confined to direct contact with lesions (FBOP, 2009b).

Signs and symptoms: Symptoms of chickenpox include fever, malaise, and eruption of a macular rash that progresses to vesicles that can be present on all parts of the body. Herpes zoster is characterized by a unilateral distribution of vesicular lesions along a nerve dermatone. Zoster is usually preceded by a prodrome of pain, numbness, or itching; the lesions usually resolve in 7–10 days. Lesions are most commonly present in the mid-thoracic to lower lumbar areas. Occasional zoster can be very severe, prolonged, disabling, and resistant to treatment (Bick, 2006a).

Patient treatment: Treatment for persons with chickenpox is primarily supportive, with emphasis on management of symptoms and prevention of secondary infection of lesions. Antiviral medications may be used for persons with zoster to shorten the duration of the outbreak; antiviral medication must be started within 72 hours of symptom onset for maximum effectiveness. Corticosteroids may be effective in reducing the duration and lessening pain, but should be avoided in those patients with immune deficiency (Bick, 2006a; FBOP, 2009b).

Prevention and control: Correctional and airborne contact precautions should be followed. Patients with Varicella symptoms should be isolated in an AII or private room, or may be cohorted with other patients with VZV infection. Close contacts of VZV-infected patients who have no proof of immunity should be quarantined and housed separately from other inmates until likelihood of infection has passed, usually about 3 weeks (FBOP, 2009b). Vaccines for chickenpox and shingles are widely available. The CDC recommends these vaccines for all health care staff and as post-exposure prophylaxis for all nonimmune persons who have significant exposures to VZV (FBOP, 2009b).

Contact investigations: Varicella infections are reportable; reporting requirements vary by state. The steps in contact investigation include: identifying, isolating, and confirming VZV infection; notifying facility managers and public health authorities; stopping inmate movement; identifing and prioritizing inmate and staff contacts; and assessing contacts for varicella symptoms or immunity (Bick, 2006a; FBOP, 2009b).

SUMMARY

Infection control in correctional settings is a daunting responsibility. Fortunately, correctional nurses do not have the sole responsibility for carrying out infection control. There are vast resources at the federal and state levels waiting to be tapped. Federal organizations like the Centers for Disease Control and Prevention and the Occupational Safety and Health Administration have experts who are willing to work with local facilities to implement infection control measures, teaching and training programs available for education and huge stores of educational materials, much

---

EXHIBIT 10.1

Useful Online Resources

http://www.apic.org
http://www.youtube.com/user/NRHNetwork
http://www.cdc.gov/correctionalhealth
http://bjs.ojp.usdoj.gov
http://www.cdc.gov/niosh/topics/correctionalhcw
http://www.cdc.gov/niosh/topics/bbp/PEPline
http://www.bop.gov/news/medresources.jsp
http://www.osha.gov/
http://www.youtube.com/user/CDCStreamingHealth
http://www.oregon.gov/DOC/OPS/HESVC/index.shtml

---

of which is free. Within corrections, the Federal Bureau of Prisons has made public their Clinical Guidelines, as have some state prison systems such as the Oregon Department of Corrections. All of these entities have placed information about their procedures on their Internet websites and invite all to use them as needed (see Exhibit 10.1).

DISCUSSION QUESTIONS

1. A food service worker was diagnosed with Hepatitis C infection. The supervisor wants to know if the inmate is "safe" to work in Food Services. What is your response to the Food Service Supervisor?
2. Compare your facility's current infection control program to elements described in this chapter and discuss the differences.
3. An inmate is diagnosed with norovirus. Several other inmates are exhibiting similar symptoms. What steps should be taken to determine if this is an outbreak?
4. Describe correctional standard precautions and isolation procedures.

REFERENCES

Altice, F. L., & Springer, S. A. (2006). HIV in the correctional setting. In *Clinical practice in correctional medicine* (2nd ed.). Philadelphia: Mosby Elsevier.

Bick, J. (2004). Hepatitis B in corrections. *Infectious Diseases in Corrections Report. 7*(10/11), 1–3. Retrieved August 31, 2011, from http://www.idcronline.org/archives/oct2004

Bick, J. (2005). Infection control in the correctional setting. *Infectious diseases in corrections report, 8*(8), 1–3. Retrieved August 31, 2011, from http://www.idcronline.org/archives/aug05

Bick, J. (2006a). Infection control in the correctional setting. In M. Puisis (Ed.), *Clinical practice in correctional medicine* (2nd ed.). Philadelphia: Mosby Elsevier.

Bick, J. (2006b). Tuberculosis in corrections. *Infectious Diseases in Corrections Report, 9*(2), Retrieved August 31, 2011, from http://www.idcronline.org/archives/feb2006

Bick, J. (2007). Methicillin-resistant *Staphylococcus aureus* in the correctional setting. *Infectious Disease in Corrections Report, 9*(14), 1–6. Retrieved August 31, 2011, from http://www.idcronline.org/archives/mar2007

Buck, J. M., Morrow, K. M., Margolis, A., Eldridge, G., Sosman, J., MacGowan, R. et al. The Project START study group. (2006). Hepatitis B vaccination in prison: The perspectives of formerly incarcerated men. *Journal of Correctional Health Care, 12*(1), 12–23.

Bureau of Justice Statistics. (2009). *Bulletin: HIV in prisons, 2007–2008* (NCJ 228307). Retrieved August 22, 2011, from http://bjs.ojp.usdoj.gov/index.cfm?ty=pbdetail&iid=1747

Centers for Disease Control and Prevention. (2003a). Prevention and control of infections with hepatitis viruses in correctional settings. *Morbidity and mortality weekly report, 52*(RR-1), 1–33. Retrieved August 22, 2011, from http://www.cdc.gov/mmwr/preview/mmwrhtml/rr5201a1.htm

Centers for Disease Control and Prevention. (2003b). Methicillin-resistant *Staphylococcus aureus* infections in correctional facilities—Georgia, California and Texas 2001–2003. *Morbidity and Mortality Weekly Report, 52*(41), 992–996. Retrieved August 22, 2011, from http://cdc.gov/mmwr/preview/mmwrhtml/mm5241a4.htm

Centers for Disease Control and Prevention. (2005).Updated U.S. Public Health Services Guidelines for the management of occupational exposures to hiv and recommendations for postexposure prophylaxis. *Morbidity and Mortality Weekly Report, 54*(RR-09). Retrieved January 19, 2012, from http://www.cdc.gov/mmwr/preview/mmwrhtml/rr5409a1.htm

Centers for Disease Control and Prevention. (2006). Prevention and control of tuberculosis in correctional and detention facilities: Recommendations from CDC. *Morbidity and Mortality Weekly Report. 55*(RR-9). Retrieved August 22, 2011, from http:www.cdc.gov/mmwr/PDF/rr/rr5509.pdf

Centers for Disease Control and Prevention. (2009). Interim guidance for correctional and detention facilities on novel influenza A (H1N1) virus. Retrieved August 1, 2011, from http://www.cdc.gov/h1n1flu/guidance/correctional_facilities.htm

Centers for Disease Control and Prevention. (2010a). *Scabies: Resources for health professionals.* Retrieved September 13, 2011, from http://www.cdc.gov/parasites/scabies/health_professionals.html

Centers for Disease Control and Prevention. (2010b). *Lice: Resources for health professionals.* Retrieved September 13, 2011, from http://www.cdc.gov/parasites/lice/health_professionals.html

Centers for Disease Control and Prevention. (2010c). *Monitoring influenza activity, including 2009 H1N1.* Retrieved September 15, 2011, from http://cdc.gov/h1n1flu/reportingqa.htm

Centers for Disease Control and Prevention. (2010d). *TB elimination: Tuberculin skin testing.* Retrieved September 27, 2011, from http://www.cdc.gov/tb

Centers for Disease Control and Prevention. (2011a). Updated norovirus outbreak management and disease prevention guidelines. *Mortality and Morbidity Weekly Report, 60*(3), 1–16.

Centers for Disease Control and Prevention. (2011b). Summary of notifiable diseases—United States, 2009. *Morbidity and Mortality Weekly Report, 58*(53). Retrieved September 7, 2011, from http://www.cdc.gov/mmwr/pdf/wk/mm5853.pdf

Conklin, T. J., Lincoln, T., & Flanigan, T. P. (1998). A public health model to connect correctional health care with communities. *American Journal of Public Health, 88*(8), 1249–1250.

Deger, G. M., & Quick, D. W. (2009). The enduring menace of MRSA: Incidence, treatment and prevention in a county jail. *Journal of Correctional Health Care, 15*(3), 174–178.

Federal Bureau of Prisons. (2008). Guidelines for Prevention and Treatment of Hepatitis A. *Federal bureau of prisons clinical practice guidelines.* Retrieved August 31, 2011, from http://www.bop.gov/news/medresources.jsp

Federal Bureau of Prisons. (2009a). Pandemic influenza plan. *Federal Bureau of Prisons Clinical Practice Guidelines.* Retrieved September 12, 2011, from http://www.bop.gov/news/medresources.jsp

Federal Bureau of Prisons. (2009b). Management of varicella Zoster virus infections. *Federal Bureau of Prisons Clinical Practice Guidelines.* Retrieved September 13, 2011, from http://www.bop.gov/news/PDFs/varicella.pdf

Federal Bureau of Prisons. (2011a). Lice and scabies protocol. *Federal Bureau of Prisons Clinical Practice Guidelines.* Retrieved September 12, 2011, from http://www.bop.gov/news/PDFs/lice_scabies.pdf

Federal Bureau of Prisons. (2011b). Stepwise approach for detecting, evaluating and treating chronic hepatitis B infection. *Federal Bureau of Prisons Clinical Practice Guidelines.* Retrieved September 12, 2011, from http://www.bop.gov/news/PDFs/hepatitis_b.pdf

Federal Bureau of Prisons. (2011c). Stepwise approach for detecting, evaluating and treating chronic hepatitis C and cirrhosis. *Federal Bureau of Prisons Clinical Practice Guidelines*. Retrieved September 12, 2011, from http://www.bop.gov/news/PDFs/hepatitis_c.pdf

Federal Bureau of Prisons. (2011d). Management of HIV Infection. *Federal Bureau of Prisons Clinical Practice Guidelines*. Retrieved September 12, 2011, from http://www.bop.gov/news/PDFs/mgmt_hiv.pdf

Federal Bureau of Prisons. (2011e). Management of methicillin-resistant *Staphylococcus aureus* (MRSA) infections. *Federal Bureau of Prisons Clinical Practice Guidelines*. Retrieved September 13, 2011, from http://www.bop.gov/news/PDFs/mrsa.pdf

Fisher, N. (2011). *Infectious Diseases Update*. Presentation at the National Conference on Correctional Health Care: Historic Times, Extraordinary Solutions. Baltimore, MD.

Hammett, T., Harmon, M. P., & Rhodes, W. (2002). The burden of infectious disease among inmates of and releases from US correctional facilities. *American Journal of Public Health, 92*(11), 1798–1794.

Hammett, T. (2006). HIV/AIDS and other infectious diseases among correctional inmates: Transmission, burden and an appropriate response. *American Journal of Public Health, 96*(6), 974–978.

Hogben, M., & St. Lawrence, J. S. (2000). HIV/STD risk reduction interventions in prison settings. *Journal of Women's Health & Gender-based Medicine, 9*, 587–592.

Johnson-Mallard, V., Lengacher, C. A., Kromrey, J. D., Campbell, D. W., Jevitt, C. M., Daley, E. et al. (2007). Increasing knowledge of sexually transmitted infection risk. *The Nurse Practitioner, 32*(2), 26–32.

Kahn, R. H., Joesoef, R., Aynalem, G., Puisis, M., Raba, J. M. et al. (2006). Overview of sexually transmitted diseases. In M. Puisis (Ed.), *Clinical practice in correctional medicine* (2nd ed.). Philadelphia: Mosby Elsevier.

Kennamer, M. (2007). *Basic infection control for health care providers* (2nd ed.). Delmar-Cengage Learning: New York.

Lane, M. E. (2006). The infection control program. In M. Puisis (Ed.), *Clinical practice in correctional medicine* (2nd ed.). Philadelphia: Mosby Elsevier.

Lincoln, T., & Miles, J. R. (2006). Correctional, public, and community health collaboration in the United States. In M. Puisis (Ed.), *Clinical practice in correctional medicine* (2nd ed.). Philadelphia: Mosby Elsevier.

Lincoln, T., Tutlhill, R. W., DePietro, S. L., Tocco, M. J., Keough, K., & Conklin, T. J. (2006). Viral hepatitis, risk behaviors, aminotransferase levels, and screening options at a county correctional center. *Journal of Correctional Health Care, 12*(4), 249–261.

Lobato, M. N., & Goldenson, J. (2006). Tuberculosis in the correctional setting. In *Clinical practice in correctional medicine* (2nd ed.). Philadelphia: Mosby Elsevier.

National Commission on Correctional Health Care. (1997). *Position statements: Management of hepatitis B virus in correctional facilities*. Retrieved September 12, 2011, from http://www.ncchc.org/resources/statements/hepB.html

Occupational Safety and Health Administration. (2007). Pandemic influenza preparedness and response guidance for healthcare workers and healthcare employers. (OSHA 3328-08). Retrieved August 22, 2011, from http://osha.gov/Publications/3328-05-2007-English.html

Parvez, F. M., Lobato, M. N., & Greifinger, R. B. (2010). Tuberculosis control: Lessons for outbreak preparedness in correctional facilities. *Journal of Correctional Health Care, 16*(3), 239–242.

Restrum, Z. G. (2005). Public health implications of substandard correctional health care. *American Journal of Public Health, 95*(10), 1689–1691.

Romero, D. V., Treston, J., & O'Sullivan, A. L. (2006). Hand-to-hand: Preventing MRSA. *The Nurse Practitioner, 31*(3), 16–23.

Schoenly, L. (2008). Infection control nursing: A critical role in disease prevention and effective intervention. *CorrectCare, 22*(2), 10–11.

Spaulding, A. C., Weinbaum, C. M., Lau, D. T. Y., Sterling, R., Seeff, L. B., Margolis, H. S. et al., (2006). A framework for management of hepatitis C in prisons. *Annals of Internal Medicine, 144*(10), 762–769.

Webb, J. A., & Czachor, J. S. (2009). MRSA prevention and control in correctional facilities in southwestern Ohio. *Journal of Correctional Health Care, 15*(4).

Zeigler, M. (2010). *Re: What is the chain of infection?* (Web log message). Retrieved August 31, 2011, from http://contagions.wordpress.com/2010/11/06/what-is-the-chain-of-infection

ELEVEN

Health and Well-Being of Juveniles

Ellyn Presley and Lorry Schoenly

With an average of nearly 93,000 juveniles in the U.S. criminal justice system (OJJP, 2006), correctional nurses must be aware of physical, emotional, psychosocial, and developmental issues affecting the delivery of health care to this population. Most offenders under the age of 18 are detained and held in facilities designed for adolescents; however, a significant number are sentenced as adults, making them a highly vulnerable segment of the prison community. Correctional nurses working with juvenile patients must consider the additional concerns common in a troubled adolescent population.

CHARACTERISTICS OF THE JUVENILE OFFENDER POPULATION

Adolescents detained in the criminal justice system require special attention, whether they are in a juvenile setting or in an adult setting. Even though they are considered a healthy population, often their first one-on-one encounter with a dental, mental health, or medical care provider is during their detention stay. In addition, many incarcerated youth present with unresolved mental health issues stemming from exposure to trauma and abuse (Cohen, Burd, & Beyer, 2006). Correctional facilities can have a harmful effect on an adolescent's health, with incarceration increasing stressors and lessening coping strategies and abilities (Schnittker & John, 2007). The intake health screening coupled with a mental health screening is crucial in capturing, identifying, and reducing those stressors.

The Survey of Youth in Residential Placement (SYRP) estimated 101,040 adolescents between the ages of 10 and 20 were in residential placement in the United States because they were arrested for, charged with, or adjudicated for an offense (Sedlak & McPherson, 2010). This reflects a custody rate of 224 youth per 100,000 in the general youth population. The same survey states 85% of all youth in residential placement in 2003 were male, with the majority (51%) age of 16 or 17. About one-third (35%) are White non-Hispanic, another third (32%) are African American, and close to one-fourth (24%) are Hispanic. An estimated 6% are identified as multiracial. Multilingual and multicultural educational material and nurses who are sensitive to diverse adolescent populations are necessary to intervene with this population. Multilingual signage is essential to inform the youth where to go with questions and concerns.

The SYRP (2003) also reported that many youth in custody (46%) said that both parents helped raise them, although this could have been in separate households. A slightly lower percentage (42%) had just one parent caring for them and 11% reported no parental care while growing up. However, at the time they were taken into custody, more youth were living with one parent (45%) than with two parents (30%), and one-fourth of youth (25%) were not living with a parent. Significantly more females than males entered custody from a no-parent living arrangement (32% of females vs. 24% of males).

Substance Abuse

Many of the adolescents who get in trouble with the law have problems with substance use, and their offense is tied to their involvement with drugs or alcohol. Criminal behavior and substance use follow a parallel course over time (Sullivan & Hamilton, 2007). Among adolescents detained for criminal offenses in 2006, 56% of boys and 40% of girls tested positive for drugs. The rate of substance abuse in the juvenile justice system is significantly higher than in the general population. Substance use is linked with continued offending and a broad range of other high-risk behaviors, such as smoking, risky sexual encounters, and violence that results in a poor educational, occupational, and psychological outcome (Chassin, 2008). For pregnant adolescents, the harm to fetal development is also a concern.

There is a marked decrease in substance use as an adolescent acquires new skills (either personal or vocational) that lead to new opportunities and offer alternative forms of validation. Once an adolescent forms a commitment to work and family, they have something to lose and therefore something to guard. Delinquent behavior and substance use problems go hand in hand in adolescence, making incarceration an important time and setting for substance abuse education programs. The vast majority of adolescents who receive substance abuse treatment participate while in a correctional setting as opposed to a community-based program (Mulvey, Schubert, & Chung, 2007). Correctional nurses have an opportunity to assist in the rehabilitation process by encouraging and supporting the skill development and validation process of substance abuse education programs in the correctional setting.

Tobacco

The majority of adult smokers started before the age of 18 (CDC, 2010a). Correctional nurses play a critical role in improving the health of incarcerated adolescents through smoking cessation information and education. Although the initiation of smoking among youth has been declining over the last two decades, nearly 20% of male and 15% of female high-school students reported being current cigarette smokers in 2009 (Centers for Disease Control, 2010a). Overall tobacco use among high schoolers, including cigars, smokeless tobacco, and bidis, is 24%.

Tobacco use is linked to other risky behaviors in the youth population. Tobacco-using youths are more likely to use alcohol, illegal drugs, attempt suicide, and engage in high-risk sexual practices (American Cancer Society, 2010). In addition, smoking youth have increased health problems, including shortness of breath, frequent headaches, worsened cold and flu symptoms, and poor lung growth and function (American Cancer Society, 2010). Discouraging the use of tobacco products can significantly improve health for incarcerated youth.

Sexually Transmitted Disease

Detained youth report more risky behaviors and initiate them at younger ages than do youth in the community, including adolescents having unprotected sex and sharing injection/piercing equipment (Elkington et al., 2008). Psychiatric disorders and substance abuse, both common in this population, exacerbate this situation (Elkington et al., 2008). In addition, females of age 15 to 19 had the highest rate of chlamydia and gonorrhea compared to any other age or sex group (Schwartz, 2010). Correctional nurses working in the juvenile justice system have the opportunity to decrease the spread of sexually transmitted diseases through screening, detection, and educational activities.

From the Experts ...

"Juvenile Corrections offers the perfect opportunity to educate a population still in their formative years. Instruction in pregnancy and STD prevention, health promotion, and the negative effects of drugs, alcohol, and tobacco on their bodies are offered through a variety of various teaching methods. Every opportunity is given to dispel myths, instill self-esteem, and encourage the adoption of a healthy lifestyle. If they choose to embrace and implement these changes, they can become productive and healthful citizens."

Cynthia Chancellor RN, BSN
Tecumseh, OK

Because most detained youth return to their communities, HIV/STI risk behaviors in delinquent youth are a community public health problem, not just a problem for the juvenile justice system. Improving the coordination between the community health systems and the juvenile justice systems providing HIV/STI intervention to youth through primary care, education, and mental health can reduce the prevalence of risky behaviors and substantially reduce the spread of HIV/STIs among young people.

Physical Development

Adolescence is a time of increased physical growth, sexual cognition, and psychosocial and brain development. Norms of physical, cognitive, sexual, and brain development can vary among individual adolescents and affect the nurse's inter-actions with them. Adolescents are acutely cognizant of their ever-changing body appearance and budding sexuality. Because of the rapid bodily changes occurring, adolescents experience a profound preoccupation with how their bodies compare to their peers. This view of their body influences all aspects of a developing adolescent. Disadvantaged youth are even less likely to have healthy foods available or make wise food choices for healthy development. Correctional nurses have an opportunity to improve nutrition and physical activity habits for these youths while in custody.

Nutritional Needs

Due to differences in body type, physical activity, and rate of growth, adolescents have differing nutritional needs. Puberty can double a person's nutritional needs for protein, calcium, zinc, and iron (Saewyc, 2011), presenting a challenge for the detained youth. The emotional distress of incarceration may cause a youth to eat too much, eat too little, and/or make unhealthy dietary choices. Caloric needs are usually based on growth rate and the level of exercise, but range between 1800 and 2400 calories per day for the adolescent (U.S. Department of Agriculture & U.S. Department of Health and Human Services, 2010). Protein needs for adolescents are 42–56 g daily. Recommended intake of calcium is 1300 mg per day; iron requirements are about 11 mg for males and 15 mg for females (U.S. Department of Agriculture and U.S. Department of Health and Human Services, 2010). Adolescents with chronic illnesses may have additional nutritional needs based on their individual health circumstances. Pregnant youth have increased needs because they are still growing and developing themselves.

A healthy diet in adolescence promotes adequate growth and helps decrease the risk of dental caries, as well as obesity, hypertension, hyperlipidemias, and other chronic health problems that can manifest in adolescence and later on in life. Correctional nurses play an important role in educating youth regarding eating well-balanced meals, making healthy food choices, and portion control. Including a measurement of body mass index (BMI) at intake health screening and periodically thereafter can alert the nurse to nutritional problems.

Obesity

With nearly one in every six adolescents being obese (Ogden, Carroll, Curtin, Lamb, & Flegal, 2010), correctional nurses are challenged to assist youth to manage their weight through wise and healthy food choices and daily exercise. Although genetics and some medical disorders can cause obesity, adolescent obesity often results from a lack of physical activity, overeating, and lack of knowledge to make healthy food choices. In addition, antipsychotic and antidepressant medications are associated with higher rates of obesity (Frincu-Mallos, 2010). Adolescents need physical activity for healthy growth and development. Physical activity can reduce the risk of obesity and has numerous benefits that extend beyond just physical health, such as reducing depression and improving self-esteem (Harvey, Hotopf, Overland, & Mykletun, 2010). Physical activity should be maximized at every opportunity. The current recommended amount of physical activity for adolescents is 60 minutes every day (CDC, 2011).

Psychosocial and Cognitive Development

An important part of adolescent psychosocial growth is developing a stronger recognition of their own personal identity, including a set of ethical values, personal morals, and greater perception of feeling of self-worth and esteem. Peer influence is a dominant psychosocial issue during adolescence. Peer group acceptance becomes essential to counter instability generated by rapid body changes, allows the development of same-sex friends that encourages them to "try out different roles," and to win the struggle for mastery as they become an independent-thinking individual. Youths are acutely cognizant of their physical appearance and social behaviors; peer group acceptance is fundamental (Saewyc, 2011).

In early adolescence (11–13 years), concrete thinking, egocentrism, and impulsive behavior are the hallmarks of this period. The inability of young adolescents to apply abstract reasoning makes it difficult for them to comprehend the relationship between high risk behavior and consequences, such as, unprotected sex and STIs. Problem-solving skills are evolving as the brain matures during early adolescence, hindering behavior changes and the ability to recognize how current behaviors influence future outcomes (Spano, 2004).

Middle adolescence (14–16 years) is characterized by increasing detachment from family and developing emotional autonomy. This is the stage where abstract reasoning begins to emerge. However, when faced with overwhelming emotions or stressful situations, the adolescent will often regress to an old familiar pattern— concrete thinking. Youth begin to comprehend the relationship between existing health behaviors and future health consequences, but can revert back to the belief that "it won't happen to me" and reengage in risky behaviors. This is a time of strong peer influence and it is often difficult for youth to make health-related choices based on knowledge rather than peer pressure (Saewyc, 2011).

Late adolescents (17–19 years) have developed skills to handle complicated social situations, are better able to control impulsive behavior, and are moving away from the influence of peer pressure. The refinement of abstract reasoning skills continues to develop during late adolescence, which allows greater understanding of health choices. This skill is especially important for adolescent females who may be engaging in high-risk sexual behaviors that could lead to STIs and pregnancy. As adolescent females begin to utilize more abstract thinking and reasoning skills, this may help them prevent risky situations, delay immediate gratification, and see the benefit of planning for a future partner and family (Spano, 2004).

Older youth are capable of using problem-solving skills to understand and implement behavior changes to reduce poor health outcomes. Adolescence is a time of enormous biological, psychosocial, and cognitive growth and development. It is important for health professionals to help the youth identify where they are on this journey called "adolescence" and how collaboratively the adolescent and nurse can determine an individualized teaching plan to reduce high-risk behaviors.

Mental Illness and Emotional Disturbance

Forty to seventy percent of the roughly one million youth referred to the juvenile justice system were reported to have comorbid mental health disorders (Kessler, 2002). Almost 48% of incarcerated adolescents suffer from an emotional disturbance (Quinn, Rutherford, Leone, Osher, & Poirier, 2005). An emotional or behavioral disorder refers to a condition in which the behavior or emotional responses of an individual school are so different from one's generally accepted age, ethnic, or cultural norm that they adversely affect performance in such areas as self-care, social relationships, personal adjustment, academic progress, classroom behavior, or work adjustment (National Association of School Psychologist, 2004). Mental illness and emotional disturbances complicate the course of confinement and contribute to behavioral management issues.

Traumatic Stress

Exposure to traumatic events and situations can overwhelm an adolescent's ability to cope with what they have experienced, causing traumatic stress (National Child Traumatic Stress Network, 2008).

Traumatic events include physical abuse, sexual abuse, domestic violence, community violence, and/or disasters. Youth exposed to traumatic events can exhibit a wide range of symptoms such as depression, anxiety, aggression, conduct problems, and defiant or oppositional behavior (Caporino, Murray, & Jensen, 2003). Traumatic stress can interfere with the youth's ability to think and learn, and can disrupt the course of healthy physical, emotional, and intellectual growth (Ford, Chapman, Hawke, & Albert, 2007).

The prevalence of youth exposed to trauma is greater in the juvenile justice system than in the community (Ford et al., 2007). Traumatic stress symptoms may worsen as a result of involvement in the juvenile justice system. Arrest, court hearings, detention, and incarceration are stressful, and stressful experiences can exacerbate trauma symptoms (Ford et al., 2007). In addition, traumatic history has been found to result in an increased use of health care and mental health services (Ford, 2005). For all these reasons, correctional nurses should recognize and be sensitive to the trauma backgrounds of detained youth. Trauma-informed care is discussed in Chapter 9, Women's Health Care.

COMMON MEDICAL CONDITIONS OF THE JUVENILE OFFENDER

A review of the health issues for incarcerated adolescents reveals several key medical conditions, of which the correctional nurses working with juveniles must be aware (Griel & Loeb, 2009). Incarcerated youth are significantly less healthy and have many unmet physical needs (Committee on Adolescence, 2011). Key conditions of greatest concern are discussed with implications for the correctional nurse. General information about chronic conditions can be found in Chapter 6, Chronic Conditions. General information about dental health can be found in Chapter 7, Dental Conditions. Information in this chapter will focus on interventions and teaching specific to the adolescent population.

Asthma

Asthma is the most common serious chronic disease in children (EPA, 2011). In 2009, over 1.7 million American children had a diagnosis of asthma, a rate of 1 in 7 (American Lung Association, 2011). Boys under 18 years of age have a 44% higher rate of asthma than girls the same age, although this trend reverses in adulthood. Asthma is found to be 43% more prevalent in Blacks than in Whites. A survey of high-school students found that 38% of those with asthma had an episode or attack in the last 12 months, occurring more often in the earlier grades than those who were seniors. These data indicate that asthma management is a major part of health care in the juvenile justice system.

Nursing Management

Early identification of asthma in the youth population is an important component of nursing care. Categorizing asthma according to degree of severity along with ongoing evaluation is recommended upon entry into the juvenile justice system (NCCHC, 2011b). Initial assessment should include a complete physical exam with focus on the respiratory system, including peak expiratory flow measurements or spirometry, if indicated. Follow-up visits should then include evaluation of asthma control at rest, with activity and during sleep; and monitoring of daily asthma control (Table 11.1).

In addition to screening and assessment, correctional nurses have an opportunity to reduce environmental factors that can exacerbate asthma symptoms. Asthma attacks can be triggered by dust mites, molds, cockroaches, and secondhand smoke (EPA, 2011). Efforts to remove or reduce these triggers from the correctional environment could improve patient health. Nurses can work with administration and housing officers to reduce these triggers in the youth's living areas.

School-based approaches to asthma management can have application in the youth detention setting. Improved knowledge of asthma and increased youth self-efficacy and self-management resulted from programs that have these four essential components (Sadof & Kaslovsky, 2011):

- Case identification of youth with asthma
- Education of all personnel on how to manage an asthma episode
- Linkage to higher-level health care when needed
- Youth self-management skills taught and tailored to the specific age and individual characteristics

TABLE 11.1   Adolescent Asthma Control Categories

The clinician should assess disease severity to initiate treatment for patients who are not currently taking long-term control medications.

COMPONENTS OF CONTROL	DEGREE OF SEVERITY			
		PERSISTENT		
	INTERMITTENT	MILD	MODERATE	SEVERE
Short-acting beta-agonist inhaler use	<2 days a week	≥2 days a week but not daily	Daily	Several times a day
Symptoms	≤2 days a week	>2 days a week but not daily	Daily	Throughout the day
Nighttime awakenings	≤2 times a month	3–4 times a month	>1 time a week but not nightly	Often, 7 times a week
Interference with normal activity	No limitation	Minor limitation	Some limitation	Extreme limitation
Lung function/ FEV	>80% predicted	>80% predicted	60–80% predicted	<60% predicted

Source: National Asthma Education and Prevention Program, Expert Panel Report 3, Summary Report, *Guidelines for the Diagnosis and Management of Asthma*, p. 44. http://www.nhlbi.nih.gov/guidelines/asthma/asthsumm.pdf

Correctional nurses can apply these principles through early screening and identification of youth with asthma. Custody officers, youth workers, and support staff need information about how to handle an asthma episode. Regular chronic care visits for medical management of asthma links juveniles to the medical system. Efforts to maximize self-management of asthma symptoms and interventions through education during the medical office visit are strongly recommended.

Patient Education

Medication understanding and compliance can be a challenge with a youthful patient. Adolescents often underestimate the severity of this chronic condition and are willing to engage in risky behaviors such as smoking, use of cocaine, and nonadherence to medication (Sadof & Kaslovsky, 2011). Patient education, particularly peer-led education programs, can be beneficial in improving compliance and decreasing risk behaviors, and supports understanding that they are not the only resident with asthma (Sadof & Kaslovsky, 2011). Consider group teaching sessions if a significant number of youths in the facility have this condition. NCCHC (2011b) suggests key elements of an individual or group education program (Exhibit 11.1). Age-specific information sheets for patient teaching can be obtained through the Centers for Disease Control and Prevention at http://www.cdc.gov/asthma/pdfs/kids_fast_facts.pdf.

EXHIBIT 11.1
Basic Education for Adolescents with Asthma

- Teach basic facts about asthma, including
  - Inhaler/spacer/holding chamber techniques
  - Role of medications
- Develop a self-management plan
- Develop an action plan for when and how to take rescue actions, especially for those with a history of severe exacerbations
- Discuss appropriate environmental control measures to avoid exposure to known allergens and irritants
- Teach self-monitoring and refer to group education, if possible
- Review and update the self-management plan
- For patients with severe persistent asthma, provide individual education and counseling

Source: From NCCHC (2011b), used with permission.

Dental Conditions

Studies of detained youth oral health needs indicate most have untreated tooth decay, poor dental hygiene, and lack of basic knowledge of how to use a toothbrush, and require dental care (Bolin & Jones, 2006; Committee on Adolescence, 2011). Over 6% are found to have immediate needs due to dental infection, tooth or jaw fracture, or severe periodontal disease with bleeding (Committee on Adolescence, 2011). The high frequency of dental concerns in the youth population requires correctional nurses to increase skill in detecting issues needing immediate attention.

Nurses also need skill in providing education regarding basic tooth hygiene issues including practice using a toothbrush and/or floss. In addition, nurses can advocate for increased dental services for detained youth.

Nursing Management

An oral evaluation should be a part of intake screening and performed no later than 7 days after admission (NCCHC, 2011a). This initial screening determines conditions of immediate need such as traumatic injury, which may have occurred during the arrest process. In addition, this screening can indicate advancing periodontal disease and other dental problems. Irreversible tissue damage from periodontal disease begins in late adolescence and early adulthood. Adolescents have a higher prevalence of gingivitis than prepubertal children or adults. Some symptoms of periodontal disease in adolescents include swollen, tender, and red gums; receding gums; constant odorous breath; loose teeth; and bleeding during brushing or flossing. Advancing periodontal disease can lead to tooth deterioration and infection (American Academy of Periodontology, 2004).

Based on the level of need found in the initial screening, schedule an oral examination with a dentist within 60 days of admission (NCCHC, 2011a). The adolescent patient whose oral health has not been monitored routinely by a dentist may have advanced caries, periodontal disease, or other oral involvement urgently in need of professional evaluation and treatment. Chronic dental conditions of drug-related gingivitis, pregnancy gingivitis, and periodontitis may also be found in this population. Fluoridated toothpaste should be provided and teeth brushing encouraged twice daily for plaque removal (American Academy of Pediatric Dentistry, 2010).

Reproductive and sexually transmitted infection: The rise in sex hormones during adolescence is suspected to be a cause of the increased prevalence of gingivitis by affecting the composition of the subgingival microflora or altering the capillary permeability and increase fluid accumulation in the gingival tissue (American Academy of Periodontology, 2004). Pregnant youths are at higher risk for several dental conditions. Untreated periodontitis has been associated with preterm and low-birth-weight infants and, if left untreated, can compromise the health of the mother and unborn child. In addition, gingivitis is aggravated by hormonal changes and exacerbated by poor plaque control and mouth breathing (American Academy of Pediatric Dentistry, 2010).

Professional dental care is necessary to assess for oral manifestations of sexually transmitted diseases. Oral sex has been implicated in the transmission of herpes, syphilis, gonorrhea, genital warts (HPV), intestinal parasites (amebiasis), and hepatitis A (CDC, 2009a). Any signs of oral infection should be referred to a dentist.

Oral piercing: Oral piercing is popular in adolescence and usually involves the tongue, lips, and cheeks. They are more common in women than men (Janssen & Cooper, 2008). Oral piercings can produce many undesired complications, including bacterial infection, pain, swelling, prolonged bleeding, and difficulty swallowing and speaking (ADA, 2004). Late complications include chipped and fractured teeth, gingival trauma, localized periodontitis, persistent difficulties in oral functions, aspiration, or swallowing oral jewelry (American Academy of Pediatric Dentistry, 2011). The piercing procedure exposes the youth to a high risk of infection because the oral cavity harbors a significant amount of bacteria. Periodontal diseases are serious infections caused by bacteria that harm gums and tissue in the vicinity of the mouth. Dental cavities or caries only affect the teeth, while periodontal disease affects the bone surrounding the tooth, the gums, and coverings of the tooth root and membrane. Plaque buildup is the main cause of gum disease. Oral jewelry is removed from the youth during the intake process. Document location of piercings in the medical record and note any signs of infection or pain at the site.

Patient Education

A personal, age-appropriate oral health education program should include oral health self-assessment, oral hygiene, consequences of tobacco and drug use, diet management, professional preventative care, and the preservation of teeth during sports. In addition, the role of carbohydrates in dental caries is well documented (American Academy of Pediatric Dentistry, 2010). Adolescents are exposed to and consume high quantities of refined carbohydrates and acid-containing beverages. Education in healthy eating habits can reduce dental decay. Tobacco use can lead to significant oral and dental conditions. Reducing smoking and other uses of tobacco can improve adolescent dental health.

Traumatic Injury and Bone Healing

Correctional nurses working with incarcerated youth must be prepared to manage traumatic injury. Risky behaviors such as physical fighting, use of firearms, and lack of attention to helmets or seatbelts are high in this population (CDC, 2010b). In addition, emphasis on physical activity during confinement may lead to sports-based injuries.

Nursing Management

Correctional nurses in juvenile facilities should have adequate supplies for emergency first-aid for traumatic injuries, including splinting materials. Muscle sprains and strain may be handled conservatively with rest for 24–48 hours and 20 minutes of icing 4 times daily (Ball, Bindler, & Cowen, 2010). Elastic compression bandaging is not recommended due to the potential for misuse. Airsplints can provide joint stability and restrict movement, which can help reduce swelling. However, any indication of deformity, inability to bear weight after walking more than five steps, or lack of healing must initiate diagnostic procedures such as x-rays of the affected body part. Children under 17 are still in a process of ossification, progressing from cartilage to bone (Wilson & Curry, 2011). Generally, bone heals faster at younger ages. Injury in the epiphyseal plate area of growing bone can lead to deformity; therefore, correctional nurses must be vigilant to manage bone injuries with attention to orthopedic follow-up and adherence to treatment plan.

Patient Education

Detention is an opportune time for healthy living instruction, including injury reduction. Provide safety teaching with all health care interventions, focusing on the immediate need. In addition, adequate amounts of vitamins A and D and calcium are needed for proper bone growth and healing (Hockenberry, 2011). Include healthy food choices that are high in calcium and vitamins in patient teaching interventions with injured youth.

Reproductive and Sexual Health

Higher rates of sexual activity are reported among incarcerated youth than the general high-school population (CDC, 2010c). In addition, incarcerated youth report lower use of condoms or other contraceptives. These risky behaviors require attention by correctional nurses working with the juvenile population. Reproductive and sexual health—combined with emotional problems and mental health disorders, unintentional injury and violence, substance abuse, and poor nutrition—form a complex set of potential challenges to an adolescents' healthy emotional and physical development. During adolescence, the body undergoes significant developmental changes involving puberty, bodily changes of sexual maturation, and the formation of sexual identity. The reproductive and health needs of adolescents differ from those of adults. Achieving sexual health involves more than preventing unplanned pregnancies and sexually transmitted infections. It includes developing the ability to form and maintain meaningful relationships with others and with one's own body. During this period of forming one's sexual identity, adolescents can experiment sexually with people of the same sex.

Experimenting with or thinking about people of the same sex may cause concerns and anxiety regarding their sexual orientation. These feelings and behaviors do not necessarily mean an individual is homosexual or bisexual. Despite increased knowledge and information available to adolescents, gay, lesbian, and bisexual youths still have many concerns. These concerns include feeling different from peers; worrying about AIDS, HIV infection, and other sexually transmitted diseases; and being rejected and harassed by others. For an adolescent discovering their sexual orientation, a correctional facility can be a frightening and dangerous place. Enforcing provisions of the Prison Rape Elimination Act offers added protection to the incarcerated adolescent. Gay, lesbian, and bisexual youth account for a significant number of deaths by suicide during adolescence (AACAP, 2006).

Cervical Cancer

About 35% of 14–19-year olds have tested positive for high-risk human papillomavirus (HPV), a virus linked to cervical cancer in women, usually over 30 (Schwartz, 2010). HPV is the most common sexually transmitted infection in the United States and usually shows few symptoms. Over time, dysplasia of the cervical tissue can develop in young women who have high-risk HPV. The early onset and increased sexual activity among incarcerated youth suggests a higher level of HPV virus in this population. Cervical cytology is generally not recommended for young women under 21 years of age, regardless of the age of onset of sexual activity, because most acquired HPV infections are in the low-risk category, and will resolve over several years without medical intervention (ACOG, 2010). Therefore, cervical cancer prevention through HPV vaccination of both sexes should be a priority.

Nursing Management. Cervical cancer, itself, is quite rare in the adolescent population. However, awareness of the risk factors of early onset sexual activity, multiple partners, lack of condom use, and development of HPV, which can cause cervical changes leading over time to cervical cancer, can be helpful for young sexually active women.

More important for this patient population is encouragement to obtain the HPV vaccination to decrease chances of cervical cancer. Correctional nurses have the opportunity to improve future health of juvenile females who are less likely to be in contact with the health care system.

The majority of states offer HPV vaccination to female juveniles in their care (Henderson, Rich, & Lally, 2010). If your facility does not offer this service to both female and male adolescents, consider pursuing approval. Vaccination during incarceration improves public health and provides protection for this vulnerable population.

Patient Education. Include information about HPV virus and vaccination opportunity with other sexually transmitted infection education. Adolescents are less future focused than adults and may not consider the risk of contracting HPV in the future.

Testicular Cancer

The lifetime chances for testicular cancer are 1 in 270 men. Fortunately, with effective treatment options, the risk of dying from this cancer is low (American Cancer Society, 2011). Still, testicular cancer is the most common form of cancer for 15- to 35-year-old men (PubMed Health, 2011). This cancer is more prevalent in White males, although Hispanic males have a moderate risk (National Cancer Institute, 2011). Correctional nurses who care for adolescents should have an understanding of testicular cancer symptoms and screening.

Nursing Management. Rather than screening all young men for testicular cancer, current recommendations are for this cancer to be considered in a differential diagnosis of pain, swelling, lumps in the testes, or fullness/heaviness in the scrotum. The U.S. Preventive Services Task Force has recommended against screening asymptomatic men for testicular cancer as it has not provided added benefit over detection through symptomatic evaluation (Lin & Sharangpani, 2010). Include questions about pain, swelling, or testicular lumps in the health assessment and document any physical findings for follow-up with a physician.

Patient Education. As with other important health information, detention is an opportunity to improve young male's understanding of health practices and body functioning. Provide information about testicular cancer and the need for self-examination. Encourage young men to seek medical attention for pain, swelling, or lumps in the genital area.

Pregnancy

Incarcerated youths have higher pregnancy rates than the general public. The Survey of Youth in Residential Placement (SYRP) found that 12% of incarcerated youth are expecting a child (combined male and female; Sedlak & Bruce, 2010). At least 2.1% of incarcerated female youth are pregnant in the juvenile justice system (Committee on Adolescence, 2011). Unhealthy lifestyles, use of tobacco, alcohol, and drugs, along with missing prenatal care, can render these adolescent pregnancies at high risk (NCCHC, 2011a). Specialized obstetric services and close medical management are warranted.

Nursing Management. As with adult pregnancy (see Chapter 9), pregnant adolescents should have regular prenatal obstetric visits. These will, most likely, require outside specialty visits. An agreement with a local obstetric service that provides a community adolescent service is ideal. Establish a strong communication system with this service and the labor/delivery unit of a community hospital.

One area of assistance correctional nurses can provide is helping the adolescent identify antenatal options for themselves and the baby. Most juvenile centers do not have live-in options for children (Committee on Adolescents, 2011). The youth will need to determine the best placement for their baby. Work with in-house social services to develop a listing of local options for support services.

Adolescent pregnancy includes additional concerns for mother and child. With the mother still growing herself, the stress of pregnancy can increase the likelihood of several conditions. Correctional nurses should, in particular, keep the following conditions in mind when assessing pregnant youth.

Anemia: Iron-deficiency anemia is a concern in all pregnancies but is a frequent outcome for pregnant adolescents. Both adolescence and pregnancy are risk factors for the condition (AHRQ, 2006). Assessment findings for anemia include fatigue, weakness, susceptibility to infection, and skin pallor. Vital signs may show tachycardia (Ricci, 2009). Laboratory testing will reveal any iron deficits. Iron supplementation is advised for anemia and this substance is a part of most prenatal vitamin combinations. Iron supplementation should be taken between meals and not with substances that interfere with absorption, such as tea, coffee, chocolate, or high-fiber items (Ricci, 2009).

Pre-eclampsia: Pre-eclampsia is a condition manifested by hypertension and proteinuria. Left untreated, it progresses to eclampsia with grand mal seizures and high mother and infant mortality (Ricci, 2009). Adolescence is a risk factor for pre-eclampsia (Ross, 2011). Progressive blood pressure readings and urine analysis for protein should be taken at each prenatal check-up. Pre-eclampsia is diagnosed at blood pressures greater than 140/90 and more than 1+ protein in a random dip stick urine sample (Ricci, 2009).

Pregnancy psychoses: Incarcerated youth have significant risk factors for initiation or exacerbation of mental illness during pregnancy and the postpartum period. Risk factors for peri-pregnancy mental illness include low socioeconomic status, lack of social support, unwanted pregnancy, and substance abuse. Higher rates of pregnancy mental health issues occur among African Americans and low-income Latinas (NIHCM, 2010).

Correctional nurses should be on special alert for increased symptoms of mental instability during and after pregnancy. Physical, emotional, and academic demands during the adolescent years contribute to vulnerability for youthful mothers (Yozwiak, 2010). Vigilant nursing care can intervene to provide additional support through referral to mental health and social services. Educating youth workers and security staff to the special needs of this population can also be helpful.

Low birth weight/premature birth: Adolescent pregnancy increases the risk of adverse birth outcomes such as low birth weight and premature birth (Chen et al., 2007). Although early research suggested that these outcomes were related to low socioeconomic status, inadequate prenatal care, and inadequate weight gain during pregnancy, these factors no longer seem to vary the outcome. Correctional nurses should consider all pregnant adolescents at risk for premature birth and low-birth-weight infants. Early preparations for delivery should be made. All staff members should be alert for initiation of labor in order to facilitate rapid transport to a local acute care setting.

Patient Education. Pregnant youth require special understanding, medical care, and education, particularly about nutrition, substance abuse, infections, and complications of pregnancy. In addition, they need to know how alcohol, tobacco, and other drugs affect their developing fetus. The American College of Obstetrics and Gynecology has patient teaching resources, including a Frequently Asked Questions guide, found at http://www.acog.org/~/media/For%20Patients/faq103.ashx. Nutrition education is of particular importance. Pregnant adolescents prone to anemia need guidance in selecting iron-rich foods such as meat, eggs, fish, poultry, green leafy vegetables, dried fruits, and peanut butter (Ricci, 2009). One in six pregnant adolescents will become pregnant again in the next year. This is an excellent time to teach pregnancy prevention, contraception, and decision-making skills about high-risk sexual situations (Ricci, 2009). Case Example 11.1 applies information from this section.

CASE EXAMPLE 11.1

Medical is notified of an incoming 15-year-old youth claiming to be 5 months pregnant. Due to her uncooperative and assaultive behavior during arrest, she arrives in handcuffs attached to a belly belt. Her charges are drug related and she appears under the influence of an unknown substance. What information will you gather during assessment and what are the important elements in a plan of care for this patient?

Sexually Transmitted Infection

Although adolescents (aged 15–24) make up only 25% of those sexually active, they acquire nearly half of all new sexually transmitted infections (STIs; CDC, 2009b). In addition, higher rates of chlamydia, gonorrhea, and syphilis exist among those admitted to juvenile correctional facilities than the general population (CDC, 2009c). Correctional nurses have an opportunity to positively affect youth sexual health while they are detained.

Nursing Management

The key to STI treatment is early detection. Intake processes should routinely screen for chlamydia and gonorrhea. CDC (2010a, 2010b, 2010c) recommendations include routine chlamydia and gonorrhea screening in juvenile detention facilities. Syphilis screening should be governed by local and institutional prevalence (CDC, 2010c). In addition, the advent of rapid oral HIV testing makes providing an opt-out HIV evaluation a logical part of routine health care as recommended by the CDC (Branson et al., 2006). Standard STI treatment involves antibiotic therapy. Stock supply of commonly ordered STI treatment antibiotics should be maintained based on frequency of use in the facility population.

Patient Education

Left untreated, STIs can lead to pelvic inflammatory disease and infertility in women. Use time in detention as an opportunity to dispel myths about STI transmission, treatment, and outcomes. Appropriate teaching materials can be obtained from the CDC at http://www.cdc.gov/std/general/. This is also a good time to discuss risky sexual behaviors and healthy habits.

COMMON MENTAL HEALTH ISSUES OF THE JUVENILE OFFENDER

Youth in the juvenile justice system have much higher rates of mental disorders than the general adolescent population. Prevalence rates vary greatly depending on the sample population, but anywhere from 50% to 100% of youth offenders have mental health or disruptive behavioral issues (Committee on Adolescence, 2011). Youth with mental disorders are found to engage in activities leading to criminal sentencing (Grisso, 2008). Correctional nurses working with this population need to understand key mental health issues and recognize behaviors that may signal a change in their mental health status in order to provide holistic care.

Behavior Management Issues

Behavior management in correctional settings can become punitive and focus on institutional goals rather than the needs of the disruptive youth (Cohen et al., 2006). Behavioral problems can arise from underlying psychosocial issues such as feelings of isolation, sadness, anger, and loss. A unified approach to behavioral issues is recommended.

Treatment of juvenile mental health disorders includes medication, psychotherapy, and psychosocial interventions. Cognitive-behavioral therapy (CBT) has shown some effectiveness in reducing future delinquency and has specifically shown results in adolescents with anxiety disorders or depression (Grisso, 2008; Weersing, Iyengar, Koloko, Birmaher, & Brent, 2006). CBT involves instruction on problem solving, non-aggressive responses, and awareness of social cues. Correctional nurses should have a full understanding of the anticipated CBT effects in order to support and model them during health care interactions.

Crisis Management

Emotional crises and aggression are common among incarcerated youth. Use of de-escalation techniques during these times has proven successful (Royal College of Nursing, 2006). Many juvenile detention programs include crisis management training for staff members. Correctional nurses should be trained in crisis management techniques used by facility staff and know the mechanisms to summon additional support when initial efforts to de-escalate a situation are unsuccessful.

Disordered Eating

Correctional nurses need to know the warning signs for anorexia nervosa and bulimia. The presentation of anorexia and bulimia is most often seen in adolescent females. Only about 10% of male adolescents present with a disordered eating problem. Anorexia nervosa is a chronic debilitating psychiatric illness in which the adolescent demonstrates an altered eating pattern and subsequent weight loss; it is a complicated mixture of physical, psychological, and emotional changes. A desire to control is an underlying component of anorexia nervosa, often beginning with a stressful event. The stress and unknown aspects of incarceration can push an adolescent into this eating disorder.

Bulimia nervosa is defined by two particular behaviors: binge eating and purging. Purging behavior can be from self-induced vomiting; or the misuse of laxatives, enemas, diuretics, and rectal suppositories. The use of excessive exercising and appetite suppressants often compensate for the binging in an effort to prevent weight gain and gain mastery over their life situations.

Treatment for eating disorders requires a team approach, including individual counseling, family counseling, working with a nutritionist or the primary care physician, and sometimes medication. Further treatment considerations can be found in Chapter 9, Women's Health Care.

Adolescent Suicide and Self-Harm

Suicide is the leading cause of death for confined youth (Committee on Adolescence, 2011). Many factors contribute to this finding, including high rates of mental disorders, emotional abuse, substance abuse, and prior suicidal behavior (Hayes, 2009). A strong suicide prevention program should be in place in all juvenile confinement programs. Unlike the adult population, youth are less likely to attempt suicide in the first 24 hours of detainment (NCCHC, 2007). However, a strong suicide screening tool should be in place to identify suicidality and begin intervention at the start of confinement. A mechanism for continued risk assessment is needed, as vigilance is necessary throughout detainment. Precipitating factors that may indicate an increased suicide risk include perceived parental abandonment, recent family member death, fear of transfer or placement, failure in a program, and recent suicide in the facility (Committee on Adolescence, 2011). With an understanding of potential causes of suicide attempts in detained youth, correctional nurses can assist in preventing adolescent suicide.

The most frequent method of juvenile suicide in confinement is hanging (Cohen, Burd, & Beyer, 2006). Correctional nurses should be prepared to provide care to hanging victims. A universal tool for cutting through the ligature to release the patient should be readily available to all staff members. Full resuscitation efforts should be initiated even if the juvenile appears lifeless.

Suicide is one form of self-harm frequently attempted by juveniles. Other self-harm actions can include nonlethal actions such as cutting and burning. Some suggest that deliberate nonlethal self-harm is a coping mechanism to deal with psychiatric distress while avoiding suicide (Mangnall & Yurkovich, 2008). Whatever the cause, self-harm actions are frequent in adolescent and college-age populations, with estimates of up to 40% (Thomas, Leaf, Kazmierczak, & Stone, 2006). Self-harm has been linked to other addictive behaviors such as drug and alcohol use. The behavior is challenging to treat and requires a multifaceted approach. Correctional nurses must deal with deliberate self-injury in an open and nonjudgmental fashion. Further information on this phenomenon can be found in Chapters 9 and 12, Women's Health Care and Mental Health, respectively. Case Example 11.2 applies information from this section.

SPECIAL JUVENILE ISSUES
Parental Consent in the Treatment of Minors

Consent for treatment of minors is of concern in juvenile health care. Laws vary among jurisdictions; therefore, correctional nurses must investigate and understand

CASE EXAMPLE 11.2

A 14-year-old male, first-time offender, with sexual assault and drug charges is detained while awaiting trial. During the first 3 months, he seems to be adjusting to confinement. Due to a disruption in school, he is sent to his room for a "time out." During the routine 15-minute room checks, he is found trying to hang himself with his T-shirt tied tightly around his neck. What red flags placed this youth at increased risk for suicidal behavior?

the legal framework in which they practice in order to know their responsibilities for informed consent in various patient situations. Generally, a juvenile's legal guardian, whether parent, court-appointed guardian, or the facility superintendent, should be informed of significant changes in health status. In addition, even when a blanket consent to treat is obtained upon admission, invasive procedures require prior written consent (NCCHC, 2011a). The juvenile's informed consent is generally required unless the treatment is of immediate necessity for patient safety, the patient does not have the capacity to understand, or the treatment is a public health concern (NCCHC, 2011a). The legal guardianship of a juvenile may change based on their placement in the legal process. For example, parental consent may be necessary when providing health care to minors in a detention facility but the court may grant primary custody to a confinement facility authority or probation officer after sentencing (Gudeman, 2009).

The Juvenile Offender in an Adult Facility

Criminal laws regarding juvenile offenses vary greatly among states. Correctional nurses working with juveniles must have a working knowledge of the juvenile justice system in the jurisdiction of care delivery to provide prudent care. An investigation of varying practices revealed that 22 states and the District of Columbia allow children as young as 7 to be tried as adults and incarcerated in adult facilities (Deitch, 2009). Social pressure and public outcry are moving states to change laws to detain these young offenders in juvenile facilities to better meet their physical, mental, psychosocial, and safety needs (Arya, 2011). Juveniles under 18 years of age end up living in adult facilities due to several reasons, including detainment for hearing, prior offenses or transfer, and waiver provisions based on the type of crime (Arya, 2011).

No matter what the reason for adult facility placement, youth in these facilities are highly vulnerable to violence, rape, and victimization (Deitch, 2009). In addition, the special health needs of juveniles may be overlooked in the course of providing a variety of health services to the primary adult population. Correctional nurses working in facilities housing juveniles should take into account the special needs of this population in delivering care services.

SUMMARY

Caring for juvenile offenders requires specialized knowledge of the physiologic, psychological, and social development issues of this age group. Risky behaviors common to this patient population lead to increased degrees of sexually transmitted infections, drug and alcohol withdrawal issues, and dental problems. Correctional nurses have great opportunity to improve the health of detained youth through healthy lifestyle education, treatment of acute conditions, and establishing connection with support services.

DISCUSSION QUESTIONS

1. Describe the physiologic, psychological, and social development issues correctional nurses need to take into account when providing care to juvenile offenders.
2. What are the most common substances abused by youth at your facility? How does the intake screening take these into account?
3. What are the most frequent chronic conditions treated at your facility? How does this compare with conditions discussed in this chapter?
4. Outline the healthy living elements of a youth education program. How does this compare with what is currently taught at your facility?
5. What behavior modification principles are used by youth workers at your facility? Do nursing staff also use them?
6. If you are working in an adult facility that houses adolescent offenders, how are their physical and psychological needs met? Identify at least three concerns that require addressing when organizing health care for juveniles in an adult facility.

REFERENCES

Agency for Healthcare Research and Quality. (2006). *Screening for iron deficient anemia.* Retrieved from http://www.uspreventiveservicestaskforce.org/uspstf06/ironsc/ironscrev.pdf

American Academy of Child and Adolescent Psychology (AACAP). (2006). *Facts for families: Gay and lesbian adolescents. No. 63.* Retrieved from http://www.aacap.org/galleries/FactsForFamilies/63_gay_and_lesbian_adolescents.pdf

American Academy of Pediatric Dentistry. (2010). *Guidelines on adolescent oral health care.* Retrieved from http://www.aapd.org/media/policies_guidelines/g_adoleshealth.pdf

American Academy of Pediatric Dentistry. (2011). *Policy on intraoral/perioral piercings and oral jewelry/accessories. Oral health policies.* Retrieved from http://www.aapd.org/media/policies_guidelines/p_pierce.pdf

American Academy of Periodontology. (2004). *Periodontal diseases of children and adolescents. Reference Manual. 33*(6). Retrieved from http://www.aapd.org/media/Policies_Guidelines/E_PeriodontalDisease.pdf

American Cancer Society. (2010). *Child and youth tobacco use: Understanding the problem.* Retrieved from http://www.cancer.org/Cancer/CancerCauses/TobaccoCancer/ChildandYouthTobacco-Use/ child-and-youth-tobacco-use-facts-and-stats

American Cancer Society. (2011). *Testicular cancer overview.* Retrieved from http://www.cancer.org/Cancer/TesticularCancer/OverviewGuide/testicular-cancer-overview-key-statistics

American College of Obstetricians and Gynecologists (ACOG). (2010). *Committee on adolescent health care opinion: Cervical cancer in adolescents: Screening, evaluation, and management.* Retrieved from http://www.acog.org/~/media/Committee%20Opinions/Committee%20on%20Adolescent%20Health%20Care/co463.ashx?dmc=1&ts=20111207T0906269160

American Dental Association (ADA). (2004). *Oral health topics: Oral piercing.* Retrieved from http://www.ada.org/3090.aspx

American Lung Association. (2011). *Trends in asthma morbidity and mortality.* Retrieved from http://www.lungusa.org/finding-cures/our-research/trend-reports/asthma-trend-report.pdf

Arya, N. (2011). *State trends: Legislative changes from 2005 to 2010 removing youth from the adult.* Retrieved from http://www.campaignforyouthjustice.org/documents/CFYJ_State_Trends_Report.pdf

Ball, J. W., Bindler, R. C., & Cowen, K. J. (2010). *Clinical handbook child health nursing: Partnering with children & families* (2nd ed.). Upper Saddle River, NJ: Pearson Education.

Bolin, K, & Jones, D. (2006). Oral health needs of adolescents in a juvenile detention facility. *Journal of Adolescent Health, 38*(6), 755–757.

Branson, B. M., Hansfield, H. H., Lampe, M. A., Janssen, R. S., Taylor, A. W., & Lyss, S. B. et al., (2006). Centers for disease control and prevention revised recommendations for HIV testing of adults, adolescents, and pregnant women in health-care settings. *MMWR Recommendations and Reports, 55*(RR-14), 1–17. Retrieved from http://www.cdc.gov/mmwr/preview/mmwrhtml/rr5514a1.htm

Caporino, N., Murray, L., & Jensen, P. (2003). Impact of different traumatic experiences in childhood and adolescence. *Emotion Behavior Disorder Youth,* (Summer), 63–64, 73–76.

Centers for Disease Control and Prevention. (2009a). *Oral sex and HIV risk.* Retrieved from http://www.cdc.gov/hiv/resources/factsheets/pdf/oralsex.pdf

Centers for Disease Control and Prevention (CDC). (2009b). *STDs in adolescents and young adults.* Retrieved from http://www.cdc.gov/std/stats09/adol.htm

Centers for Disease Control and Prevention (CDC). (2009c). *STDs in persons entering corrections facilities.* Retrieved from http://www.cdc.gov/std/stats09/corrections.htm

Centers for Disease Control and Prevention (CDC). (2010a). Tobacco use among middle and high school students—United States, 2000—2009. *Morbidity and Mortality Weekly Report (MMWR), 59*(33), 1063–1068. Retrieved from http://www.cdc.gov/mmwr/preview/mmwrhtml/mm5933a2.htm

Centers for Disease Control and Prevention (CDC). (2010b). Youth risk behavior surveillance—United States, 2009. *Morbidity and Mortality Weekly Report, 59*(SS-5), 1–36. Retrieved from http://www.cdc.gov/mmwr/pdf/ss/ss5905.pdf

Centers for Disease Control and Prevention (CDC). (2010c). *Sexually transmitted diseases treatment guidelines, 2010: Special populations.* Retrieved from http://www.cdc.gov/std/treatment/2010/specialpops.htm

Centers for Disease Control and Prevention (CDC). (2011). *Physical activity for everyone: How much exercise do children need?* Retrieved from http://www.cdc.gov/physicalactivity/everyone/guidelines/children.html

Chassin, L. (2008). Juvenile justice and substance use. *The Future of Children, 18*(2), 165–183.

Chen, X. K., Wen, S. W., Fleming, N., Demissie, K., Rhoads, G. G., & Walker, M. (2007). Teenage pregnancy and adverse birth outcomes: A large population based retrospective cohort study. *International Journal of Epidemiology, 36*(2), 368–373.

Cohen, M. D., Burd, L., & Beyer, M. (2006). Health services for youth in juvenile justice programs. In M. Puisis (Ed.), *Clinical practice in correctional medicine* (2nd ed.). Philadelphia: Mosby Elsevier.

Committee on Adolescence. (2011). American Academy of Pediatrics policy statement: Health care for youth in the juvenile justice system. *Pediatrics, 128*(6), 1219–1235. Retrieved from http://pediatrics.aappublications.org/content/128/6/1219.full.pdf+html

Committee on Adolescents. (2011). Policy Statement: Health care for youth in the juvenile justice system. *Pediatrics, 128*(6), 1219–1235.

Deitch, M. (2009). *From time out to hard time: Young children in the adult criminal justice system.* Austin, TX: The University of Texas at Austin, LBJ School of Public Affairs. Retrieved from http://www.utexas.edu/lbj/archive/news/images/file/From%20Time%20Out%20to%20Hard%20Time-revised%20final.pdf

Elkington, K. S., Teplin, L. A., Mericle, A. A., Welty, L. J., Romero, E. G., & Abram, K. M. (2008). HIV/sexually transmitted infection risk behaviors in delinquent youth with psychiatric disorders: A longitudinal study. *Journal of the American Academy of Child Adolescent Psychiatry, 47*(8), 901–911. Retrieved from http://www.ncbi.nlm.nih.gov/pmc/articles/PMC2754224/pdf/nihms129073.pdf

Ford, J. D. (2005). Treatment implications of altered neurobiology, affects regulation and information processing following child maltreatment. *Psychiatry Ann, 35,* 410–419.

Ford, J. D., Chapman, J. R., Hawke, J., & Albert, D. (2007). *Trauma among youth in the juvenile justice system: Critical issues and new directions. Research and program brief.* National Center for Mental Health and Juvenile Justice. Retrieved from http://www.ncmhjj.com/pdfs/Trauma_and_Youth.pdf

Frincu-Mallos, C. (2010). Psychotropic medications linked to increased rates of obesity. *Medscape Medical News.* Retrieved from http://www.medscape.com/viewarticle/718087

Griel, L. C., & Loeb, S. J. (2009). Health issues faced by adolescents incarcerated in the juvenile justice system. *Journal of Forensic Nursing, 5,* 162–179.

Grisso, T. (2008). Adolescent offenders with mental disorders. The future of children. *Juvenile Justice, 18*(2), 143–164.

Gudeman, R. (2009). Consent to medical treatment for youth in the juvenile justice system: California law: A guide for health care providers. *National Center for Youth Law/Youth Health Rights Initiative.* Retrieved from http://www.youthlaw.org/fileadmin/youthhealth/youthhealthrights/ca/Juv._Justice_Consent_Manual_11-09.pdf

Harvey, S. B., Hotopf, M., Overland, S., & Mykletun, A. (2010). Physical activity and common mental disorders. *The British Journal of Psychiatry, 197,* 357–364. Retrieved from http://bjp.rcpsych.org/content/197/5/357.full.pdf

Hayes, L. M. (2009). Characteristics of juvenile suicide in confinement. *Juvenile Justice Bulletin,* February.

Henderson, C., Rich, J., & Lally, M. (2010). HPV vaccination practices among juvenile justice facilities in the United States. *Journal of Adolescent Health, 46*(5), 495–498.

Hockenberry, M. (2011). Communication and physical assessment of the child. In M. Hockenberry, & D. Wilson (Eds.), *Wong's nursing care of infants and children* (9th ed.). St. Louis, MO: Elsevier/Mosby.

Janssen, K. M., & Cooper, B. R. (2008). Oral piercing: An overview. *The Internet Journal of Allied Health Science and Practice, 6*(3), 1–3. Retrieved from http://ijahsp.nova.edu/articles/vol6num3/pdf/cooper.pdf

Kessler, C. (2002). Need for attention to mental health of young offenders. *Lancet, 359,* 1956–1957.

Lin, K., & Sharangpani, R. (2010). Screening for testicular cancer: An evidence review for the U.S. prevention services task force. *Annals of Internal Medicine, 153*(6), 396–399. Retrieved from http://www.annals.org/content/153/6/396.full.pdf

Mangnall, J., & Yurkovich, E. (2008). A literature review of deliberate self-harm. *Perspectives in Psychiatric Care, 44*(30), 175–184.

Mulvey, E. P., Schubert, C. A., & Chung, H. L. (2007). Service use after court involvement in a sample of serious adolescent offenders. *Children and Youth Services Review, 29*(4), 518–544.

National Association of School Psychologist. (2004). *Position statement on students with emotional and behavioral disorders.* Retrieved January 18, 2011, from http://www.ici.umn.edu/products/impact/182/over.html

National Cancer Institute. (2011). *SEER state fact sheet: Testis.* Retrieved from http://seer.cancer.gov/statfacts/html/testis.html

National Child Traumatic Stress Network. (2008). *Child welfare trauma training toolkit.* Retrieved January 19, 2011, from http://www.nctsnet.org.nccts/asset.do?id=1340

National Commission on Correctional Health Care (NCCHC). (2007). *Position statement: Prevention of Juvenile suicide in correctional settings.* Retrieved from http://www.ncchc.org/resources/statements/juvenile_suicide.html

National Commission on Correctional Health Care (NCCHC). (2011a). *Standards for health services in juvenile detention and confinement facilities.* Chicago, IL: Author.

National Commission on Correctional Health Care (NCCHC). (2011b). *Guidelines for disease management in correctional settings: Adolescent asthma.* Retrieved from http://www.ncchc.org/resources/guidelines/Adolescent_Asthma2011.pdf

National Institute for Health Care Management (NIHCM). (2010). *Identifying and treating maternal depression: Strategies & considerations for health plans.* Retrieved from http://nihcm.org/pdf/FINAL_MaternalDepression6-7.pdf

OJJP. (2006). *Office of Juvenile Justice and Delinquency statistical briefing book.* Retrieved from http://www.ojjdp.gov/ojstatbb/corrections/qa08201.asp?qaDate = 2006

Ogden, C. L., Carroll, M. D., Curtin, L. R., Lamb, M. M., & Flegal, K. M. (2010). Prevalence of high body mass index in US children and adolescents, 2007–2008. *Journal of the American Medical Association, 303,* 242–249

PubMed Health. (2011). *Testicular cancer: Causes, incidence and risk.* Retrieved from http://www.ncbi.nlm.nih.gov/pubmedhealth/PMH0002266/

Quinn, M. M., Rutherford, R. B., Leone, P. E., Osher, D. M., & Poirier, J. M. (2005). Youth with disabilities in juvenile corrections: A national survey. *Exceptional Children, 71,* 339–345.

Ricci, S. S. (2009). *Essentials of maternity, newborn, and women's health nursing* (2nd ed.). Philadelphia: Wolters Kluwer/Lippincott Williams & Wilkins.

Ross, M. G. (2011). *Eclampsia.* Retrieved from http://emedicine.medscape.com/article/253960-overview#a1

Royal College of Nursing. (2006). Violence clinical practice guidelines: The short-term management of disturbed/violent behaviour in in-patient psychiatric settings and emergency departments. London: Royal College of Nursing. Retrieved from http://www.rcn.org.uk/__data/assets/pdf_file/0018/109800/003017.pdf

Sadof, M., & Kaslovsky, R. (2011). Adolescent asthma: A developmental approach. *Current Opinion in Pediatrics, 23,* 373–378. Retrieved from http://www.medicalhomeinfo.org/downloads/pdfs/MHCCPA-Sadof.Kaslovsky_AdolescentAsthma.pdf

Saewyc, E. M. (2011). Health promotion of the adolescent and family. In M. J. Hockenberry & D. Wilson (Eds.), *Wong's nursing care of infants and children* (9th ed.). St. Louis, MO: Elsevier Mosby.

Sedlak, A. J., & McPherson, K. (2010). Survey of youth in residential placement: Youth's needs and services. SYRP Report. Rockville, MD: Westat.

Schwartz, S. (2010). *Adolescent reproductive and sexual health. Fact for policymakers.* National Center for Children in Poverty. Retrieved from http://www.nccp.org/publications/pdf/text_931.pdf

Schnittker, J., & John, A. (2007). Enduring stigma: The long-term effects of incarceration on health. *Journal of Health and Social Behavior, 48,* 16.

Sedlak, A. J., & Bruce, C. (2010). Youth's characteristics and backgrounds. *Juvenile Justice Bulletin,* NCJ227730. Retrieved from https://www.ncjrs.gov/pdffiles1/ojjdp/227730.pdf

Spano, S. (2004). *Research facts and findings: Stages of adolescent development.* Ithaca, NY: Cornell University Family Life Development Center. Retrieved from http://www.actforyouth.net/resources/rf/rf_stages_0504.pdf

Sullivan, C. J., & Hamilton, Z. K. (2007). Exploring careers in deviance: A joint trajectory analysis of criminal behavior and substance use in an offender population. *Deviant Behavior, 28,* 497–523.

Thomas, J., Leaf, M., Kazmierczak, S., & Stone, J. (2006). Self-injury in correctional settings: "Pathology" of prisons or of prisoners? *Criminology and Public Policy, 5*(1), 193–202.

U.S. Department of Agriculture. (2010). *Report of the Dietary Guidelines Advisory Committee on the dietary guidelines for Americans, 2010.* Retrieved from http://www.cnpp.usda.gov/DGAs2010-DGACReport.htm

U.S. Department of Agriculture, U.S. Department of Health, Human Services. (2010). *Dietary guidelines for Americans, 2010* (7th ed.). Washington, DC: U.S. Government Printing Office. Retrieved from http://www.health.gov/dietaryguidelines/dga2010/DietaryGuidelines2010.pdf

United States Environmental Protection Agency (EPA). (2011). *Asthma fact sheet.* Retrieved from http://www.epa.gov/asthma/pdfs/asthma_fact_sheet_en.pdf

Weersing, V. R., Iyengar, S., Koloko, D. J., Birmaher, B., & Brent, D. A. (2006). Effectiveness of cognitive-behavioral therapy for adolescent depression: A benchmarking investigation. *Behavioral Therapy, 37,* 36–48.

Wilson, D., & Curry, M. (2011). The child with musculoskeletal or articular dysfunction. In M. Hockenberry, & D. Wilson (Eds.), *Wong's Nursing Care of Infants and Children* (9th ed.). St. Louis, MO: Elsevier/Mosby.

Yozwiak, J. A. (2010). Depression and adolescent mothers: A review of assessment and treatment approaches. *Journal of Pediatric and Adolescent Gynecology, 23*(3), 172–178.

TWELVE

Mental Health

Rosanne E. Harmon

P risons, jails, and detention facilities house 3 times more mentally ill individuals than all in-patient psychiatric facilities in the United States (Torrey, Kennard, Eslinger, Lamb, & Pavle, 2010). Nursing assessment in the correctional setting considers the patient's mental status, as well as potential for suicide, harm to self and/or others, assault, and abuse. Indications and timeframes for referral to mental health providers are reviewed, as well as the nurses' role in patient safety during suicide watch, seclusion, and restraint. Other aspects of nursing practice that contribute to mental health treatment include patient education, symptom counseling, honoring informed consent and refusal, and assisting the patient with medication adherence.

MENTAL ILLNESS IN CORRECTIONAL SETTINGS
Incidence and Trends

Over the last 20 years, the number of mentally ill entering the criminal justice system has risen to the extent that more than half of all inmates have mental health issues (Glaze & James, 2006). In this same timeframe, the percentage of mentally ill inmates has tripled. Forty percent of individuals with serious mental illness have been in jail or prison, and correctional institutions have become the new mental hospitals in almost all communities (Torrey et al., 2010).

According to the results of a recent national survey; the mentally ill are more likely to reoffend once released, resulting in high rates of readmission or recidivism. The length of time that mentally ill individuals are incarcerated is typically longer than those who are not mentally ill. The mentally ill are more vulnerable to assault and victimization while incarcerated and, because of common cognitive impairments, are likely to present management problems, resulting in rule infractions and disciplinary issues. Finally, the mentally ill have higher rates of suicide than those who are not (Torrey et al., 2010).

Special Populations

Mental health problems are more common among female inmates than male inmates. The Bureau of Justice (BJS) estimates 60%–75% of female inmates have mental health problems. The BJS data includes substance abuse and so is considered a relatively high estimate; however other published studies have found rates of severe mental illness among women in jails and prisons to be higher than rates for men. In addition to higher incidence of mental illness, women are also more likely to have a co-occurring substance abuse disorder (Cloyes, Wong, Latimer, & Abarca, 2010; Steadman, Osher, Robbins, Case, & Samuels, 2009).

Skowyra and Cocozza (2007) reported that the prevalence of mental disorders among youth in the juvenile justice system is 70%. They also found that more than 60% of these youth also suffer from a co-occurring substance abuse disorder. Finally, from this same report, 20% of these youth experience mental illness so severe that their functional ability is impaired (Skowyra & Cocozza, 2007).

Nurses' Role in Mental Health Care

The availability and complexity of mental health services vary from one correctional facility to another. In some systems, nurses work as part of a mental health team including providers such as advanced practice nurses and psychiatrists, so a basic understanding of the various mental illnesses and how they are treated is adequate. In other systems, more limited access to mental health professionals requires nurses to exercise more judgment in the identification, treatment, and referral of mentally ill persons (Race, Yousefian, Lambert, & Hartley 2010).

It is clear from the high prevalence rates that all nurses working in corrections will care for people who are mentally ill. The American Nurses Association (ANA) acknowledged this as a distinguishing feature of the population served by nurses in the correctional setting when defining the scope and standards of practice for correctional nurses (2007). As much as it is desirable to have mental health professionals available, it is not possible for nurses to avoid treating the mentally ill, no matter how large or small the facility may be. Nurses interact with the mentally ill at intake screening, at sick call, during medication administration, in chronic disease clinics, in emergencies, at "man down" calls, and during rounds in isolated housing or segregation. Every nurse should be competent in basic mental health practice, including distinguishing normal from abnormal thoughts and behavior, communicating respectfully and in a clear and nonthreatening manner, responding appropriately and nonjudgmentally to aberrant behavior, and collaborating with mental health and custody professionals in the interest of the patient's well-being (Smith, 2005). Due to their frequent interactions and assessments, nurses are at the center of the decision tree in determining patient access to mental health services (Smith & Smith, 2006; Tann, 2010).

IDENTIFICATION AND TREATMENT OF MENTAL ILLNESS

The courts have helped define what is considered to be a major or serious mental illness: "A mental health need is 'serious' if it has caused significant disruption in an inmate's everyday life and...prevents his functioning in the general population

TABLE 12.1   Mental Illnesses Encountered in the Correctional Setting

MENTAL HEALTH CONDITION	SPECIFIC CONDITIONS INCLUDED
Psychotic disorders	Hallucinations Delusions Schizophrenia Other thought disorders
Mood disorders	Bipolar disorder Depression
Personality disorder	
Traumatic brain injury (TBI)	
Post Traumatic Stress Disorder (PTSD)	

without disturbing or endangering others or himself" (Rold, 2006, p. 525). Inmates entering the correctional system may have all types of mental health conditions. The most serious conditions that mental health resources focus on in the correctional setting are listed in Table 12.1.

Psychotic Disorders

Psychosis is an abnormal condition of the mind, generally defined as having lost touch with reality. Fifteen percent of prisoners and 24% of jail detainees met the symptom criteria for a diagnosis of psychotic disorder in the most recent BJS report (Glaze & James, 2006). The main symptoms of psychosis are hallucinations, delusions, and thought disturbance. The patient might present with one of these symptoms or any combination of them. Since the presentation can vary widely from person to person, recognizing and describing the symptoms can help identify and determine the cause of the psychosis. When assessing patients who display symptoms of psychosis, the key points are:

■   What is the onset or symptom history?
■   Does delirium better explain the symptoms?

Because psychotic-like symptoms can result from a medical illness or injury (some of these are outlined in Table 12.2), the presence of hallucinations, delusions, or thought disturbance does not necessarily mean that the patient has a mental illness. Nurses may see psychotic symptoms in a patient in medical crisis, such as a high fever or an adverse response to medication. Medical or toxicological reasons for psychosis should always be considered while providing care for a patient presenting with these symptoms. The nurse needs to establish a thorough history of symptoms and conditions from both a psychiatric and a medical perspective—and always consider potential differential diagnoses—before coming to any diagnostic conclusions about the patient. Serious deficits in attention, orientation, and memory suggest delirium or dementia rather than a primary psychotic illness (McLafferty, 2007).

Hallucinations

Hallucinations are sensory perceptions that have been created by the mind. They are seen, heard, or otherwise sensed when not present or actually occurring at the time. The *DSM-IV-TR* defines hallucinations as "a sensory perception that has the

TABLE 12.2   Medical Conditions That Can Cause Mental Status Changes

SOURCE	DISEASES
Cardiopulmonary	Anoxia, congestive heart failure, hypoxia, myocardial infarction, severe hypertension, vasculitis
Chemical/drug exposure	Exposure to lead or mercury; alcohol and illicit substance intoxication or withdrawal
Central Nervous System	Aneurysm, dementia, encephalopathy, head trauma, hydrocephalus, multiple sclerosis, Parkinson's disease, seizure, tumor
Infection	Herpes, HIV, pneumonia, rheumatic fever, sepsis, syphilis, urinary tract infection
Medication	Anticholinergic side effects, neuroleptic malignant syndrome, serotonin syndrome, steroid use, toxic doses/levels of medications
Metabolic/endocrine	Adrenal disease, diabetes, electrolyte imbalance, hepatic disease, hyperglycemia, hypoglycemia, parathyroid disease, porphyria, renal disease, thiamine deficiency, thyroid disease, vitamin B12, deficiency, Wilson disease

Source: From Harmon and Bomberger (2010).

compelling sense of reality of a true perception but that occurs without external stimulation of the relevant sensory organ" (First, 2000).

Auditory hallucinations are reported by 75% of patients diagnosed with schizophrenia but also occur in 10%–15% of those without a psychiatric illness (Nicolson, Mayberg, Pennell, & Nemeroff, 2006). Reports of visual hallucinations in patients with schizophrenia vary widely in the studies and range from 16% to 72%. Visual hallucinations tend to involve vivid scenes with family members, religious figures, and animals (Teeple, Caplan, & Stern, 2009). Visual hallucinations described by people with psychotic disorders are usually of normal-sized people and are seen in color. Reports of seeing shadows, lights, or objects (such as bugs) are usually not associated with a psychotic disorder; these are more likely associated with substance abuse or a neurological disease (Resnick & Knoll, 2005). Olfactory, gustatory, and tactile hallucinations are less common in psychotic disorders and more often related to medical conditions or substance use (Lewandowski, DePaola, Camsari, Cohen, & Ongur, 2009; Urban & Rabe-Jablonska, 2007).

Nurses should note the quality and content of hallucinations described by the patient. Questioning for details and listening to how the hallucinations are reported will help in determining the diagnosis. Documenting the content of hallucinations and presentation of the patient, clearly and objectively, provides valuable information for the mental health professional receiving the referral. The nursing assessment provides information that helps rule out delirium and may lead to identification of a medical cause. Even a schizophrenic patient can present with delirium induced by a medical condition quite separate from the mental illness. Delirium is characterized by an acute onset with an oft-changing course; it affects attention, organization, consciousness, and other aspects of cognition. This speed of onset, impaired cognition, and compromised consciousness is not often seen in psychotic disorders.

Delusions

Delusions are defined in the *DSM-IV-TR* as a "persistent false belief held in the face of strong contradictory evidence" (First, 2000). Delusions can range from the almost plausible to the very bizarre. A common delusion in patients with psychotic disorders is the sense of external forces controlling their feelings, actions, or thoughts. Nurses are advised to avoid directly challenging patients' delusions because the patient will incorporate the challenge and reinforce it into the delusion as described in Case Example 12.1.

CASE EXAMPLE 12.1

An inmate believed that a device had been implanted in his elbow and it was controlled by government officials. The inmate would behave normally until the device was "activated" by government officials; this caused extreme pain at whatever location on his body the device was located. The inmate was so distraught by the pain that correctional staff brought him to the clinic for evaluation. No physical cause for the patient's intermittent complaints of extreme pain could be found. After many visits to the clinic, a physician recommended having a radiograph taken of the patient's elbow as a way of convincing the patient that there was nothing wrong. The patient refused to have the x-ray taken because the device had been moved by the government to avoid detection. The patient also requested copies of his medical record because he believed that government officials modified the content to hide the evidence.

Discussion Questions:

1. What approach will you take with this patient when asked next time to evaluate his complaint of pain?
2. What is a patient care experience you have had with symptoms of hallucination or delusions?
3. What information helped you most in caring for the patient with hallucinations or delusions?

Other Thought Disorders

A thought disorder is a disruption in the form or organization of thinking. Because speech is used to express thought, a patient who is unable to think in logical ways will have abnormal communication. The patient believes that what they are saying makes sense, but actually they are incoherent to others. There are many types of speech and thought patterns that characterize thought disorders; the terminology and description of some of the most common are listed in Table 12.3.

Antipsychotic Medications

Medications used to treat patients diagnosed with psychotic disorders are often referred to as antipsychotics. The "typicals" or "first-generation antipsychotics" include Haldol, Prolixin, and Thorazine. Newer medications (such as Risperdal, Abilify, Geodon, Zyprexa, Seroquel, and Invega) are referred to as "atypicals" or

TABLE 12.3   Common Terms and Descriptions of Symptoms of Thought Disorder

TERM	DESCRIPTION
Blocking	Interruption of train of speech before completion
Circumstantiality	Speech that is highly detailed and much delayed at reaching its goal
Clanging	Excessive rhyming and/or alliteration
Distractible speech	Changing the subject mid-point in response to a stimulus
Echolalia	Echoing own or other's speech. May involve repeating only the last few words or last word of the sentences, may only be once, or may be repetitious
Evasive interaction	Attempts to express ideas and/or feelings are evasive or diluted
Flight of ideas	A sequence of loose associations that moves quickly from one idea to another
Loose associations	Ideas slip off track on to another
Neologism	New word formations
Perseveration	Persistent repetition of words or ideas
Pressured speech	Increase in the amount or rate of speech and/or difficult to interrupt
Tangential	Replies in an oblique, tangential, or irrelevant manner
Word approximations	Words used in a new and unconventional way
Word salad	Words are strung together in an incomprehensible manner

Source: From Tann (2010).

"second-generation antipsychotics." These two classes of medication are chemically different from each other and have different side effects.

The side effects of these antipsychotics can range from mild to life threatening. Preventing or minimizing extrapyramidal symptoms (EPS) is the primary concern with typical or first-generation antipsychotics. Weight gain and other metabolic changes are more common with the atypical or second-generation antipsychotics and increase the patient's risk for diabetes and cardiovascular disease (Ucok & Gaebel, 2008). When starting these medications, emphasizing weight management has shown to be effective in preventing weight gain (Dixon, Perkins, & Calmes, 2009). Weight, body mass index, serum lipids, and fasting glucose should be monitored and patients counseled on diet and exercise.

Side effects that require urgent medical attention are extrapyramidal symptoms (EPS), neuroleptic malignant syndrome (NMS), and tardive dyskinesia (TD).

- EPS includes muscle spasms of the face and neck, restlessness, and Parkinson-like movements. These symptoms are very uncomfortable and stigmatizing. The patient should be referred urgently to the health care provider, who may prescribe a lower dose, switch to another antipsychotic, or add another medication.
- NMS is a rare but significant adverse reaction to antipsychotic medication. It can rapidly progress to a life-threatening condition, and nurses need to be vigilant in identifying its symptoms. Any patient on a neuroleptic medication who presents with an elevated temperature and muscle rigidity, especially when accompanied

by diaphoresis, any change in consciousness, and/or inability to maintain self-care, must be referred to a provider immediately. No further doses of neuroleptic medication should be given until the patient is thoroughly evaluated medically.

■ TD is a debilitating movement disorder characterized by repetitive, involuntary, purposeless movements particularly of the face, mouth, and limbs, although any muscle in the body may be affected. These involuntary movements increase with stress and can impair social relationships. The incidence of TD varies with the type of medication, the dose, and the duration. The first-generation antipsychotics are more likely to cause this disorder. The incidence increases with higher doses. The longer a person is on these medications, the more likely they are to develop TD.

While milder side effects usually dissipate after a few days of initial prescription or dosage increase, often will cause a patient to discontinue the medication. Nurses administering medication and conducting sick call can help patients by identifying side effects, providing information, and supporting adherence. Nurses can also identify when patients need to be referred for provider follow-up to discuss concerns about medication. These steps can greatly influence the patient's adherence and will likely improve the patient's outcome.

The ongoing goals in the care of patients on antipsychotic medications include use of the lowest-possible dose, use of medications with less potential to produce TD, and use of other medications to provide symptom relief. Administration of the Abnormal Involuntary Movement Scale (AIMS) to identify TD symptoms is recommended in the plan of care, usually administered every 3–6 months. Nurses may administer this tool but should have some training from a mental health clinician in the observation and evaluation of movement disturbance seen in persons with TD (Rush, 2000).

Ongoing treatment for patients with psychotic disorders resembles treatment for other chronic medical conditions. Regularly scheduled visits with mental health providers, structured daily activity, supportive lifestyle education, skills training, sheltered living, and work are the other components of ongoing care for these patients. The use of psychotherapy as a way to support the person and manage their chronic illness has also been shown to improve the overall outcome (Dixon et al., 2009; Challoner & Newton, 2010).

Mood Disorders

Mood disorders are pervasive and sustained emotion beyond the normal range of intensity, out of proportion to life circumstances, that interfere with normal daily functioning. The primary categories of mood disorder are bipolar disorder and major depression (First, 2000).

Bipolar Disorder

Bipolar disorder is a brain disorder that causes unusual shifts in mood, energy, activity levels, and ability to carry out day-to-day tasks. Previously, this was known as manic-depressive disorder. Bipolar disorder often develops in the late teens or early adult years. It was once thought rare in youths, but 20% of adults with bipolar disorder began experiencing symptoms during their adolescence (Bernstein, 2010).

In the 2006 BJS report, nearly half of the inmates interviewed reported symptoms meeting the criteria for mania within the last year. While this data should be viewed with caution because substance abuse was not ruled out, it is still significant (Glaze & James, 2006). The overall prevalence of bipolar disorder in the United States is 4.4% (Merikangas et al., 2011). A retrospective review of prisoners incarcerated in Texas over a 6-year period found that inmates with bipolar disorder were 3.3 times more likely to have been incarcerated 4 or more times (Baillargeon, Binswanger, Penn, Williams, & Murray, 2009). The risk of reincarceration was the highest for prisoners with bipolar disorder. Bipolar disorder is not always easy to spot when it starts. The symptoms may seem like separate problems and not be recognized as parts of a larger problem. Some people suffer for years before they are properly diagnosed, with some estimates as long as 10 years (Bowden, 2001).

Treatment for bipolar disorder includes medication and psychotherapy for preventing relapse and reducing symptom severity. The best-known medication for treatment of bipolar disorder is lithium, although anticonvulsants (such as Depakote and Lamictal), the atypical antipsychotics, and antidepressants are also used. Nurses need to be vigilant in observing for toxicity in patients prescribed lithium by routinely monitoring blood levels and watching for the gastrointestinal symptoms of nausea, vomiting, and diarrhea, which can progress to neurological symptoms, including seizures and coma. Because lithium is cleared primarily through the kidneys, anything that influences fluid levels needs to be factored in when assessing patients for side effects. Dehydration from flu, diuretics, or excessive heat can change a normal range blood level to toxic. Nurses need to communicate with housing and work assignment officers to ensure that a patient taking lithium has access to water and is protected from exposure to high temperatures in the housing or work setting. Any inmate taking lithium who seeks medical attention for flu-like symptoms and tremors should be referred immediately for evaluation of lithium toxicity. In making the referral, nurses should report how much lithium the patient is taking, document when the last blood level was assessed (and what that result was), and describe the patient's hydration and neurological status. This information is obtained by interviewing the patient, reviewing the chart, and completing a focused physical assessment.

In addition to pharmacological treatment, psychoeducation may be offered to assist patients with bipolar disorder to identify stresses that may trigger episodes, to develop coping skills, and identify signs that additional assistance is needed to manage risk behaviors or suicidal thoughts.

Depression

The most common psychiatric disorder, depression, continues to be a major cause of illness and disability throughout the world. In the United States, recent samples estimate a lifetime depression prevalence of 16.2%; the prevalence rate for symptoms reported within the last year was 6.6% (Shim, Baltrus, Ye, & Rust, 2011). In the most recent BJS study, 23% of state prisoners and 30% of jail inmates reported symptoms of major depression (Glaze & James, 2006).

Major depressive disorder is characterized by an all-encompassing low mood, accompanied by low self-esteem and the loss of interest or pleasure in normally enjoyable activities. Major depression significantly affects a person's family and personal relationships, work or school life, sleeping and eating habits, and general health. According to the Centers for Disease Control and Prevention (CDC), 80% of persons with depression reported some difficulty in their daily functioning due to symptoms; of these respondents, 35% of men and 22% of women rated their symptoms as severe enough to markedly impair their ability to work, interact with others, or take care of daily household chores (Pratt & Brody, 2008). Depressed people may be preoccupied with or ruminate over thoughts and feelings of worthlessness, inappropriate guilt or regret, helplessness, hopelessness, and self-hatred. In severe cases, depressed people may have symptoms of psychosis (First, 2000). It is not uncommon for the presenting symptom of depression to be increased irritability, anger, or aggression. Separating this from behavioral acting out is a challenge in the correctional setting. Training staff, both security and clinical, to identify and refer any inmate who displays unusual behavior, especially if they have a history of mental health problems, is critical to early diagnosis and treatment of depression.

Treatment for depression in the correctional setting most commonly incorporates medication and psychotherapy. There are several categories of antidepressant medication, including selective serotonin reuptake inhibitors (SSRIs), serotonin norephinephrine reuptake inhibitors (SNRIs), and tricyclics (TCA). Patients should be informed that it may take several weeks before any change in symptoms and 6–12 weeks for the full effect of antidepressant medication to occur. Patients should be encouraged to continue taking the antidepressant even if they are frustrated with the slow pace of improvement. About half of all people prescribed antidepressants will experience side effects; especially in the first week or so. Usually these dissipate in a couple of weeks. Patients should be counseled to talk with their mental health prescriber about the side effects and not to stop taking these medications abruptly since dosages need to be tapered to avoid having an adverse reaction.

People respond differently to the antidepressants, and some will have to try more than one before finding the one that works for them. Adding a second antidepressant, incorporating one of the atypical antipsychotics, or switching to another antidepressant have all been found effective in achieving symptom relief when the original treatment was not effective (Blier, 2005; American Psychiatric Association [APA], 2010).

While medication can reduce the symptoms of depression, psychotherapy will help patients address the problems that the depression causes in their daily lives. Cognitive behavioral therapy helps patients change behavior that contributes to negative thoughts. An example would be learning how to be less sedentary or isolated while experiencing the therapeutic effect of social interaction. Interpersonal psychotherapy helps patients improve relationship skills by focusing on the patient's awareness and understanding of their interaction in relating to others.

Personality Disorders

Personality disorders are pervasive patterns of behavior that often cause serious personal and social difficulties, as well as general functional impairment. They are significant for the enduring and inflexible symptoms over the lifetime. Approximately 1 in 10 people in the United States meet the criteria for personality disorder (Lamont & Brunero, 2009; Lenzenweger, Lane, Loranger, & Kessler, 2007). People with personality disorder are heavy users of health care, mental health, and other social support systems (Vaughn et al., 2010). Many patients with a psychotic or mood disorder have a personality disorder as well (Lamont & Brunero, 2009; Lenzen-weger, 2008).

A large part of the day-to-day interaction that correctional nurses have is with inmates who display suspiciousness, hostility, self-centeredness, and social withdrawal; behavior consistent with personality disorder. In the New York State prison system, a study of patients being treated by mental health clinicians reported that one fifth to one third also had a personality disorder (Rotter, Way, Steinbacher, Sawyer, & Smith, 2002). Similar findings were reported from a study of inmates on mental health caseloads while in prison: 27.4% had a co-occurring personality disorder (Wolff, Maschi, & Bjerkie, 2004). In a study of the prevalence of mental illness among persons admitted to the jail system in Connecticut, 34.6% met criteria for antisocial personality disorder (predominately men), while 12% of men and 23% of women met the criteria for borderline personality disorder (Trestman, Ford, Zhang, & Wiesbrock, 2007).

Individuals with severe, function-impairing personality disorders comprise a large proportion of inmates who are considered by nurses to be "difficult to manage," with their persistent need for attention and high utilization of services. Nurses describe the characteristics of "difficult" patients as those who self-harm, act in violence toward others, sabotage treatment, and are unable to form an alliance or constructive relationship with care providers (Lamont & Brunero, 2009). These inmates are generally viewed as manipulative and problematic, therefore causing great amounts of frustration and anger. Remaining professional and managing the emotional response of staff when working with patients who have personality disorders requires a team effort (Swift, 2009). Nurses should ask for help from mental health staff when responding to patients who are "difficult to manage." Information about the origin and function of the patient's behavior should be provided so that the nurse can develop realistic expectations, ways to manage negative internal thoughts, and retain a therapeutic response to the patient (Bland, Tudor, & Whitehouse, 2007). Nurses who excel in working with patients who have personality disorder are those who apply their experience and knowledge while holding a positive attitude about the patient; they have a moral commitment to patient care, are skilled interpersonally, and can stay rational in the midst of conflict (Talkes & Tennant, 2004).

Psychotherapy is the primary form of treatment for personality disorders. The most common psychotherapy is cognitive behavioral therapy (CBT), which combines both cognitive and behavior therapies to help participants identify unhealthy, negative beliefs and behaviors and replace them with healthy, positive ones. Dialectical behavior therapy (DBT), developed by Marsha Linehan, a psychologist and researcher at the University of Washington, has shown to be effective in treating patients with personality disorder, particularly those with borderline personality disorder, suicidal tendencies, or self-destructive aims (Oldham, 2005). DBT teaches behavioral skills to help tolerate stress, regulate emotions, and improve interpersonal relationships. Shelton, Sampl, Kesten, Zhang, and Trestman (2009) assert that "offenders, with mental health disorders, whether incarcerated or in the community, are at an increased risk for behavior problems that may cause harm to self or others"(p. 788). DBT, when adapted for the correctional setting, can be useful in managing life-threatening and aggressive behaviors (Berzins & Trestman, 2004). Medications from all mental health categories are often prescribed to help manage the affective symptoms of personality disorders such as depression, psychosis, impulsivity, and aggression (Lubit, 2010; Oldham, 2005).

Traumatic Brain Injury

It is estimated that 25%–87% of the inmate population has a history of traumatic brain injury (TBI), compared to 8.5% of people in the free community (CDC, n.d.). The long-term effects of TBI are memory problems, inability to focus, and poor impulse control. These deficits make inmates with TBI more likely to act out in anger or irritation and they are at great risk of forgetting rules of prohibited conduct, not remembering where they should be or by when, forgetting that they cannot go into certain areas, and not following instructions given by correctional officers. Shiroma et al. (2010) note a significant association between inmates with a TBI and increased behavioral infractions. A number of studies link psychiatric disorders to a TBI, including Vaishnavi, Rao, and Fann's (2009) estimate that 40% of those with a TBI have a resulting psychiatric disorder. The psychiatric disorders after a TBI most often reported are depression and anxiety disorders (Slaughter, Fann, & Ehde, 2003).

The cognitive, behavioral, and psychiatric consequences of TBI are a clinical management problem for medical and mental health staff in correctional facilities. It is important to recognize the significant impact that memory challenges, pain, headaches, and concentration have on quality of life for these patients. In the correctional setting, an inmate who has suffered a brain injury may not even be identified as having TBI, especially if the injury was mild. Three quarters of all TBI diagnosed is classified as mild, and those who do not seek treatment go undiagnosed (Curtis, 2010). While recently there has been more emphasis on the identification of inmates with a history of TBI, not everyone is identified.

With such a high percentage of inmates with TBI history, nurses should be vigilant for signs of reduced thinking speed, confusion, reduced concentration and attention, and impaired cognition during the initial health assessment upon admission. The nurse should also look for scars on the face and head, physical disability with coordination or one-sided weakness, and difficulty with speech or following direction. These inmates will often react with anger, aggression, or verbal disrespect to cover their cognitive deficits, as do TBI patients in other settings. In the face of such symptoms, it is reasonable to assume a cognitive impairment of some kind, adjust nursing interactions accordingly, and evaluate the patient's response.

From the Experts ...

"The key to successful nursing care of the patient with a traumatic brain injury is to acknowledge the impact of the injury and then use of tools that mitigate and manage the effect of cognitive deficits."

Barbara B. Curtis, RN, MSN
Olympia, WA

TBI treatment focuses on symptom management and compensation for cognitive deficits. As with other special needs patients, custody staff need to be aware of inmates who have TBI and need to know how to best interact and manage the offender's behavior to help avoid disciplinary infractions. The communication with custody staff also needs to address risks for and management of impulsive behavior,

TABLE 12.4 Strategies for Managing TBI Inmates

SYMPTOM	STRATEGY
Attention deficit	Have inmate repeat instructions back Have the inmate write down the instruction Allow the inmate extra time to complete the task Reduce distractions
Memory deficit	Explain slowly, step by step Put instructions in writing Provide examples, ask inmate to give an example Encourage questions
Slow verbal or physical response	Give directions clearly Repeat directions as necessary Allow additional time to respond
Irritability or anger	Avoid arguing with the inmate Try to rephrase the issue or problem Break the instruction into smaller parts Reinforce positive behavior
Uninhibited or impulsive behavior	Calmly state that the behavior is not acceptable Redirect the inmate Seek advice from mental health professionals

Source: From Curtis (2010).

including violence, sexual activity, and suicide or self-harm. Some examples of suggestions that staff can incorporate into their interactions with inmates who have TBI that help to manage symptoms in the correctional setting are listed in Table 12.4.

Post-traumatic Stress Disorder

Post-traumatic stress disorder (PTSD) is a type of anxiety disorder and can occur after someone goes through a traumatic event like combat, assault, or disaster. Most people after a trauma have some stress reactions. If the reactions an individual experiences remain over a period of time or disrupt daily life, they may be diagnosed with PTSD (First, 2000). The National Center for PTSD recommends that health care providers routinely screen individuals for trauma-related symptoms for the following reasons: prevalence of the disorder, negative effects on health, increased utilization of services, and low self-report of symptoms by patients (Hamblen, 2009). Intrusive memories, avoidance or emotional numbing, and anxiety are the main symptoms. Typical questions for PTSD screening are the following: Have you had nightmares about it or thought about it when you did not want to? Have you tried hard not to think about it or went out of your way to avoid situations that remind you of it? Are you constantly on guard, watchful, or easily startled? Do you feel numb or detached from others, activities, or your surroundings? A "yes" answer to even a couple of these questions should trigger a referral for a mental health evaluation (Prins et al., 2003). Prevalence of PTSD in the incarcerated population is higher than in the general population and women are disproportionately affected (Goff, Rose, Rose, & Purves, 2007). Treatment of PTSD often includes therapy and medication, particularly antidepressants and anxiolytics.

SELF-HARM, SUICIDE, AND DECLINE IN MENTAL STATUS DURING INCARCERATION

In 1969, Elisabeth Kübler-Ross introduced a model for understanding grief associated with death in the book *On Death and Dying* (Kübler-Ross, 1969). Since then, this model has been used to understand the emotional reaction of people experiencing trauma and emotional distress at any time in life. The stages that people experience in preparing for death are denial, anger, bargaining, depression, and acceptance (Kübler-Ross, 2005). Arrest, trial, conviction, and incarceration are traumatic, distressing, and result in loss. Therefore, inmates may express anger, manipulate to achieve secondary gain, and fail to follow through with expectations. It may be helpful to remember that these behaviors can also be part of a grieving cycle. For those inmates who are experiencing grief or adjustment issues, nurses should consider these negative actions as a part of the grief process, rather than solely personality faults. Thus, the nurse can help the inmate accept the consequences of incarceration and begin to seek realistic solutions for their future.

Certain points during incarceration are recognized as having greater risk for mental decline or suicide. In a jail setting, the first 24–48 hours is a period of high risk for self-harm. Known high-risk times are at booking or admission, with new legal problems such as additional charges or denial of parole, and upon placement in disciplinary or isolated housing settings. Other stressors, that staff might not know of, include loss of relationships, death in the family, or other bad personal news (Hayes, 2011). Even good news, like a pending release after years of incarceration, can be overwhelming.

Mentally ill inmates are at high risk for self-harm when they are transferred from one setting to another, either to a new cell or to a different institution. It is important for nurses to be aware of any inmate who has poor coping skills and to be vigilant for his or her safety during stressful times such as intake, sentencing, interpersonal events, isolation, or segregation. Custody staff are likely to be aware of recent events in an inmate's life, as well as changes in mental status and behavior that may indicate poor coping. Nurses should build sound working relationships with custody staff to ensure that any changes in attitude or behavior are immediately brought to the nurse's attention.

Isolation is another aspect of incarceration that has the potential to contribute to a decline in an inmate's mental status. Inmates may experience anxiety, depression, despair, and psychotic-like symptoms when they are isolated for prolonged periods of time. Without social support or psychological stimulus, inmates with mental illness may experience rapid decline in mental status when placed in isolation. Mental health experts and national standard-setting organizations such as the National Commission on Correctional Health Care (NCCHC) and the American Correctional Association (ACA) recommend that seriously mentally ill inmates should not be placed in isolation unless no other setting is appropriate—and then only for the shortest amount of time possible. These standards require monitoring of all inmates placed in segregation for signs of mental deterioration and very close clinical supervision of mentally ill inmates in this setting (ACA, 2002; NCCHC, 2008). The observations and information gathered by each of the staff who interact with the inmate during medication passes, mental health checks, rounds, and activities of daily living (ADLs) such as showering, eating, and sleeping are critical in identifying changes in mental status so that timely, responsible treatment intervention is provided (Way, Sawyer, Barboza, & Nash, 2007).

NURSING ASSESSMENT AND REFERRAL

Because the practice of correctional nursing includes care of mentally ill patients, nurses need training to accurately complete the mental health portions of intake screening and the initial health assessment, and have knowledge and skill in assessing mental status and suicidality (American Nurses Association, 2007). These nursing assessments identify inmates who are mentally ill or emotionally fragile so that they can be managed safely and receive appropriate treatment during incarceration.

In preparing to interview an inmate, the nurse should review any records that are available to establish a baseline and identify any previous mental health diagnoses the inmate may have been given. Create a safe, private area to meet with the inmate, and try to be at the same eye level. The first steps in building rapport are clearly identifying yourself and describing the purpose of the interview. Ask open-ended questions that allow the inmate to do the majority of the talking. Listen carefully, and do not rush through the interview process. These steps ensure a more thorough interview that yields the quality of information that will often make a difference in determining the urgency for mental health referral and intervention.

Intake Screening

The American Psychiatric Association (APA) recommends mental health screening upon intake at a correctional facility because it is the "primary means by which staff can determine which inmates require more specialized mental health assessment or evaluation, as well as treatment. Unless inmates are identified as potentially needing mental health treatment, they will not receive it" (Ford, 2007, p. 3). The NCCHC and the ACA adopted accreditation standards that support the APA recommendation for universal mental health screening at reception into a correctional facility or system (ACA, 2002; NCCHC, 2008).

Mental health screening is often a part of the initial health screening and assessment done by nurses and is discussed in Chapter 14, Health Screening. Referral guidelines for inmates identified with current or past history of mental illness are also discussed in this chapter. No screening tool can accurately identify 100% of inmates with mental health needs, and screening does not replace a comprehensive mental health evaluation. These screening tools give the nurse a guide for assessment of emotional instability and thought disorders, as well as past mental health treatment and medication. Nurses should rely on their observation and judgment and make a referral for further mental health assessment, even if the inmate's answers to the screening questions do not by themselves indicate a referral is necessary.

Mental Status Assessment

A mental status assessment should be completed whenever the patient's affect or behavior is incongruent with the circumstances of the encounter and the setting. The purpose of a mental status assessment is to determine the likely nature of a patient's illness, whether it is a thought or mood disorder, delirium, withdrawal, or other organic process. The nurse gleans information directly from the patient through interview and observation of their behavior during the interview. The components of the mental status assessment are listed in Table 12.5. Mental status is assessed during many different types of patient care encounters such as sick call, routine clinic appointments, rounds in segregation, inpatient care, and emergencies.

TABLE 12.5   Mental Status Assessment

COMPONENT	FACTORS ASSESSED	METHOD
Appearance	Dress: appropriate, attention to detail, well-groomed, cleanliness	Observation
	Hygiene: grooming, cleanliness, age-appropriate appearance	Observation
Behavior	Expression: general presentation, body posture, eye contact	Observation
	Motor activity: restlessness, pacing, wringing of hands, rigidity, slow or no movement	Observation
Speech	Rate: fast, slow, appropriate	Observation
	Tone: normal, loud, monotone, soft	Observation
	Manner: normal, pressured, hesitant, slurred, emotional	Observation
	Content: appropriate, expansive, nonsensical	Observation
Cognition	Orientation: time, place, person, situation, stable or fluctuating	Interview
	Memory: short-term, long-term	Interview
	Attention: spell a word backwards, subtract serial sevens from 100	Interview
	Insight: awareness of illness or need for treatment, treatment adherence, recognition of consequences	Interview
Mood and affect	Mood: patient description of how they feel: depressed, anxious, angry, fearful, etc.	Interview
	Affect: appropriate to situation, expressive, blunted, labile, etc.	Observation
Thoughts	Form: logical, flow, relevance, detail, complete	Interview
	Content: suicidal, homicidal, obsessions, compulsions, phobias, delusions	Interview
Perception	Hallucinations: audio, visual, tactile, gustatory, olfactory	Interview

Source: From Snyderman and Rovner (2009); Tann (2010).

The first step in a mental status exam is assessing the inmate's general appearance and presentation:

- Grooming such as cleanliness, clothing condition, and hair tidiness, and if there is a noticeable change from the inmate's usual appearance;
- Orientation to person, place, and date;
- Signs of distress such as restlessness, evasiveness, or excessive animation; and
- Engagement in the interview, good eye contact, or noted avoidance.

These initial signs can help determine which way to proceed. If the inmate presents as well-groomed and oriented, with good eye contact and a calm presentation, there might not be any indication for further mental health assessment. If the patient's presentation is abnormal, given the circumstances, further assessment is warranted.

The second step is to note any difficulties of general intelligence and evaluate the inmate's ability to articulate their concerns and needs. The nurse notes whether the inmate is able to grasp concepts and problem solve, and if the inmate's judgment seems adequate. Finally, the nurse evaluates the logic and coherence of the inmate's speech and thought content. The nurse should try to elicit a description from the inmate regarding the specifics of any hallucinations or delusions, if present, and ascertain the inmate's potential for self-harm or violence toward others.

The facility should have well-established timeframes and procedures for mental health referral since mental health expertise for evaluation and treatment is a minimal expectation of an adequate health care delivery system (Rold, 2006). Guidelines to use in establishing referral timeframes are that psychiatric emergencies are referred and seen immediately, urgent problems are seen within 24–48 hours of the referral, and routine problems are seen within no more than 2 work weeks of the referral (Smith & Smith, 2006). Psychiatric emergencies include "acute psychotic episodes and exacerbation of a chronic mental illness, cutting or other self-injurious behavior, medical sequelae of psychiatric conditions, serious suicide attempts, and violent behavior" (Schwartz-Watts & Frierson, 2006, p. 306). Urgent problems are mentally ill inmates experiencing symptoms that will require new or changed orders, medication orders that will expire before the next visit, or who are experiencing a change (housing reassignment, etc.) that increases the risk of suicide or self-harm.

Suicide Risk Assessment

The NCCHC and ACA require all correctional facilities to have a comprehensive program to prevent suicide, including training of staff in suicide risk factors, screening procedures to identify at-risk inmates, and referral to mental health professionals for evaluation and treatment (NCCHC, 2008; ACA, 2002, 2010). The nurse will often initiate suicide precautions based on assessment after a notification from custody staff about warning signs or statements made by the inmate.

The nurse should keep in mind that someone who has attempted suicide in the past is more likely to do so again (Hayes, 2010), and that having a family member commit suicide or witnessing a suicide increases the suicidal risk factor (Goldsmith, Pellmar, Kleinman, & Bunney, 2002). Stresses related to the correctional setting that contribute to the suicide potential include unanticipated sentencing or disciplinary decisions, pressure from other inmates (intimidation, extortion, sexual assault), and shame of incarceration (Blitz, Wolff, & Shi, 2008; Hayes, 2010). There is strong evidence that having a mental disorder places a person at considerably higher risk of suicide than the general population (Hayes, 2010). Mental health symptoms may impair a person's ability to utilize adequate coping skills, especially in the face of stressors such as assault, extortion, relationship problems, or deaths. Direct questions regarding ideation, plan, preparations, and determination can assist in determining the level of intervention needed for the inmate's safety. There is almost always ambivalence regarding suicide, so exploring positive reasons for living during the interview is encouraged. Being familiar with the risk factors, comfortable asking the necessary questions, and clearly documenting findings greatly assist in identification and timely referral of inmates at risk of suicide to mental health professionals (Cox & Lawrence, 2010).

If there are findings from the assessment that indicate potential for suicide or the inmate vocalizes suicidality at any time during incarceration, suicide precautions must be initiated and an immediate referral made to a mental health professional. When mental health staff is not on site, the nurse will be notified by correctional staff of an inmate who is at risk; the nurse will see the inmate to assess suicide risk and contact the mental health professional. Data collected by the nurse will be used by the mental health professional to determine the level of suicidal risk, as well as the type of intervention and supervision to be implemented. These procedures are intended to provide for the safety of the inmate until treatment strategies and services such as counseling, medication, and program housing options are determined and put into place, with regular treatment follow-up to reduce further risk of suicide.

NURSING CARE

Nursing care includes monitoring patients who are on suicide watch, in seclusion, or restraint because their behavior puts themselves or others at risk of harm. It includes responding to incidents of suicide, intentional injury, or self-harm. Nursing care of mentally ill inmates also includes administering medication, supporting the patient's adherence to treatment, and monitoring effectiveness. It also includes making arrangements to ensure that the patient's care continues upon release from incarceration and return to the community.

Suicide Watch

Inmates who are placed on suicide watch will be reassessed by nursing staff intermittently. The purpose is to reassess ongoing suicide risk and to identify changes in the inmate's medical or psychiatric condition that need intervention. This encounter also provides the inmate an opportunity for therapeutic communication and may decrease the effects of isolation. Asking open-ended questions, giving the inmate full attention, and keeping an open mind help the nurse focus on the central ideas the inmate is communicating. Asking clarifying questions to explore the inmate's situation will assist in identifying the significance of the inmate's thoughts and feelings. Asking explicit questions about suicide and validating the person's right to view suicide as a rational solution through normalizing statements can aid in a more accurate suicide assessment because the inmate may be more forthcoming in responding to the nurse's inquiry. An inquiry of "tell me what is happening with you right now" is more likely to elicit an informative response than a statement like "You don't feel like killing yourself, do you?" The nurse should also ask for and consider information from custody staff in the periodic nursing assessment. The nurse communicates the results of the assessment to health and mental health personnel on the team, documents in the health record, and acts on nursing care needs that have been identified.

From the Experts . . .

"In correctional facilities, nurses are frequently the primary support for incarcerated individuals when these individuals perceive their lives as out of control. This provides nurses with the opportunity for life-long impact in the lives of our patients."

Scott Haynes, PMHNP
Aurora, OR

Seclusion and Restraint

When a mentally ill inmate is combative or attempting to self-harm, a nurse will be involved in the application and use of seclusion and restraint. The primary goal for therapeutic seclusion and restraint is patient safety; further harm should not be caused through this intervention. Over the years, restraints have been used less and less frequently because of the potential for harm to the patient and the development of effective alternatives to manage this type of behavior (Champion, 2007). The NCCHC standards (2008) provide clear guidelines regulating the use of restraints. These include an order by a physician or other qualified health care professional, documented 15-minute checks of the restrained inmate by health services staff, and range-of-motion (ROM) exercises every 2 hours.

Seclusion and restraint should be used for the shortest possible time in keeping with current community practice. When placing an inmate in seclusion or restraint, the nurse is the communicator between the provider who ordered restraint, the mental health team, and custody staff. The nurse's role is to continually assess the patient and notify the provider when restraints are no longer needed. It is also the nurse's responsibility to notify the provider if additional intervention is needed to prevent any further harm.

Responding to Suicide and Self-Harm

When an inmate harms themselves, it is a medical emergency and will be responded to according to facility policy and procedure. The ACA and NCCHC require that staff who have direct inmate contact be trained in first aid and CPR (ACA, 2002; NCCHC, 2008) and can respond to medical emergencies. Nurses are likely to be the first medical responder and need to be skilled in responding to suicide and self-injury and managing the resuscitation effort.

Correctional staff has a responsibility to secure the area in addition to initiating first aid and calling for emergency assistance. When nursing staff arrive at the scene there should be little or no delay in accessing the patient. Since all the details of what happened may not be known, custody staff may delay response until adequate back-up has arrived and may ask that the area not be disturbed to preserve evidence. If a nurse is unable to reasonably access the patient or apply timely and responsive life-saving measures, the nurse needs to be insistent and notify their chain of command. Case Example 12.2 describes an incident like this. Emergency response drills are useful in identifying these conflicts and providing opportunity for resolution well before an actual situation comes up.

Less understood is the self-harm behavior that may or may not be intended as a suicide attempt. Because the motivations behind it may be mixed and (with repeated acts) the suicidal intent may vary over time, self-harm must always be treated seriously. Types of self-harm include cutting, burning, head-banging, swallowing objects, self-suffocation, inserting objects into wounds, overdosing, and other forms of dangerous behaviors. Self-harm is a sign of emotional distress or poor coping response. Self-harm may or may not be associated with a mental illness, personality disorder, or learning disability (Paton & Jenkins, 2002). Self-harm behavior presents one of the most difficult dilemmas for all staff in the correctional setting, often causing anxiety, frustration, or anger (Fagan, Cox, Helfand, & Aufderheide, 2009).

Managing one's own emotions while tending to the inmate is often more difficult than the treatment itself. Whether or not there is a physical injury that requires

CASE EXAMPLE 12.2

An inmate in the maximum custody unit that houses the mentally ill is not responsive to the officer during rounds. The nurse is called for a medical emergency and arrives on the unit to find the officer standing outside the cell door. The nurse knows that the inmate is on a mental health caseload and takes medication for depression. The nurse observes the inmate to be in a sitting position hunched over on the edge of the bed. He does not respond to the nurse's inquiry to him. He appears to have shallow, irregular respirations, is pale in color, and diaphoretic.

When the nurse asks the officer to pop the cell door, the officer tells the nurse that they must wait until adequate back-up is available. The officer has called in a "use of force" request and is waiting for the team to arrive.

Discussion Questions:

1. What is the procedure for response to medical emergencies like this?
2. What steps should the nurse take while waiting to go into the cell?
3. How long should the nurse wait?

emergency treatment, it is important that the nurse respond succinctly and treat the inmate with respect. Self-harm is only seldom and never exclusively caused by a wish to get attention or for manipulative reasons (Paton & Jenkins, 2002). Behavioral approaches to managing patients who self-harm have proven successful, especially when they are targeted to the needs of the individual patient; involve excellent collaboration between correctional, health, and mental health staff; and involve both flexible and strategic interventions (Fagan et al., 2009).

Whenever there is a serious self-harm incident or completed suicide, it is a stressful time for all involved. Emotions of anxiety, guilt, and anger are common, as everyone questions whether they were the one who missed the signs and symptoms or whether procedure was properly followed. Debriefing allows for open discussion and expression of emotions, so that staff does not carry misplaced guilt, feelings of being ostracized, or anxiety about what others might be thinking. Health care staff often is turned to at these times due to their training and experiences with traumatic events. The nurse can assist in demobilizing or de-escalating with a brief intervention to help those involved in the incident transition back to their posts. This can include letting those involved discuss the incident, their reactions, and the coping skills to use in order to return to their routine. The nurse might also help identify staff that might need to be relieved from regular duties until further counseling can be arranged. Communication with the supervisor and staff is needed to provide support for the individuals involved. It is important, however, that the nurse called upon to fill this counseling role also seeks out some personal counseling (Hayes, 2008).

Medication Administration

Psychotropic medications are most often administered by nurses in correctional facilities rather than patients taking medication on their own, as they would if they were living in the community. The reliance on nurse administered medication in correctional settings is for two reasons: first, a concern that these medications will be traded, sold, or stolen and, second, to prevent accidental or intentional overdose. A key benefit of this method is the frequent interaction with nurses, allowing for early identification of side effects or other issues. However, this approach requires mentally ill inmates to go get their medication once or more each day, and if it conflicts with other important activities (meal times, work, visitation, etc.) or exposes the inmate to bad weather, fatigue, or the stigma of being identified as mentally ill, adherence to prescribed treatment will drop.

There is a growing practice of allowing some inmates to self-administer their mental health medications (especially those that have limited potential for misuse). Because managing medication is a skill needed for success in the community, many argue that this skill should be fostered among the mentally ill who are incarcerated, especially in preparation for release. The benefit of self-administered medication is the confidentiality it affords, as well as the promotion of greater self-sufficiency and responsibility for self-care (Velligan et al., 2010).

Washington v. Harper made way for inmates to be treated involuntarily if certain conditions were met. One of these conditions is in an emergency, when there is clear danger to the patient of self-harm or danger to staff due to the patient's aggressive behavior (1990). Emergency treatment is considered a short-term solution only until the patient is admitted for mental health treatment and an ongoing treatment plan established. On rare occasions, a patient may refuse treatment that has been recommended and explained by the provider. In certain situations, involuntary treatment may be ordered after an administrative due-process hearing and review.

The nurse should be clear that an emergency exists or an involuntary order is in place before giving medication against the inmate's will. It is likely that the nurse will need to administer the medication in an injection form, at least initially. When an inmate is agitated and resisting treatment, the custody staff is involved in securing the inmate so an injection can be safely given. This experience can vary widely from dramatic to quietly resigned compliance. Often, after the initial injection or two, the inmate decides to comply with oral medication or accepts the injection without incident. Frequently, after a simple discussion with the nurse about what needs to happen and what the options are, the inmate will take the medication voluntarily. A little extra time to calmly and proactively discuss the situation and dispel the fear the inmate may have can minimize the drama.

Monitoring Treatment

A major problem with mental health treatment is patient adherence with the prescribed medication regime. Poor adherence contributes to increased symptoms, high economic costs, hospitalizations, and poor outcomes. With mental illness, poor adherence also contributes to disturbed and sometimes violent behavior. Compliance is improved with patient education about the need for treatment and the possible side effects of the medication, access to treatment, and support for mental health treatment among staff and peers. Likewise, contributing to poor adherence is a lack of understanding regarding need for treatment and management of side effects (Gray, Bressington, Lathlean, & Mills, 2008). A recent review of the literature suggested that five factors contribute to medication adherence in the incarcerated mentally ill. These are personal characteristics, prior medication use, insight, environment, and side effects (Shelton, Ehret, Wakai, Kapetanovic, & Moran, 2010). This review suggests incorporating this information into patient teaching to increase medication adherence.

There are many approaches to identify, track, and report nonadherence. Some facilities have policies that require every mental health patient be identified and referred for one missed dose, while others call for weekly monitoring of those identified as the most critical. Long and time-consuming medication lines do not often permit much time for patient education regarding the need for consistent medication treatment. One suggestion is to keep handy a list of patients with the most critical need for monitoring. Mental health staff can generate this list, and the nursing staff can then check their medication administration register at a separate time from medication line, when they have more time to devote to monitoring. Inmates who are not taking ordered medication need referral to mental health staff to provide counseling and education regarding medication adherence. In most cases, the refusal of medication or treatment would suggest a different degree of need for monitoring, as it might be symptomatic of a much larger mental health concern.

Most mental health medications carry side effects and potential risks. The standard of care for mental health patients calls for regular monitoring for intended and unintended effects. Managing the medical aspects of psychiatric treatment is much like that for other chronic diseases. Providers use clinical guidelines to determine lab and other diagnostic tests and monitoring to manage the ongoing care of mentally ill patients. Nurses may be responsible for monitoring symptoms according to an algorithm and collaborating with the provider for changes in the plan of care as necessary based upon results.

Discharge Planning

It is critical to remember that the correctional facility is a part of the community. When the inmate with mental illness arrives in the local jail or prison, there is often a community provider or mental health facility that has been caring for this person before they arrived in custody. Likewise, when the inmate with mental illness is released from custody, they will return to the community with the same level of need for care. The ACA (2002) and NCCHC standards (2008) stipulate that follow-up care be addressed for those especially diagnosed as severely mentally ill. Follow-up appointments, mental health care summaries, and help with applications for entitlement programs and medication assistance are often the keys for successful reentry into society and reducing the recidivism rate.

Policies will vary from system to system but should generally include identifying the inmates who will need services upon discharge, developing an individualized discharge plan for each inmate, connecting with community resources and making the follow-up appointments, providing a summary of care on each inmate for the community provider, and assuring that release medications are ordered. The nurse is often responsible for transcribing or copying health information for the community provider, giving the inmate the information about appointments for follow-up that have been made and providing release medications or a prescription.

SUMMARY

The incidence of mental illness in the criminal justice system requires that correctional nurses are experts in the identification and care of patients with mental illness. Correctional nurses are knowledgeable of the presenting signs and symptoms of major mental illnesses, familiar with recommended approaches to treatment, can engage and support the patient in treatment, and care for their illness or condition. Correctional nurses provide leadership and direction in managing the initial response to psychiatric emergencies and coordinate care among correctional, health, and mental health professionals to ensure patient safety.

DISCUSSION QUESTIONS

1. What are some of the medical reasons for disordered behavior?
2. Why is the prevalence of mental illness increasing in corrections?
3. What are the key points for nurses providing care for the mentally ill in corrections?

REFERENCES

American Correctional Association. (2002). *Performance based standards for correctional health care in adult correctional institutions*. Alexandria, VA: Author.

American Correctional Association. (2010). *2010 Standards supplement*. Alexandria, VA: Author.

American Nurses Association. (2007). *Corrections nursing: Scope & standards of practice*. Silver Spring, MD: Author.

American Psychiatric Association. (2010, November). *Practice guidelines: Treatment of patients with major depressive disorder* (3rd ed.). Retrieved August 4, 2011, from American Psychiatric Association: http://www.psychiatryonline.com/pracGuide/pracGuideTopic_7.aspx

Baillargeon, J., Binswanger, I. A., Penn, J. V., Williams, B. A., & Murray, O. J. (2009). Psychiatric disorders and repeat incarcerations: The revolving prison door. *American Journal of Psychiatry, 166,* 103–109.

Bernstein, B. E. (2010). *Pediatric bipolar affective disorder*. Medscape Reference. Retrieved February 11, 2011, from http://emedicine.medscape.com/article/913464

Berzins, L. G., & Trestman, R. L. (2004). The development and implementation of dialectical behavior therapy in forensic settings. *International Journal of Forensic Mental Health, 3*(1), 93–103.

Bland, A., Tudor, G., & Whitehouse, D. M. (2007, October). Nursing care of inpatients with borderline personality disorder. *Perspectives in Psychiatric Care, 43*(4), 204–212.

Blier, P. (2005). Atypical antipsychotics for mood and anxiety disorders: Safe and effective adjuncts? *Journal of Psychiatry Neuroscience, 30*(4), 232–233.

Blitz, C. L., Wolff, N., & Shi, J. (2008). Physical victimization in prison: The role of mental illness. *International Journal of Law and Psychiatry, 31*(5), 385–393.

Bowden, C. L. (2001). Strategies to reduce misdiagnosis of bipolar depression. *Psychiatric Services, 52,* 51–55.

Centers for Disease Control and Prevention. (n.d.). *Traumatic brain injury in prisons and jails: An unrecognized problem*. Retrieved December 31, 2011, from Centers for Disease Control and Prevention: http://www.cdc.gov/traumaticbraininjury/pdf/Prisoner_TBI_Prof-a.pdf

Challoner, K. R., & Newton, E. J. (2010). *Neuroleptic agent toxicity*. Medscape Reference. Retrieved February 19, 2011, from http://emedicine.medscape.com/article/815881

Champion, M. K. (2007). Seclusion and restraint in corrections: A time for change. *Journal of the American Academy of Psychiatry and the Law, 35*(4), 426–430.

Cloyes, K., Wong, B., Latimer, S., & Abarca, J. (2010, March 1). Women, serious mental illness and recidivism: A gender-based analysis of recidivism risk for women with SMI released from prison. *Journal of Forensic Nursing, 6*(1), 3–14.

Cox, J., & Lawrence, J. (2010). Suicide prevention in correctional settings. In A. Ruiz, J. Dvoskin, C. Scott, & J. Metzner (Eds.), *Manual of forms and guidelines for correctional mental health* (pp. 121–154). Arlington: American Psychiatric Publing, Inc.

Curtis, B. (2010). *Traumatic brain injury and the offender*. Washington Department of Corrections, Health Services, Olympia.

Dixon, L., Perkins, D., & Calmes, C. (2009, September). *Guideline watch (September 2009): Practice guideline for the treatment of patients with schizophrenia*. Retrieved August 2, 2011, from American Psychiatric Association: http://www.psychiatryonline.com/pracGuide/PracticePDFs/Schizophrenia_Guideline%20Watch.pdf

Fagan, T., Cox, J., Helfand, S., & Aufderheide, D. (2009). Self-injurious behavior in correctional settings. *Journal of Correctional Health Care, 16*(1), 48–66.

First, M. B. (Ed.) (2000). *Diagnostic and statistical manual of mental disorders* (4th ed., *DSM-IV-TR*™, 2000). Washington, DC. American Psychiatric Association. Retrieved December 30, 2011, from http://online.statref.com.proxy.heal-wa.org/document.aspx?fxid=37&docid=405

Ford, J. T. (2007). *Mental health screens for corrections*. Washington, DC: U.S. Department of Justice, Office of Justice Programs, National Institute of Justice.

Glaze, L. E., & James, D. J. (2006, September). Mental health problems of prison and jail inmates. *Bureau of Justice Statistics (BJS) Special Report*. Retrieved from http://bjs.ojp.usdoj.gov/content/pub/pdf/mhppji.pdf

Goldsmith, S., Pellmar, T., Kleinman, A., & Bunney, W. (2002). *Reducing suicide: A national imperative*. Washington, DC: National Academies Press.

Goff, A., Rose, E., Rose, S., & Purves, D. (2007). Does PTSD occur in sentenced prison populations? A systematic literature review. *Criminal Behaviour and Mental Health, 17*, 152–162.

Gray, R., Bressington, D., Lathlean, J., & Mills, A. (September 2008). Relationship between adherence, symptoms, treatment attitudes, satisfaction, and side effects in prisoners taking antipsychotic medication. *Journal of Forensic Psychiatry & Psychology, 19*(3), 335–351.

Hamblen, J. (2009). *What is PTSD? National Center for PTSD*. United States Department of Veterans Affairs. Retrieved January 25, 2012, from http://www.ptsd.va.gov/professional/ptsd101/course-modules/what-is-ptsd.asp

Harmon, R., & Bomberger, R. (2010). *Delusions, hallucinations or little green men: Detection of malingered psychosis*. National Conference on Correctional Health Care. Las Vegas. National Commission on Correctional Health Care.

Hayes, L. M. (2008). Guide to developing and revising suicide prevention protocols. *Standards for Mental Health Services in Correctional Facilities*. Chicago National Commission on Correctional Health Care.

Hayes, L. M. (2010). *National study of jail suicide 20 years later*. Washington, DC: U.S. Department of Justice, National Institute of Corrections.

Hayes, L. M. (2011). *Guiding principles to suicide prevention in correctional facilities*. Baltimore: National Center on Institutions and Alternatives. http://www.ncianet.org/services/suicide-prevention-in-custody/publications/guiding-principles-to-suicide-prevention-in-correctional-facilities/

Kübler-Ross, E. (1969). *On death and dying*. London: Routledge.

Kübler-Ross, E. (2005). *On grief and grieving: Finding the meaning of grief through the five stages of loss*. London: Simon & Schuster.

Lamont, S., & Brunero, S. (2009). Personality disorder prevalence and treatment outcomes: A literature review. *Issues in Mental Health Nursing, 30*, 631–637.

Lenzenweger, M. (2008). Epidemiology of personality disorders. *Psychiatric Clinics of North America, 31*(3), 395–403.

Lenzenweger, M. F., Lane, M. C., Loranger, A. W., & Kessler, R. C. (2007). *DSM-IV personality disorders in national comorbidity survey replication*. *Biological Psychiatry, 62*(6), 553–564.

Lewandowski, K. E., DePaola, J., Camsari, G. B., Cohen, B. M., & Ongur, D. (2009). Tactile, olfactory, and gustatory hallucinations in psychotic disorders: A descriptive study. *Annals Academy of Medicine Singapore, 38*(5), 383–385.

Lubit, R. H. (2010). *Borderline personality disorder*. Medscape Reference. Retrieved from: http://emedicine.medscape.com/article/913575

McLafferty, F. (2007). Delirium part one: Clinical features, risk factors and assessment. *Nursing Standard, 2129*, 35–40.

Merikangas, K. R., Jin, R., Kessler, R. C., Sampson, L. S., Viana, M. C., Andrade, L. H. et al. (2011). Prevalence and correlates of bipolar spectrum disorder in the World Mental Health Survey Initiative. *Archives of General Psychiatry, 68*(3), 241–151.

National Commission on Correctional Health Care (NCCHC). (2008). *Standards for mental health services in correctional facilities.* Chicago, IL: Author.

Nicolson, S. E., Mayberg, M. D., Pennell, P. B., & Nemeroff, C. B. (2006). Persistent auditory hallucinations that are unresponsive to antipsychotic drugs. *American Journal of Psychiatry, 163,* 1153–1159.

Oldham, J. (2005, March). *Guideline watch: Practice guideline for the treatment of patients with borderline personality disorder.* Retrieved August 7, 2011, from American Psychiatry Association: http://www.psychiatryonline.com/content.aspx?aID=148745

Paton, J., & Jenkins, R. (2002). *Mental health primary care in prison.* London: Royal Society of Medicine.

Pratt, L. A., & Brody, D. J. (2008). *Depression in the United States household population, 2005–2006.* Centers for Disease Control and Prevention. Retrieved from http://www.cdc.gov/nchs/data/databriefs/db07.htm

Prins, A., Ouimette, P., Kimerling, R., Cameron, R. P., Hugelshofer, D. S., Shaw-Heger, J. et al. (2003). The primary care PTSD screen (PC-PTSD): Development and operating characteristics. *Primary Care Psychiatry, 9,* 9–14.

Race, M. M., Yousefian, A., Lambert, D., & Hartley, D. (2010). Mental health services in rural jails. *Maine Rural Health Research Center,* Working Paper #42. Retrieved from http://www.ruralhealthresearch.org

Resnick, P. J., & Knoll, J. (2005). Faking it: How to detect malingered psychosis. *Journal of Family Practice, 4*(11), 13–25.

Rold, W. J. (2006) Legal considerations in the delivery of health care services in prisons and jails. In M. Puisis (Ed.), *Clinical practice in correctional medicine* (pp. 520–528). Philadelphia: Moseby Elsevier.

Rotter, M., Way, B., Steinbacher, M., Sawyer, D., & Smith, H. (2002). Personality disorders in prisoners: Aren't they all antisocial? *Psychiatric Quarterly, 73,* 337–349.

Rush, J. A. (2000). *Handbook of psychiatric measures.* Washington, DC: American Psychiatric Association.

Schwartz-Watts, D., & Frierson, R. (2006). Crisis stabilization in correctional settings. In M. Puisis (Ed.), *Clinical practice in correctional medicine* (pp. 306–316). Philadelphia: Elsevier.

Shelton, D., Ehret, M. J., Wakai, S., Kapetanovic, T., & Moran, M. (2010). Psychotropic medication adherence in correctional facilities: A review of the literature. *Journal of Psychiatric and Mental Health Nursing, 17,* 603–613.

Shelton, D., Sampl, S., Kesten, K. L., Zhang, W., & Trestman, R. L. (2009). Treatment of impulsive aggression in correctional settings. *Behavioral Sciences and the Law, 27,* 787–800.

Shim, R. S., Baltrus, P., Ye, J., & Rust, G. (2011). *Prevalence, treatment, and control of depressive symptoms in the United States: Results from the national health and nutrition examination survey, 2005–2008.* Retrieved from http://www.medscape.com/viewarticle/735685

Shiroma, E. J., Pickelsimer, E. E., Ferguson, P. L., Gebregziabher, M., Lattimore, P. K., Nicholas, J. S. et al. (2010). Association of medically attended traumatic brain injury and in-prison behavioral infractions: A statewide longitudinal study. *Journal of Correctional Health Care, 16*(4), 273–286.

Skowyra, K. R., & Cocozza, J. L. (2007). *Blueprint for change: Improving the system response to youth with mental health needs involved with the juvenile justice system.* Retrieved July 29, 2011, from National Center for Mental Health and Juvenile Justice: http://www.ncmhjj.com/Blueprint/pdfs/ProgramBrief_06_06.pdf

Slaughter, B., Fann, J. R., & Ehde, D. (2003). Traumatic brain injury in a county jail population: Prevalence, neuropsychological functioning and psychiatric disorders. *Brain Injury, 17*(9), 731–741.

Smith, S. (2005). Stepping through the looking glass: Professional autonomy in correctional nursing. *Corrections Today.* Retrieved from http://www.allbusiness.com/public-administration/justice-public-order/982858

Smith, H., & Smith, L. (2006). Correctional-based mental health services: Designing a system that works. In M. Puisis (Ed.), *Clinical Practice of Correctional Medicine* (2nd ed., pp. 292–305). Philadelphia: Elsevier.

Snyderman, D., & Rovner, B. W. (2009, October 15). Mental status examination in primary care: A review. *American Family Physician, 80*(8), 809–814.

Steadman, H., Osher, F., Robbins, P., Case, B., & Samuels, S. (2009, June). Prevalence of serious mental illness among jail inmates. *Psychiatric Services, 60*(6), 761–765.

Swift, E. (2009, November). Borderline personality disorder: Aetiology, presentation and therapuetic relationship. *Mental Health Practice, 13*(3), 22–25.

Talkes, K., & Tennant, A. (2004). The therapy seesaw: Achieving therapuetically balanced approaches to working with emotional distress. *British Journal of Forensic Practice, 6*(3), 3–12.

Tann, I. (2010). Nursing skills for managing the mentally ill in corrections. *Correctional Health Care Perspectives: What We Know.* Portland: American Correctional Health Services Association.

Teeple, B. S., Caplan, J. P., & Stern, T. A. (2009). Visual hallucinations: Differential diagnosis and treatment. *The Primary Care Companion to the Journal of Clinical Psychiatry, 11*(1), 26–32.

Torrey, E., Kennard, A., Eslinger, D., Lamb, R., & Pavle, J. (2010, May). *More mentally ill persons are in jails and prisons than hospitals: A survey of the states.* Retrieved July 29, 2011, from http://www. treatmentadvocacycenter.org/storage/documents/final_jails_v_hospitals_study.pdf

Trestman, R. L., Ford, J., Zhang, W., & Wiesbrock, V. (2007). Current and lifetime psychiatric illness among inmates not identified as acutely mentally ill at intake in Connecticut's jails. *Journal of the American Academy of Psychiatry and the Law, 35*(4), 490–500.

Ucok, A., & Gaebel, W. (2008, February). Side effects of atypical antipsychotics: A brief overview. *World Psychiatry: Official Journal of the World Psychiatric Association (WPA), 7*(1), 58–62.

Urban, M., & Rabe-Jablonska, J. (2007). Olfactory dysfunctions in patients with schizophrenia. (2002). *Psychiatria Polska, 41*(4), 503–512.

Vaishnavi, S., Rao, V., & Fann, J. R. (2009). Neuropsychiatric problems after traumatic brain injury: Unraveling the silent epidemic. *Academy of Psychosomatic Medicine, 50*, 198–205.

Vaughn, M., Fu, Q., Beaver, D., DeLisi, M., Perron, B., & Howard, M. (2010, December 1). Are personality disorders associated with social welfare burden in the United States? *Journal of Personality Disorders, 24*(6), 709–720.

Velligan, D. I., Weiden, P. J., Sajatovic, M., Scott, J., Carpenter, D., Ross, R. et al. , (2010, September). Strategies for addressing adherence problems in patients with serious and persistent mental illness: Recommendations from the Expert Consensus Panel. *Journal of Psychiatric Practice, 16*(5), 306–324.

Washington v. Harper, 494 U.S. 210 (1990).

Way, B. B., Sawyer, D. A., Barboza, S., & Nash, R. (2007). Inmate suicide and time spent in special disciplinary housing in New York state prison. *Psychiatric Services, 58*, 558–560.

Wolff, N., Maschi, T., & Bjerkie, J. (2004). Profiling mentally disordered prison inmates: A case study in New Jersey. *Journal of Correctional Health Care, 11*(1), 5–29.

THIRTEEN

Pain Management

Catherine M. Knox

THE CHALLENGE OF PAIN

*P*ain is often the reason inmates request attention to a health complaint (LaMarre, 2006) and reducing the volume of inmates seen for complaints of pain is one of the reasons given for creating guidelines to treat pain (Mollina, 2006; Reichert, 2010). In assessing a patient's complaint of pain, correctional nurses are advised to compare the subjective description to objective findings. Even then, the extent and significance of the patient's pain may be impossible to verify. Complicating the assessment and treatment of pain is that inmates in jail and prison also have extremely high rates of substance abuse and dependence (James & Glaze, 2006). The circumstances caused by imprisonment, such as separation from family and other emotional and physical support systems, may create and certainly exacerbate pain. Some correctional health care experts suggest that the challenges of treating pain in the correctional setting are more similar than different from the general community and that the correctional setting provides some advantages not available in other settings (Lubelczyk, 2008; Puerini, 2011).

Pain is also the most common reason people in the general community seek health care (National Pharmaceutical Council [NPC] and the Joint Commission on Accreditation of Healthcare Organizations [JCAHO], 2005). The Institute of Medicine (IOM, 2011) reports that a third of adults in the United States experienced chronic pain in the last 3 months. Health care providers in the community also express concern about the inability to precisely diagnose or confirm the intensity and quality of pain reported by patients (Beck, 2011).

The importance and controversies of adequately addressing pain emerged over 30 years ago in a study that found over 70% of hospitalized medical patients were undertreated for pain (Marks & Sachar, 1973; Wells, Pasero, & McCaffery, 2008).

Since then, studies continue to document the tremendous amount of pain experienced by patients in all types of settings, including nursing homes, outpatient, and surgical care (IOM, 2011; Registered Nurses Association of Ontario [RNAO], 2002, Supplement 2007; Wells et al., 2008). Similar findings were reported in a study of patients who had cancer in the Texas prison system (Lin & Mathew, 2005).

Unrelieved pain causes anxiety and depression; it also predisposes a patient to an exaggerated response to subsequent pain experiences (Wells et al., 2008). Other complications of inadequate pain relief are sleep disturbance and functional decline and impairment of the endocrine, pulmonary, cardiovascular, gastrointestinal, and immune systems. These complications add to the patient's experience of pain (Grose & Shub, 2010; Helms & Barone, 2008).

Explanations for inappropriate or ineffective treatment of pain by health care professionals includes the influence of regulatory agencies on prescribing patterns (Johnson, Todd, & Moulton, 2007), lack of knowledge or interest by health care providers in pain control, failure by health care providers to assess pain, failure in communication between the patient and health care providers, and concerns of both the patient and the prescriber about addiction (Daykin, 2006; Ferrell, McCaffery, & Rhiner, 1992; IOM, 2011). In correctional settings, additional barriers to adequate treatment not already identified include the safety and security issues of misuse, and diversion and lack of inmate credibility (Lin & Mathew, 2005; Lubelczyk, 2008; Puerini, 2011; Reichert, 2010).

In the last decade, some states have established requirements for continuing education of nurses in the subject of pain (Michigan Department of Licensing and Regulatory Affairs, 2009; Oregon State Board of Nursing, 2011), developed guidelines for nurses in the assessment and treatment of pain (Nursing Care Quality Assurance Commission, 2011), and disseminated position statements about the role of nurses and other health professionals in assessing and managing pain (Oregon Pain Management Commission, n.d.; Nursing Care Quality Assurance Commission, 2011). For example, California law stipulates that pain is the fifth vital sign and sets expectations for nurses to assess pain whenever other vital signs are taken (California

CASE EXAMPLE 13.1

Mr. Long is well known to the nursing staff in a correctional facility because he is followed regularly in chronic care clinic for his hepatitis C. On Saturday, the nurse assigned to sick call reviews a new request from Mr. Long. He has written, "I saw a specialist for possible cancer and am pending a CT scan. The doctor gave me a prescription for Tylenol # 3 but I don't get it often enough and I am in pain." The nurse called the on-call provider and obtained a verbal order that was documented in the record as *Motrin 600 mg. 1 tab p.o. tid prn for chest pain × 90 days. Patient may carry.* The nurse documented on the patient's request slip that a medication refill was ordered and could be picked up on Monday.

Discussion Questions:

1. To what extent were the nursing actions taken consistent with the
    *   Nurse practice act in your state?
    *   The ANA Scope and Standards of Practice for Correctional Nurses?
2. Describe the patient advocacy that took place in this example.

Board of Registered Nursing, 2000). In addition to standards established by regulatory agencies, accreditation organizations such as The Joint Commission (formerly known as JCAHO) and the National Commission on Correctional Health Care (NCCHC) have established standards recommendations for pain management (NCCHC, 2011; The Joint Commission, 2011).

Nurses working in correctional settings must be sure that their practice is consistent with state professional regulations as well as the standards of accreditation organizations. Standards of practice such as those established by the American Nurses Association (ANA, 2007) for correctional nursing also serve as guidelines for nursing practice in the care of patients in pain. Nurses who fail to practice consistent with these standards are at risk of practice violation and potential litigation for negligence (D'Arcy, 2005; Johnson et al., 2007). An example of a nurse's response to a patient in pain is provided in Case Example 13.1 and can be compared to the standards for practice set by the state board of nursing, the NCCHC, and the ANA.

DEFINITION AND DESCRIPTION OF PAIN

A simple and widely used definition of pain in clinical practice is "whatever the experiencing person says it is, existing whenever the experiencing person says it does" (Pasero & McCaffery, 2011, p. 21). The International Association for the Study of Pain (IASP, 2011) defines pain on its website as "an unpleasant sensory and emotional experience associated with actual or potential tissue damage or described in terms of such damage." The IOM defined pain "as a complex condition involving numerous areas of the brain; multiple two-way communication pathways in the central nervous system (from the site of pain to the brain and back again); and emotional, cognitive, and environmental elements—a complete, interconnected apparatus" (2011, pp. 15–16). The key concept in understanding pain is that it is a subjective sensation unique to the individual, and it may or may not have an etiology (Helms & Barone, 2008; S. Shelton, personal correspondence, March 16, 2011).

Biological Dimension of Pain

Nociceptors are the nerve endings in tissue that respond to stimuli corresponding to tissue damage or threat of tissue damage (Patel, 2010). The information provided by activation of the nerve fibers is transmitted to the spinal cord and from there to the brain, where the stimulus is perceived, interpreted, and made meaningful. The biological origins of pain include

- Inflammation of the nerves
- Injury to nerves and or nerve endings and formation of scar tissue
- Invasion of nerves by cancer
- Injury to the spinal cord, thalamus, or cerebral cortex
- Abnormal nerve activity perceived by the cortex as pain (Helms & Barone, 2008; Patel, 2010).

The interpretation of painful stimuli by the cerebral cortex is influenced by the person's affect, expectations, memory, and learned behaviors. The combination of biological, psychological, and sociocultural influences results in a matrix of pain perception unique to each individual (Helms & Barone, 2008). Thoughts, ideas, fears, and emotions are processed at an electrochemical level just as information supplied from damaged tissue is processed in the brain. Pain can originate or be a result from any of these processes as well as their interaction (Butler & Moseley, 2003). Thus, the IASP (2011) emphasizes that "Pain is always subjective . . . ."

A model used by a colleague in correctional health care to explain the phenomenon of pain is that of a sphere comprised of layers like an onion. Each layer (as depicted in Figure 13.1) can be modified by any of the other layers within the sphere as well as the environment around the sphere. What can be observed by others is an incomplete view of all of the factors that influence the patient's experience of pain (S. Shelton, personal correspondence, March 16, 2011).

Sociocultural Dimensions of Pain

Women report more frequent and/or severe pain and have a lower threshold and tolerance for painful stimuli than men (Charlton, 2005). Women also employ more active coping strategies with chronic painful conditions (Mailis-Gagnon, 2010). There is no scientific evidence that pain perception or sensitivity varies as a result of age (Helms & Barone, 2008). Older adults are less likely to have their pain effectively managed because of inadequate assessment of pain, concern about drug–drug interaction, and reluctance to prescribe opiates (Mohn-Brown, Burke, & Eby, 2010;

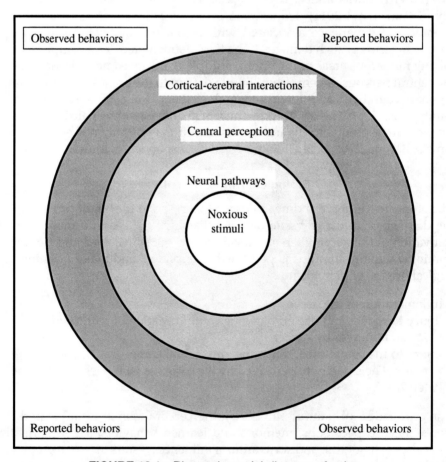

FIGURE 13.1   Biopsychosocial diagram of pain.

Source: From S. Shelton, personal correspondence, March 16, 2011.

Rutledge & Caple, 2010). Pain in older adults is often accompanied by reduced coping ability, sleep disruption, and functional decline (McLennon, 2007). Family cohesion and support has a significant positive impact on pain perception in adolescents (Rutledge & Caple, 2010). Women, the elderly, and juveniles are relatively small populations among all those incarcerated in the United States; age and gender account for some of the incidence and variation in the experience of pain among patients in the correctional setting.

Numerous studies demonstrate that minorities in the United States are at risk of inadequate pain control (Ezenwa, Ameringer, Ward, & Serlin, 2006; Lasch, 2002; Meghani & Houldin, 2007). Minorities are over-represented among correctional populations. In a clinical update, the IASP identified the most important variable in inadequate treatment of minority patients was a difference in staff perception of the patient's pain intensity (Lasch, 2002). Cultural factors related to pain include language used to describe pain, lay remedies for pain, social roles, and perceptions of the health care system (Lasch, 2002).

Psychosocial Dimension of Pain

Anxiety, fear, depression, and anger are all emotional reactions to painful experiences and condition an individual's response to subsequent painful experiences (Charlton, 2005). Patients with chronic pain are 4 times more likely to be depressed and/or anxious, a third of pain patients have comorbid depression, and clinical depression is one of the results of chronic pain (Adams & Field, 2001; Field & Adams, 2001; Charlton, 2005; Mollina, 2006). A study by the Bureau of Justice Statistics found that nearly one fourth of all inmates in jail and one third in prison reported symptoms of major depression (James & Glaze, 2006).

Marital discord, family violence, and abuse contribute to the likelihood of pain and its exacerbation as well as sustaining pain and eventual disability (Charlton, 2005). Adolescents and adults who have experienced sexual abuse and other traumatic injury may manifest greater sensitivity to all subsequent painful experiences (Helms & Barone, 2008). The first chapter described the high rates of sexual abuse and trauma among the incarcerated population, particularly women (Belknap, 2006; Glaze, 2004; Kelly, Parlaz-Dieckmann, Chang, Collins, 2010). The Bureau of Justice Statistics also reported that more than half of all persons in jail described growing up in a single household and nearly a third had a parent or guardian who abused alcohol or drugs (Glaze, 2004).

Types of Pain

Pain is classified into several different types based upon etiology, as described in Table 13.1. There is usually a well-defined reason for and onset of acute pain. It is often characterized by redness, increased local temperature, or swelling, as well as signs of autonomic nervous system activity including rapid heartbeat, rapid shallow respirations, increased blood pressure, diaphoresis, pallor, and dilated pupils (Helms & Barone, 2008). Acute pain usually ends after the underlying cause is treated or has been resolved.

Chronic pain no longer serves the purpose of protecting tissue from damage. It may be continuous or intermittent and is of sufficient duration and intensity to adversely affect well-being, level of function, and quality of life (Jacobson, 2001). Complaints of chronic pain are common among patients in correctional settings

TABLE 13.1   Types and Characteristics of Pain

TYPE OF TISSUE	STRUCTURES INVOLVED	DESCRIPTION OF PAIN	EXAMPLES
Somatic Transmitted by nociceptors in cutaneous or deep tissue	Skin, muscle, blood vessels, connective tissue, bone	Sharp, cutting burning, throbbing, aching, and gnawing. Well localized	Laceration, fracture, surgical procedures, wound complications, low back pain, PVD
Visceral Transmitted by autonomic fibers in organs	Organs and linings of body cavities	Dull, deep, aching, and colicky. Poorly localized. Nausea, vomiting, hypotension, weakness. Pain may be referred to a cutaneous site supplied by the same segment of spinal system	Appendicitis, colitis, liver metastases, myocardial infarction
Neuropathic	Peripheral nervous system, spinal cord and central nervous system	Sharp, burning, shooting. May be associated with numbness, tingling, and itching sensation. May include pain with nonpainful stimuli (i.e., touch) or exaggerated response to painful stimuli	Diabetic neuropathy, shingles, post-stroke, multiple sclerosis, phantom limb

Source: From Mohn-Brown et al. (2010); Helms and Barone (2008).

(Lubelczyk, 2008; Mollina, 2006; NCCHC, 2011; Puerini, 2011). Table 13.2 compares the features of acute and chronic pain.

Assessment

The saying "pain, the fifth vital sign" was suggested as a way to remind nurses to assess pain whenever the other vital signs were taken. When nurses assess pain regularly, use of the nursing process ensures that the nurse will intervene to relieve pain when it is present and advocate for change or additions to the treatment plan if relief is not achieved (Daykin, 2006; Helms & Barone, 2008; Wells et al., 2008).

Nursing assessment of *acute pain* is focused on collecting subjective and objective information that assists in diagnosis and monitoring the patient's condition to prevent adverse effects of treatment intervention and minimize discomfort and side effects. Reassessment should include the intensity of pain present, the degree of relief obtained as a result of the intervention, barriers to treatment effectiveness, side effects from medication, and extent to which sleep, mood, and activity is affected. The outcome of nursing care for patients with acute pain is uncomplicated recovery from the illness or injury causing the pain.

TABLE 13.2   Features of Acute and Chronic Pain

CHARACTERISTIC	ACUTE	CHRONIC
Relief of pain	Highly desirable	Highly desirable
Dependence or tolerance to medications	Unusual	Common
Psychiatric component	Not usual	Often significant
Organic cause	Common	Not common
Environmental or family contribution	Minimal	Significant
Insomnia	Unusual	Common
Treatment goal	Cure	Improve function

Source: From Mollina (2006).

Acute pain should be reassessed by a nurse after every pain intervention to evaluate effectiveness. In an ambulatory or outpatient setting, the correctional nurse may instruct the patient to stay in the clinic area or to return to the clinic if pain is not reduced within a certain time period. The nurse also informs the patient about what to expect in terms of the pain experience, time frames for relief, side effects and how they can be prevented or managed, as well as the process of healing. These steps help the patient manage anxiety and fear and may prevent some subsequent requests for health care attention.

In the inpatient setting, reassessment of pain should take place according to the interval set in the patient's treatment plan and after any intervention to reduce pain. Any new report of pain or pain that is increasing in intensity should also be assessed. Unexpected pain associated with symptoms of hypotension, tachycardia, or fever requires immediate assessment and communication with the patient's health care provider (RNAO, 2002, Supplement 2007).

Care of *chronic pain* patients is improved when managed using the collaborative care model that incorporates the patient as a member of a multidisciplinary team (Institute for Clinical Systems Improvement [ICSI], 2009, 2011). The NCCHC recommends use of the chronic care model and correctional health care programs have already begun to adopt this approach (G. Burrow, personal communication, January 20, 2012; Mollina, 2006; NCCHC, 2011; Puerini, 2011). The assessment of chronic pain is more comprehensive and is done to determine the mechanisms of pain that are operative, identify factors contributing to pain as well as barriers to treatment, and to engage the patient in a therapeutic relationship (ICSI, 2009, 2011).

The information to be elicited in an assessment of a patient with chronic pain is listed in Exhibit 13.1. With the exception of the physical examination, it is within the scope of nursing practice for the registered nurse to collect any of this information. The initial assessment of chronic pain is time consuming but can be gathered over several encounters and by different members of the treatment team. The patient can also be asked to provide information in advance via questionnaire. The outcome for treatment and management of chronic pain is maintenance or improvement in the patient's functionality and well-being (ICSI, 2009, 2011; Puerini, 2011).

In the correctional setting, nurses sometimes struggle with the emphasis on the patient's subjective report of pain and are advised to supplement this with data gained from observation of the patient. The weakness of observational data is that

EXHIBIT 13.1
Components in the Assessment of Chronic Pain

Pain: each area where the patient has pain should be described in terms of location, intensity, quality, onset, duration, variation, methods of pain relief used, what makes it better/worse. May include asking patient to rate pain intensity several ways, such as current pain, worst pain, least pain, average pain, and tolerable over the last week or some other standard time period.

Pain history: onset and progression of pain(s), treatments, and response to treatment. May also include review of records.

Physical exam: focused especially on the pain described in the history and in current pain assessment to identify correctable physical problems, determine the type of pain, as well as contributory factors. May include diagnostic testing or review of prior diagnostic tests.

Functional assessment: has pain affected sleeping, appetite, getting out of the bunk, going to the toilet/shower and to meals, hygiene, going to the yard, exercise/activity, hobbies or other interests, mood and relationships with others.

Psychological assessment: presence of depression and/or anxiety, other psychiatric diagnoses and treatment, history of substance abuse and treatment or recovery status, physical/sexual abuse, coping skills and patterns.

Social history: work performed, job satisfaction, relationship with others at work, reasons for not working. Involvement in programming (GED, workforce training, anger management, etc.) including attendance, completion, relationships with participants and supervisors. Pending legal issues, expected release date, disciplinary history.

Patient knowledge and expectations: degree of pain relief expected and acceptable, type of treatment requested and expected effect, role of the patient in participating in treatment, specific functional improvements sought and time frame for accomplishment.

Source: From ICSI (2009, 2011); RNAO (2002, Supplement 2007); McLennon (2007); Mackintosh and Elson (2008).

it is filtered by the nurse's own beliefs and experiences. The same is true with observations provided by custody staff. There are many possible explanations for discrepancy between the patient's description of pain and the objective signs and symptoms. These may include misunderstanding terminology or lack of knowledge, cultural factors, secondary gain, and denial, as well as effective use of relaxation or other coping skills. The NCCHC (2011) recommends including the patient's self-report in the assessment of chronic pain.

The quality of subjective data can be improved as communication with the patient is improved (Daykin, 2006). Referring to Figure 13.1, only the patient can describe the knowledge, feelings, and perceptions that act on and are influenced by the experience of pain. Listening to concerns and communicating a desire to help the patient be more comfortable are core dimensions of improved pain control. Skilled communication may reveal causes of discomfort or symptoms that are contributing to underlying pain that can be alleviated (Wells et al., 2008).

Factors That Contribute to the Pain Experience and Barriers to Treatment

The next step in the treatment of chronic pain is identification of the factors that contribute to the patient's pain and the barriers to treatment. Contributory factors are things that exacerbate, amplify, or perpetuate pain but are not causal. Contributory factors can be modified to improve pain control and are the focus of treatment intervention. Barriers are things that interfere with a thorough assessment and/or completing treatment. Barriers may be impossible or very difficult to overcome. Identifying barriers provides a realistic basis for predicting treatment progress. An example of a barrier specific to corrections may be the unpredictable release or transfer of the patient. Table 13.3 lists some common contributing factors and barriers for treatment of chronic pain in the correctional setting.

Some factors are listed as both a barrier and a contributing factor. For example, the patient's expectations for pain relief and functionality may be a barrier because they are unrealistic. If these expectations can be modified, perhaps as a result of the influence and advice from the nurse or another trusted provider, they contribute less to the anger, hopelessness, and frustration that is part of the chronic pain experience (Bialosky, Bishop, & Cleland, 2010).

Other barriers to assessment and treatment of chronic pain that are systemic in correctional settings and are not patient specific include the availability of mental health consultation and treatment, availability of cognitive behavioral programming, formulary restrictions, property or canteen limitations and restrictions, physical plant limitations, unskilled or disinterested health care providers, and general access to health care resources in correctional facilities (Mollina, 2006; Puerini, 2011).

TABLE 13.3   Pain: Barriers and Contributing Factors in the Correctional Setting

BARRIERS	CONTRIBUTING FACTORS
Passive or low motivation	Other physical health problems
Poor communication	Poor posture or use of body mechanics
Unrealistic expectations	Unrealistic expectations
History of substance or sexual abuse	Activity restrictions or limitations
Poor work history	Poor physical strength and stamina
Poor treatment compliance in the past	Insomnia
Language	Passive or low motivation
Culture	Depression, anxiety, other mental illness
Family support	Job dissatisfaction
Depression, anxiety, other mental illness	Poor relationships
Peer pressure	Coping skills
Disciplinary consequences, pending sentence or other legal issues	Knowledge about pain, anatomy, medications, etc.
Program or assignment conflicts	Financial resources
Release date	Living conditions (noise, distances, safety)
Transfers	Grief or loss

COMPREHENSIVE PLAN OF CARE

Elements that should be addressed in the plan of care for all chronic pain patients are the patient's personal goals and expectations, sleep, hygiene, physical activity, stress management, and pain reduction. In the correctional setting, use of a comprehensive treatment plan for chronic pain provides a basis for broadening the discussion with the patient from demands for medication and other forms of treatment with limited duration of effectiveness (Lubelczyk, 2008; Mollina, 2006; Puerini, 2011). An example of a patient treatment plan and record is provided in Figure 13.2. This form was adapted from material developed by the pain management program at the Santa Clara County Jail (Mollina, 2006). The use of a record increases the patient's involvement in treatment, which improves pain control; it also provides important information about coping patterns that can be reinforced or modified (Keefe, Somers, & Kothadia, 2009; RNAO, 2002, Supplement 2007).

The components of a nursing follow-up visit include vital signs (including weight), pain assessment, review of the record kept by the patient, medication adherence and side effects, and any unscheduled episodes of care. Intervals for follow-up may need to be shortened to eliminate the need to complain about pain in order to get attention from the nurse or provider (Puerini, 2011). If a patient is not progressing but has been compliant with the plan of care, then treatment should be adjusted accordingly. If the patient is not adhering to the plan of care, the contributory factors and barriers should be reassessed and the plan adjusted accordingly (ICSI, 2009, 2011). Case Example 13.2 provides an opportunity to apply material reviewed in this chapter.

CASE EXAMPLE 13.2

Ms. Farleigh is a 48-year-old woman who is seen in the chronic care program for low back pain associated with a work injury that occurred several years before this incarceration. She received supplemental medical benefits and was cared for by the Kaiser system prior to incarceration. She reports her pain as a 9, on a scale from 1 to 10, and it is unchanging in intensity. She is able to shower, dress, walk to meals, and comply with security orders. She has problems sleeping and has worries about her family, especially a teenaged daughter living alone as a result of the mother's incarceration. Her treatment plan incorporates an exercise plan, a mild anti-inflammatory medication, and use of heat with stretching exercises done in cell.

Discussion Questions:

1. What are the factors that are likely to contribute to this patient's pain?
2. What are the barriers to treatment if this woman were incarcerated at a facility you are familiar with?

Symptom Management

The use of medicine, particularly analgesics, is the primary focus in managing acute pain; nonpharmacologic approaches are supplementary. In managing chronic, non-cancer pain, nonpharmacologic approaches are essential to improve function and reduce pain (JCAHO & NPC, 2005).

From the Experts . . .

"After reviewing so many lawsuits about pain, I started talking with our health care team about involving the patient from the beginning, forming a partnership so that the patient knew what they were getting, why, and the goals for treatment."

Gayle F. Burrow, RN, BSN, MPH, CCHP-RN (Retired)
Portland, OR

Week of:							
Goal 1: Functional ability will be improved by (specify)							
	Sunday	Monday	Tuesday	Wednesday	Thursday	Friday	Saturday
Goal 2: Decrease pain by (specify)							
Daily Pain Rating: No pain at all 0 1 2 3 4 5 6 7 8 9 10 Worst pain imaginable							
Least							
Worst							
Average							
Goal 3: Improve sleep by (specify)							
Daily rating of accomplishment: Accomplished 0 1 2 3 4 5 6 7 8 9 10 Not Accomplished							
List action							
List action							
Goal 4: Increase physical activity by (specify)							
Type							
# of minutes							
What activities were affected by pain: Not affected 0 1 2 3 4 5 6 7 8 9 10 Unable to do							
Appetite							
Shower							
Yard/activity							
Work							
Program							
List any specific activity missed because of pain (work, school, meals, visit, program, etc.)							
1.							
2.							
3.							
Goal 5: Manage stress by (specify)							
(List activity)							
# of minutes							
(List activity)							
# of minutes							
(List activity)							
# of minutes							
Describe any important events (family, friends, work, school, program, legal etc.)							
1.							
2.							
Describe improvements noted in functional ability by the end of the week:							

FIGURE 13.2 Patient plan and daily record.

Source: From Mollina (2006); Institute for Clinical Systems Improvement (2009, 2011).

Pharmacologic

Analgesics include acetaminophen, nonsteroidal anti-inflammatory drugs (NSAIDS), and opioids. Acetaminophen is used for initial treatment of mild pain and if combined with other agents (NSAIDS and opioids) to treat mild to moderate pain. It does not have the gastric side effects of NSAIDS. Nurses should caution patients with liver or renal disease in the use of acetaminophen. NSAIDS are used for mild to moderate pain, and when combined with an opioid are used to treat moderate to severe pain. NSAIDS are most effective with somatic or visceral pain (see Table 13.1), but less so with neuropathic pain. Risks include gastritis and bleeding; caution should be used in recommending NSAIDS with older adults, diabetics, and patients with bleeding disorders and liver disease (RNAO, 2002, Supplement 2007; Wells et al., 2008).

Self-care instructions and nursing protocols used in correctional settings commonly use acetaminophen and/or NSAIDS for many health problems that involve pain, particularly soft tissue injuries, strains, sprains, toothache, and headache. Patients should be cautioned by nurses not to go above the recommended dosage, not to combine NSAIDS, and to get more specific instructions from their provider for pain relief if they have hepatitis, diabetes, kidney or liver disease, have ulcers, or have a bleeding disorder.

Opiates are used to relieve moderate to severe pain. Their use is indicated in the short-term management of acute pain and they may be appropriate in treatment of chronic pain when first-line approaches are not effective. Clinical guidelines used in correctional health care settings are designed to provide evidenced-based support for providers to prescribe opiates when appropriate, as well as to reduce demands for pain medications from patients when they are not clinically indicated (Puerini, 2011; Reichert, 2010).

When opiates are included in the plan of care, the expectations of the patient with regard to treatment adherence, side effects, and monitoring should be specified in the written plan, along with documentation of the risks and benefits for informed consent (Bittner, Marcus, Tenzer, & Romito, 2010). In addition to goals for functionality and pain, monitoring is likely to include tracking medication compliance closely, crushing medication and mouth checks to prevent hoarding or diversion, and periodic urine drug screening (Reichert, 2010; Rossi & Kenney, 2010).

Antidepressants are another drug group effective in treatment of pain, particularly tricyclic antidepressants (TCA) and serotonin/norepinephrine reuptake inhibitors (SSRIs) (ICSI, 2009, 2011; JCAHO & NPC, 2005). The use of antidepressant medication enhances the analgesic effects and also addresses symptoms of anxiety, depression, and insomnia which frequently accompany pain (ICSI, 2009, 2011; Mackintosh & Elson, 2008). Nurses should advise the patient that it may take 2–3 weeks before they notice a difference.

Anticonvulsants relieve neuropathic pain, particularly pain described as "shooting" or "pins and needles." Their mechanism of action is to reduce the excitability of neurons and the resulting irritation of nerve stimulation (Mackintosh & Elson, 2008). It may take 2–3 weeks before the patient reports symptom relief. Side effects are sedation and dizziness (ICSI, 2009, 2011). Topical analgesics also relieve neuropathic pain, particularly products that contain lidocaine or capsaicin.

Muscle relaxants are used to address *acute* musculoskeletal pain but are not recommended for treatment of chronic musculoskeletal pain. Benzodiazepines may be used to treat anxiety and muscle spasms associated with acute pain, but are not indicated in the management of chronic pain (ICSI, 2009, 2011).

Nonpharmacologic Approaches

There is strong evidence to support the combination of pharmaceutical and non-pharmaceutical interventions in managing pain. The Institute for Clinical Systems Improvement (ICSI) reviewed the literature and published the fifth edition of evidence-based guidelines for chronic pain in 2011. The RNAO similarly reviewed the literature and published a best practice guideline for assessment and management of acute and chronic pain in 2002, which was updated in 2007. Both these guidelines report evidence-based support for the use of acupuncture and cognitive behavioral strategies. They also found increasing evidence for the use of relaxation, music, massage, and heat and cold (RNAO, 2002, Supplement 2007; ICSI, 2011).

Cognitive behavioral strategies use operant conditioning to change behavior related to pain. As the way the patient thinks and feels changes, pain is decreased or becomes more tolerable, and functionality improves. The ICSI (2009, 2011) identified several cognitive behavioral strategies that are simple to implement in the primary care setting. These would be appropriate to include in the collaborative chronic care model advocated by the NCCHC (2011) for management of chronic pain. The strategies are to:

1. Inform the patient that pain management is complicated and that effective treatment involves their active participation.
2. Convey to the patient a desire to work with them to manage their pain and that their experience of pain is important to know about.
3. Identify and de-couple the factors that reinforce pain behavior so that a patient does not have to complain of pain to see a health care provider, take medication, or stop an activity.
4. Introduce increased activity and functionality (going to school, programming, or work) incrementally that is not dependent upon pain level.

In suggesting nonpharmacologic approaches to patients, nurses need to be careful to avoid undermining the patient's preferred technique for pain relief or expectations regarding pain relief from a particular technique. Patient expectations very much determine the extent of relief they will achieve from a particular intervention, and nurses can influence those expectations both positively and negatively (Bialosky et al., 2010; Wells et al., 2008).

The following techniques do not require special training or certification and can easily be used in the correctional setting by patients as part of a chronic pain plan.

Diaphragmatic breathing is the slow inhale/exhale of breath using the diaphragm to extend and slow breathing. Done in a relaxed position with eyes closed, the length of inhale and exhale should be the same and slowly reach 6–8 breaths a minute.

Progressive muscle relaxation is a method of slowly tightening and relaxing different muscle groups to reach a state of deep relaxation. Audiotapes or scripts can be used to guide a patient through this process. The speed and depth of the relaxation response increase with practice.

Imagery is imagining a pleasant or relaxing scene from the past. Imagination may be enhanced with auditory (audio tape, music) and visual input to progress through a series of pleasant scenes to a deep state of relaxation. Imagery reduces autonomic arousal by diverting attention away from painful stimuli. Imagery has been very helpful in helping burn patients and others tolerate repeated painful procedures such as dressing changes. Several sessions of imagery work are necessary before pain relief will occur (ICSI, 2009, 2011; RNAO, 2002, Supplement 2007).

Journaling is writing in an emotional way over a period of days. Journaling helps organize and resolve complex emotional experiences that contribute to pain. Patients write about something that is influencing their life and causing emotional upset for 15–20 minutes a day without regard for spelling, punctuation, or grammar. The patient is likely to begin to sense relief and resolution after a week of writing (American Pain Foundation, 2011; Esterling, L'Abate, Murray, & Pennebaker, 1999; Pennebaker & Seagal, 1999). The patient does not need to share the material or even review it themselves, and in a correctional setting can be encouraged to tear it up or mail it outside the facility, if privacy or victimization is a concern.

Physical Activity

Fitness and physical rehabilitation is a key aspect of managing chronic pain and patients should be engaged in selecting the type of exercise program and goals. Favorable outcomes in reducing low back pain with exercise were reported when patients had good two-way communication with their provider, who explained the relationship between exercise, functionality, and pain while accepting and validating the patient's experience (Slade, Molloy, & Keating, 2009). There is no evidence that supports any one type of exercise program over another (ICSI, 2009, 2011). Activities can include endurance, strengthening, balance, and flexibility, so even correctional facilities without access to physical therapy expertise can include exercise in a patient's plan of care.

Goals for exercise should start within the patient's pain capacity and increase in intensity according to a gradual schedule that is not pain dependent. Patients should be advised in the use of heat and cold, relaxation, and other cognitive techniques to manage pain during activity (ICSI, 2009, 2011). Some correctional nursing experts report no problems providing access to exercise and use of heat and cold (personal correspondence, H. Villanueva, January 19, 2012; M. Krahn, January 19, 2012; J. Kerns, January 19, 2012; P. Morris, January 20, 2012; M. Raines, January 23, 2012). Others cite these as a significant problem in the correctional setting (personal correspondence, L. Nash, January 19, 2012; K. Alves, January 19, 2012; B. Pinney, January 19, 2012; P. Voermans, January 20, 2012; M. LaMarre, January 22, 2012). Several of these nurses commented on the leadership and perseverance necessary to gain acknowledgment of the safety and effectiveness of these interventions not only with patients, but also health care providers and correctional colleagues (personal communication, M. Krahn, January 19, 2012; P. Morris, January 20, 2012).

Patient Information and Education

One of the most important roles that nurses have with patients is to provide information, education, resources for more information, and counseling for behavioral change. When nurses anticipate a patient's anxiety and potential for pain, they can provide information about what to expect and how to cope, which in turn helps reduce pain experienced by the patient. The content areas nurses assist pain patients with include:

- Anatomy and pathophysiology of the disease, injury, or illness causing pain.
- The biopsychosocial dimensions of pain.

From the Experts ...

"Starting these programs takes time, effort, and buy-in from all of the stake-holders, but it is well worth the effort."

Mary Krahn, RN, CCHP
Portland, OR

- Physical activity that provides exercise, increases flexibility, balance, and strength.
- Medication use, side effects, and misuse/abuse.
- How to use the pain record and any other expectations for the patient about their role in the plan.
- Reinforce other activities the patient is participating in, such as learning to use meditation, relaxation, and so on (Mollina, 2006).

PATIENT ADVOCACY?

In pain care, the nurse has a duty to prevent or relieve suffering; to do so requires knowledge of the patient's needs or wishes and to act on the patient's behalf when the patient is unable to do so themselves. Advocacy also involves ensuring that the patient is informed to make decisions about his or her health care and then respecting those decisions. Standard 12 of the Scope and Standards of Practice for Corrections Nursing states, "Serves as a patient advocate and assists patients in developing skills for self-advocacy..." (ANA, 2007, p. 40).

The evidence the nurse uses to advocate for change in the patient's plan of care comes from the synthesis of data gathered from the assessment and evaluation of the patient's response to each intervention or a new complaint of pain. This evidence includes

- Intensity of pain using a pain scale standardized for use with the patient
- Changes in severity scores in the last day
- Change in severity and quality of pain following administration of analgesic and adjuvant medications and length of time relief is achieved
- Amount of regular and breakthrough pain in the last day
- Patient's goals for pain relief
- Effect of unrelieved pain upon the person's functionality
- Absence or presence of side effects or toxicity
- Data regarding contributing factors or barriers that modify the plan of care (RNAO, 2002, Supplement 2007).

SUMMARY

Each of us has experience with pain; yet, each of our experiences differs from others'. The scientific knowledge about how pain is experienced has increased tremendously and so has the evidence about how pain is appropriately treated and managed.

Managing pain in the correctional setting has many of the same challenges providers in the community face. There are also advantages; the opportunity to build a therapeutic relationship to coach our patients over the term of their incarceration and the ability to monitor closely how our patients are doing in managing pain as they carry out their daily activities and adjust treatment accordingly. We can choose to employ the best scientific evidence to treat and manage our patients and they may get better. If we ignore the evidence, our patients' complaints of pain will still be as prevalent and may become more incessant.

DISCUSSION QUESTIONS

1. What aspect of pain management is most difficult or challenging for you? What would make this easier for you?
2. Provide an example of a dismissive or judgmental statement made by a nurse to a patient complaining of pain. What effect(s) do you think it had on the quality of information obtained by the nurse assessing the patient's pain?
3. How would you tell a patient about chronic pain and the approach to treating the condition?

REFERENCES

Adams, N., & Field, L. (2001). Pain management 1: Psychologiocal and social aspects of pain. *British Journal of Nursing, 10*(14), 903–911.

American Nurses Association. (2007). *Corrections nursing: Scope and standards of practice.* Silver Spring, MD: NursesBooks.org.

American Pain Foundation. (2011). Journaling for pain relief. *Pain Community News, 11*(4), 10–11.

Beck, M. (2011, July 5). Diagnosing a patient as a faker. *The Wall Street Journal.*

Belknap, J. (2006). *The invisible woman: Gender, crime, and justice.* Belmont, CA: Wadsworth/Thompson Learning.

Bialosky, J., Bishop, M., & Cleland, J. (2010, September). Individual expectation: An overlooked, but pertinent, factor in the treatment of individuals experiencing musculoskeletal pain. *Physical Therapy, 90*(9), 1345–1355.

Bittner, B., Marcus, D., Tenzer, P., & Romito, K. (2010). *Using opioids in the management of chronic pain patients: Challenges and future options.* Retrieved March 22, 2011, from American Academy of Family Physicians: http://www.aafp.org/online/en/home/publications/otherpubs/afpmonographs/opioidschronicpain/masthead.html

Butler, D. S., & Moseley, G. L. (2003). *Explain pain.* Adelaide: Noigroup Publications.

California Board of Registered Nursing. (2000, February 27). *Pain assessment: The fifth vital sign.* Retrieved March 4, 2011, from Department of Consumer Affairs, Board of Registered Nursing: http://www.rn.ca.gov/pdfs/regulations/npr-b-27.pdf

Charlton, J. (2005). *Core curriculum for professional education in pain.* Retrieved March 5, 2010, from International Association for the Study of Pain: http://www.iasp-pain.org/AM/Template.cfm?Section=Home&Template=/CM/ContentDisplay.cfm&ContentID=1978

D'Arcy, Y. (2005, April). Pain management standards, the law, and you. *Nursing 2005, 17.*

Daykin, S. (2006). Pain management. In P. Pratt (Ed.), *Fundamental aspects of caring for the acutely ill adult* (p. 165). London, England: Quay Books.

Esterling, B. A., L'Abate, L. L., Murray, E. J., & Pennebaker, J. W. (1999). Empirical foundations for writing in prevention and psychotherapy: Mental and physical health outcomes. *Clinical Psychology Review, 19*(1), 79–96.

Ezenwa, M., Ameringer, S., Ward, S., & Serlin, R. (2006). Racial and ethnic disparities in pain management in the United States. *Journal of Nursing Scholarship, Third Quarter,* 225–233.

Ferrell, B. R., McCaffery, M., & Rhiner, M. (1992). Pain and addiction: an urgent need for change in nursing education. *Journal of Pain Management, 7*(2), 117–124.

Field, L., & Adams, N. (2001). Pain management 2: The use of psychological approaches to pain. *British Journal of Pain, 10*(15), 971–974.

Glaze, L. (2004) Profile of jail inmates, 2002. *Bureau of Justice Statistics.* Retrieved from http://bjs.ojp. usdoj,gov/index.cfm?ty=pbdetail&iid=1118

Grose, S., & Shub, T. (2010, September 10). *Pain management: An overview.* Glendale: Cinahl Information Systems.

Helms, J., & Barone, C. P. (2008, December). Physiology and treatment of pain. *Critical Care Nurse, 28*(6), 38–49.

Institute for Clinical Systems Improvement. Fourth Edition. (2009, November). *Assessment and management of chronic pain.* Retrieved February 27, 2011, from http://www.icsi.org/pain_chronic_assessment_and_management_of_14399/pain_chronic_assessment_and_ management_of_guideline_.html

Institute for Clinical Systems Improvement. Fifth Edition. (2011, November). *Assessment and management of chronic pain.* Retrieved April 14, 2012, from http://www.icsi.org/pain_chronic_assessment_and_management_of_14399/pain_chronic_assessment_and_management_of_guideline_.html

Institute of Medicine. (2011, June 29). *Relieving pain in America: A blueprint for transforming prevention, care, education, and research.* Retrieved August 2, 2011, from http://www.iom.edu/Reports/2011/Relieving-Pain-in-America-A-Blueprint-for-Transforming-Prevention-Care-Education-Research.aspx

International Association for the Study of Pain (IASP). (2011). *Pain.* IASP Taxonomy. Retrieved January 22, 2012, from http://www.iasp-pain.org/AM/Template.cfm?Section=Pain_Definitions#Pain

Jacobson, L. M. (2001). General considerations of chronic pain. In J. Loeser, S. Butler, R. Chapman, & D. Turk (Eds.), *Bonica's management of pain* (3rd ed., pp. 105–106). Philadelphia: Lippincott Williams &Wilkens.

James, D., & Glaze, L. (2006, September). *Mental health problems of prison and jail inmates.* Retrieved March 3, 2011, from Bureau of Justice Statistics: http://bjs.ojp.usdoj.gov/content/pub/pdf/mhppji.pdf

Johnson, S., Todd, K., & Moulton, B. (2007). Chronic pain and healthy communities: Legal, ethical, and policy issues in improving the public's health. Public health and the law. *Journal of Law, Medicine & Ethics, 35,* 69–71.

Keefe, F., Somers, T., & Kothadia, S. (2009, October). Coping with pain. *Pain: Clinical Updates, XVII*(5), 1–5.

Kelly, P. J., Parlaz-Dieckmann, E., Chang, A. L., & Collins, C. (2010). Profile of women in a county jail. *Journal of Psychosocial Nursing, 48*(4), 38–45.

LaMarre, M. (2006). Nursing role and practice in correctional facilities. In M. Puisis (Ed.), *Clinical practice in clinical medicine* (p. 421). Philadelphia: Mosby Elsevier.

Lasch, K. (2002, December). Culture and pain. *Pain Clinical Updates, X*(5).

Lin, J., & Mathew, P. (2005, May 29). Cancer pain management in prisons: A survey of primary care practitioners and inmates. *Journal of Pain & Symptom Management, 29*(5), 466–473.

Lubelczyk, R. (2008). Managing chronic pain: It doesn't have to be so painful. *National Conference on Correctional Health Care.* Chicago: National Commission on Correctional Health Care.

Mackintosh, C., & Elson, S. (2008). Chronic pain: Clinical features, assesment and treatment. *Nursing Standard, 23*(5), 48–56.

Mailis-Gagnon, A. (2010). Ethnocultural and sex differences in pain. In A. Kopf, & N. Patel (Eds.), *Guide to Pain Management in Low Resource Settings* (pp. 27–31). Seattle: International Association for the Study of Pain.

Marks, R. M., & Sachar, E. J. (1973). Undertreatment of medical inpatients with narcotic analgesics. *Annals of Internal Medicine, 78*(2), 173–181.

McLennon, S. (2007). Evidence-based guideline: Persistent pain management. *Journal of Gerontological Nursing, 33*(7), 5–14.

Meghani, S., & Houldin, A. (2007). The meanings of and attitudes about cancer pain among African Americans. *Oncology Nursing Forum, 34*(6), 1179–1186.

Michigan Department of Licensing and Regulatory Affairs (2009). Continuing education requirements for Michigan nurses. Retrieved January 22, 2012, from http://www.michigan.gov/
documents/cis_fhs_bhser_nurse_cebroc_67748_7.pdf

Mohn-Brown, E. L., Burke, K. M., & Eby, L. (2010, May 18). *Medical-surgical nursing care–3rd Ed.,
Unit II, Chapter 8 Caring for clients in pain.* E. Mohn-Brown, K. Burke, & L. Eby (Eds.), Retrieved
February 27, 2011, from STAT! Ref Online Electronic Medical Library: http://online.statref.
com.proxy.heal-wa.org/document.aspx?fxid=187&docid=95

Mollina, F. (2006). Creating something from nothing: Pain management treatment program in a
county jail setting. *Updates in correctional health care.* Las Vegas: National Commission on
Correctional Health Care.

National Commission on Correctional Health Care (2011). *Position statements: Management of
chronic pain.* Retrieved January 16, 2012, from http://ncchc.org/resources/statements/chronic_
pain.html

Nursing Care Quality Assurance Commission. (2011). Pain Management. Washington State
Department of Health. Retrieved January 22, 2012, from http://www.doh.wa.gov/hsqa/Pro-
fessions/PainManagement/Default.htm

Oregon Pain Management Commission. (n.d.). *Pain management module.* Retrieved March 4, 2011,
from Oregon State Government, Department of Human Resources: http://www.oregon.
gov/OHA/OHPR/PMC/module/Module.pdf

Oregon State Board of Nursing. (2011). *Pain CE Requirement.* Retrieved January 22, 2012, from
Oregon State Board of Nursing: http://www.oregon.gov/OSBN/pain_management.shtml

Pasero, C., & McCaffery, M. (2011). *Pain assessment and pharmacologic management* (1st ed.). St. Louis,
MO: Mosby Elsevier.

Patel, N. (2010). Physiology of pain. In A. Kopf, & N. Patel (Eds.), *Guide to pain management in
low-resource settings* (pp. 13–17). Seattle: International Association for Study of Pain.

Pennebaker, J. W., & Seagal, J. D. (1999). Forming a story: The health benefits of narrative. *Journal of
Clinical Psychology, 55*(10), 1243–1254.

Puerini, M. T. (2011, March 11). *Chronic pain and the incarcerated patient.* Oregon chapter of the
American Correctional Health Services Association. Cottage Grove.

Registered Nurses Association of Ontario. (2002, Supplement 2007). *Assessment and management of
pain.* International Affairs and Nursing Best Practice Guidelines Program. Toronto: Author.

Reichert, E. (2010). Pain management: Basics & interventions unique to the inmate population.
Updates in Correctional Health Care. Nashville: National Commission on Correctional Health
Care.

Rossi, A. F., & Kenney, J. D. (2010). *Guidelines for opioid therapy to treat pain in Washington State prisons.*
Las Vegas: National Commission on Correctional Health Care.

Rutledge, D., & Caple, C. (2010, June 18). *Evidence—based care sheet: Pain assessment in special
populations.* Retrieved February 26, 2011, from Cinahl Information Systems: Glendale.

Slade, S., Molloy, E., & Keating, J. (2009). "Listen to me, tell me": A qualitative study of partnership
in care for people with non-specific chronic low back pain. *Clinical Rehabilitation, 23,* 270–280.

The Joint Commission. (2011, January). *Facts about pain management.* Retrieved March 3, 2011, from
The Joint Commission: http://www.jointcommission.org/assets/1/18/Pain_Management.pdf

The Joint Commission on Accreditation of Healthcare Organizations and the National Pharmaceutical Council. (2005, May). *Pain: Current understanding of assessment, management and treatments.*
Retrieved March 21, 2011, from National Pharmacuetical Council: http://www.ampainsoc.
org/ce/enduring/downloads/npc/section_4.pdf

Wells, N., Pasero, C., & McCaffery, M. (2008, April). In R. Hughes (Ed.), *Improving the quality of care
through pain assessment and management.* Retrieved March 2011, 2011, from Patient Safety and
Quality: An Evidence-Based Handbook for Nurses, Rockville, MD. http://www.ahrq.gov/
qual/nurseshdbk/: http://www.ncbi.nlm.nih.gov/books/NBK2658/

FOURTEEN

Health Screening

Catherine M. Knox

*H*ealth screening is performed by correctional nurses many times every day (American Nurses Association, 2007). Screening takes place upon arrival at the facility, before inmates are assigned work duties, upon placement in segregated housing, before admission to certain treatment programs, and for many other reasons.

Using the results of screening, nurses make triage decisions critical to the health and safety of the detainee. Sometimes, these decisions also contribute to the health and safety of other detainees and personnel at the facility. The best triage decisions are made when nurses establish rapport with each individual and are skilled in obtaining information and observing nonverbal cues.

HEALTH SCREENING

Screening is a method used to identify certain characteristics, features, or problems among many people. The outcome of screening is that people are cleared efficiently, adverse events are prevented, and specialized resources are reserved (Knox, 2010).

Underidentification and Overidentification

The problems most often encountered with screening are underidentification and overidentification. Underidentification is when people who should have been identified by screening were not. An example of this would be when the intake screening does not identify someone with mental illness. The result is that the mentally ill person is cleared to population when they should have been referred for mental health assessment and evaluation. Overidentification is when people are identified by screening when, in fact, they should have been cleared. An example of this would be when nearly all the detainees screened at intake are identified as having mental illness. If this happens, mental health resources are tied up evaluating detainees who are healthy or who do not need mental health resources. There are many reasons that cause "under" or "over" identification to occur. It may be that the tool is incorrect for the purpose, the identification criteria are unclear, or it may not be appropriate to screen for the characteristic (Raffle, 2011).

Balancing Accuracy and Efficiency

The screening method used needs to be accurate enough to identify the condition but not tie up resources, like time and personnel, unnecessarily. Using the mental health example again, all detainees could receive a full mental health evaluation at intake. This approach results in more accurate identification of mentally ill persons but requires staffing intake with mental health professionals. Devoting the time of mental health professionals to evaluate all detainees at intake, even those who are healthy, may not be the best use of this valuable resource.

Alternatively, nurses can conduct mental health screening while assessing each detainee for medical problems and then refer those individuals with symptoms or history of mental illness to mental health professionals. This method takes less time to complete and the skills and resources of mental health experts are reserved to evaluate those most likely to need mental health services.

The National Commission on Correctional Health Care (NCCHC), the American Correctional Association (ACA), and the American Psychiatric Association (APA) support the use of nonmental health professionals to conduct initial screening (ACA, 2002; NCCHC, 2008a, 2008b, 2011; Spiers, Pitt, & Dvoskin, 2006). Factors such as time, resources, prevalence of the condition, and consequences are all considerations in deciding how precise identification needs to be (Raffle, 2011).

SCREENING IN THE CORRECTIONAL SETTING

Reception, transfer, and movement of inmates are major activities in correctional facilities. Health screening takes place so that inmates are not placed in situations, settings, or assignments that jeopardize their health, safety, or mental well-being. There are several different kinds of health screening that nurses perform, as listed in Table 14.1, including intake or reception screening, mental health screening, clearance for work or program assignment, and screening for contraindications to restraint or placement in segregation. The nurse should be familiar with the purpose of each type of screening, the timeframes for completion, the decisions that are made, and how these are documented. The nurse should also be trained in the tool or process used to conduct each type of screening.

TABLE 14.1 Types of Health Screening

TYPE OF SCREENING	EXAMPLES
Intake	Reception, transfer, return from court
Work assignment	Food service, labor camp, fire crew, asbestos removal
Program assignment	Substance abuse treatment, school, boot camp
Mental health	Reception, transfer, return from court
Restraint and segregation	Segregation, administrative segregation, maximum custody

Medical Clearance

Virtually all correctional jurisdictions conduct some form of receiving or intake screening. It can be a two- or three-step process. The first part is referred to as medical clearance. It's purpose is to identify anyone who has emergent medical or psychiatric needs and to arrange for the person to receive immediate evaluation and treatment. The ACA requires that those who are unconscious, semiconscious, bleeding, or in obvious need of medical attention be referred immediately, before any other intake processing takes place (ACA, 2002).

The National Commission on Correctional Health Care (NCCHC, 2008a, 2008b, 2011) allows nurses or correctional officers to perform medical clearance if they have been trained to identify signs and symptoms of an impending emergency. Medical clearance is very rudimentary and quickly completed; the detainee may still be in the squad car, in the sally port at the entrance to the facility, or stepping off the transport bus. The ACA (2002) requires that any detainee who needs emergency medical attention be cleared medically before any other intake processing takes place. The other steps in the intake process, such as identification and property inventory, take place only when detainees are medically cleared.

Initial Health Screening

The second step in intake screening is to gather health information about the detainee. The nurse accomplishes this by interview, observation, and a brief physical assessment. The purpose of this step in screening is threefold:

1. To identify persons who have urgent health needs, arrange to continue their care, and ensure that they are assigned housing that is appropriate for their condition.
2. To identify persons who have contagious disease and prevent transmission to others within the facility.
3. To make timely, appropriate referrals for further attention to nonurgent health conditions that require additional evaluation and treatment (Burrow, Knox, & Villanueva, 2006).

Health screening should be initiated as soon as possible after the person's arrival at the facility. Medical and psychiatric emergencies are prevented when receiving screening is accomplished soon after admission. Prompt screening also identifies contagious conditions early and reduces transmission of preventable diseases. The guidance provided by the NCCHC is that it should be "conducted within minutes of arrival"; and that it "... should take place no more than two to four hours after admission" (Kistler & Chavez, 2011, p. 7).

Many of the persons detained or received at correctional facilities are likely to have health problems that will require further evaluation and treatment while they are incarcerated. Persons in jails and prisons have rates of chronic and communicable disease that exceed rates for the same disorder in the community. They also have very high rates of substance abuse, violent injury, and trauma. Lastly, they are likely not to have accessed or had access to health care prior to incarceration other than for emergent disease (Burrow et al., 2006; Hammett, 2006; Maruschak, 2008; Wilper et al., 2009). The content of receiving screening is therefore directed to identifying disease that must be treated during the person's detention or incarceration.

The areas of assessment included in initial health screening are listed in Table 14.2. The amount of detail included in initial health screening varies depending upon the

TABLE 14.2 Content Included in Initial Health Screening

HISTORY	CURRENT PROBLEMS	OBSERVATION	DIAGNOSTIC DATA
Illnesses	Illness	Level of consciousness	Vital signs, including pain
Injury	Injury	Mental status	Tuberculosis testing
Chronic disease	Disability	Behavior	STD screening
Disability	Hospitalization	Appearance	Pregnancy screening
Hospitalization	Current health care provider	Skin condition	If diabetic: blood glucose
Use of medication	Allergies	Movement or gait	If asthmatic: peak expiratory flow
Infectious disease	Symptoms or report of chronic disease	Breathing	Visual acuity
Psychiatric treatment inpatient/outpatient	Dental problems	Oral cavity	Auditory acuity
Suicidal attempts	Current medications	Medication reconciliation	
Alcohol and other drug use	Symptoms or report of infectious disease		
Withdrawal symptoms	Assistive devices/ special equipment		
Immunizations	Psychiatric treatment (inpatient/outpatient)		
Tobacco use	Suicidal ideation		
Family history of cancer, coronary disease, CVA, suicide	Current mental health provider		
Prior incarcerations	Tobacco use		
Victimization or assault	Alcohol and other drug use		
	Withdrawal symptoms		
	Current or recent pregnancy		
	Last menstrual period		

Source: Burrow et al. (2006); Raba (2006); Spiers et al. (2006); National Commission on Correctional Health Care, Prisons, & Jails (2008), Juvenile Detention and Confinement Facilities (2011).

type of facility (jail, detention center, prison), the characteristics of population being received (women, juveniles, etc.), local rates for infectious disease (syphilis, etc.), the type of personnel performing the screening, and the timeframe for when detainees are seen for more comprehensive examination. Preprinted screening forms ensure that all needed information is collected and documented in a standardized manner.

Role of the Nurse

In some facilities, correctional officers perform initial health screening. To ensure complete and thorough screening, the officers should be trained in the use of the tool and how to gather information (ACA, 2002; NCCHC, 2008a, 2008b, 2011). The threshold for identification of persons with health problems must be very clear and set low to ensure that people who need health care attention are not missed (Raba, 2006). The officer must refer to a nurse for further assessment, anyone who answers "yes" to any of the intake questions, or whose condition is at all questionable. A nurse must be available at all times that admissions are received to promptly see anyone referred by the correctional staff in order to meet the requirement that receiving screening is completed within acceptable timeframes. Only individuals who answer "no" to all questions and about whom the officer has no concerns can be cleared without seeing a nurse. Finally, the nurse is expected to review the health screening forms of all individuals cleared by correctional officers the next day, to ensure that no one with a health problem is missed (Burrow et al., 2006).

So many of the detainees have health issues and must be referred by correctional staff that it is usually more efficient to have nurses conduct intake screening. While the threshold for referral still needs to err in favor of referring people with health problems, nurses are effective at intake screening because they have been trained professionally to recognize disease and know how to make decisions about who should receive what kind of follow-up, by whom, and by when (Burrow et al., 2006).

Each nurse's competency to conduct assessments should be verified during initial orientation and periodically thereafter. Nurses may benefit from refresher training, especially ways to streamline the interview and hands-on physical assessment. In addition, nurses need training in the specific procedure and tools used for health screening at the facility or by the system. This ensures that screening is conducted in a consistent manner and the findings or results are reliable. Training should also include the timeframes for accomplishing screening and referral, recognition of the presenting symptoms for the most common as well as high-risk health problems, what actions the nurse takes as a result of screening, and how it is documented.

Setting for Initial Screening

The setting in which the initial health screening takes place greatly contributes to the quality and completeness of information gained from a detainee, youth, or sentenced person (Raba, 2006). If the encounter takes place in a setting where others can overhear what the person is saying, or they can be seen by others being interviewed, concerns about privacy may create disincentive to provide accurate information. Providing auditory or visual privacy is sufficient for the interview; visual privacy should be provided for the examination (Burrow et al., 2006).

The nurse may not be able to arrange for complete auditory and visual privacy and it may not be appropriate in every case. Nurses should, however, be aware of the factors in the environment and circumstances that contribute to withholding health information or providing misinformation and consider these when making disposition decisions.

The quality of information obtained during the receiving screening interview is also diminished when the area is noisy; there are distracting activities and general confusion or when detainees are treated disrespectfully. When someone has a hearing, language, other disability, or does not speak the language, the nurse must make arrangements to provide assistance in conducting the interview so that the questions and answers are understood. Assistance is not adequate if privacy and confidentiality are sacrificed as a result.

Introductory Phase of the Screening Encounter

The initial health screening encounter can be broken down into three parts: the introduction, the working phase, and closure. The introduction is used to initiate the professional relationship with the detainee and build rapport. The nurse introduces himself or herself; then describes the purpose of the screening, the kind of information that is sought, what the information is used for, and who else has access to the information obtained.

The nurse's appearance, use of language, and nonverbal behavior during the introduction can either facilitate or undermine the quality of the remaining interaction and therefore the usefulness of information gathered from the detainee. Techniques to build rapport are listed in Exhibit 14.1. Nurses interested in improving their interview technique should consider asking a peer to use this list of behaviors to observe them interview one or more detainees and provide feedback on areas that could be improved.

Once the nurse has finished the introduction, one asks permission to proceed with screening. Someone who refuses receiving screening may have a problem with the process, such as those discussed in the previous section on the setting for screening. The nurse should attempt to find out why the person is refusing receiving screening. If there is a privacy concern, a communication barrier, or a disability, the nurse may be able to resolve it by providing clarification, additional information, translation, or another type of accommodation. An individual who still refuses receiving screening should be placed in observation until it can be determined that they do not have a health problem that will put themselves or others at risk if cleared (Anno, 2001). Nursing staff should complete receiving screening promptly when anyone who has refused previously indicates they are ready.

EXHIBIT 14.1
Techniques to Build Rapport During Screening Interviews

- Professional appearance
- Focus on the other person
- Neutral or friendly facial expression
- Allow silence so the other person can reflect and respond to each question
- Eye contact that is neither excessive nor insufficient
- Ask questions without reading verbatim
- Avoid use of leading or biased questions
- Avoid body language (distance, standing, posturing) that appears judgmental or superior
- Not distracted, preoccupied, or rushed during the interview

Collecting Subjective and Objective Information

The working phase takes place after the person agrees to proceed with receiving screening. It consists of collecting both subjective and objective information as listed in Table 14.2 using a standardized form or process. The nurse gathers additional information to amplify any positive answers to the interview questions or when objective data collected indicates a possible health problem that will require follow-up. Amplification questions are used to have the detainee describe who, how, what, where, when, and why of a symptom or history of a health condition.

The nurse also reviews any written information that may have accompanied the detainee may be available on a database, or available from another commonly used source. Examples of additional information that may be available include a transfer summary from another facility, various databases kept by a state or county (e.g., people on a mental health caseload, narcotic registry, and immunization records), and electronic health records. It is useful to know whether the individual has health coverage, the name of their health care provider(s), and, if taking medication, where they have prescriptions filled. The patient should be asked to sign a release so that the nurse can initiate a request for records from previous providers. Obtaining information promptly about health care preceding detention facilitates continuity of care for the patient during transition to the correctional setting.

Triage

Triage refers to the decisions made by the nurse based upon the subjective and objective information gathered about the individual. The first decision is if the person is healthy and can be cleared for release to general population in the jail, prison or detention facility. For those who can not be cleared to general population, the next step in triage is to determine what arrangements are necessary to continue the person's health care from the time they leave the reception area until the initial health assessment takes place. The timing of the initial health assessment can vary from immediately, to few days, or up to 2 weeks later, depending upon practices at a particular facility. If the detainee is taking medication, the nurse verifies the prescription with the pharmacy or prescribing provider and then contacts the correctional facility's provider (physician, nurse practitioner, or physician's assistant) to get orders to continue medications. If the detainee had a pending medical appointment, the nurse finds out what the appointment is for, when it is scheduled to take place, and determines if it will take place as scheduled, if it will be rescheduled, or other arrangements made (chemotherapy, dialysis, etc.). If the person appears ill or injured and needs more urgent health care attention, the nurse makes arrangements for the person to be seen within the next few hours by a provider (medical, mental health, or dental staff). Triage is the nurse's determination of what kind of provider needs to see the person and how soon they need to be seen. Guidelines for nurses to use in making triage decisions are listed in Table 14.3. These are general guidelines and do not take the place of specific guidelines established by the facility medical director.

Once the detainee's ongoing health care has been taken care of, the nurse next decides whether any special housing or equipment will be required and communicates this to custody personnel. These decisions include whether the detainee should be placed in medical housing for observation, detoxification, infection

TABLE 14.3   Guidelines for Referral from Receiving Screening

PATIENT CONDITION	REFERRED TO	TIMEFRAME	PURPOSE
Unwilling or unable to answer questions	Physician	Immediate	Arrange to observe and protect self and others until assessment completed
Active treatment for chronic disease	Midlevel Provider	End of workday	Immediate treatment orders
Active treatment for psychiatric disease	Psychiatrist	End of workday	Immediate treatment orders
Symptoms of active TB or other communicable disease	Physician	Immediate	Immediate treatment orders, housing, and precautions
Acute psychiatric symptoms	Psychiatrist	Immediate	Immediate treatment orders, housing, and precautions
Emergent dental problem	Dentist	Within 1 workday	Evaluation and treatment
Physical disability and/or prosthetic device	Midlevel provider	End of workday	Arrange housing, authorization for prosthetic, or substitute device
Current prescription	Midlevel provider	End of workday	Orders to continue treatment if medically necessary
IDDM	Physician	Within 1 workday	Health assessment, treatment plan, and orders
Asthma	Midlevel provider	Within 1 workday	Health assessment, treatment plan, and orders
Other diabetics	Midlevel provider	Within 1 workday	Health assessment, treatment plan, and orders
Hypertension	Midlevel provider	Within 1 workday	Health assessment, treatment plan, and orders
Epilepsy	Midlevel provider	Within 1 workday	Health assessment, treatment plan, and orders
HIV	Midlevel provider	Within 1 workday	Health assessment, treatment plan, and orders
Unstable vital signs	Midlevel provider	Within 1 workday	Health assessment, treatment plan, and orders

Source: This material was published in Clinical Practice in Correctional Medicine, 2nd Ed., Burrow et. al. Nursing in the primary care setting, page no 433. Copyright Elsevier (2006).

control, or supportive care. The detainee may need to be placed on suicide watch or, if there is a risk of being victimized (i.e., an underdeveloped juvenile sentenced as an adult), special housing arrangements need to be made. The nurse will also determine if a specific kind of bed assignment (lower bunk, lower tier, etc.) or assistive devices (cane, wheelchair, brace, etc.) are needed and if the detainee has medication that is to be kept with them (nitro, inhaler, etc.).

From the Experts . . .

"Communication is a MUST at intake . . . . communication to custody (in order to provide the right housing assignment—low bunk, low tier), communication to public health—to followup on public health issues, communication with providers to ensure the patient is taken care of and medications are continued, or appointments are completed in timely manner."

Lilia L. Nash, RN, MBA/HCM, PHN, CCHP
San Quentin, CA

Documentation and Communication

These decisions are then communicated to custody personnel so that classification, housing, and program decisions maintain the person's health and safety during the period of incarceration or detention. This communication must take place in a manner that preserves the patient's confidentiality (ACA, 2002; NCCHC, 2008a, 2008b, 2011). Usually, there is a formal mechanism such as a specific form or an electronic notification that is used for this communication.

All aspects of receiving screening are documented by the nurse in the detainee's health record; this includes subjective information obtained during interview, objective signs and symptoms, triage decisions, treatment that has been initiated, and the plan for subsequent care. Documentation in the health record is in addition to written communication that is forwarded to custody personnel. The documentation of receiving screening is the first step in creating the health record of the detainee kept during detention or incarceration. It is often referred to as a baseline against which the patient's health status is compared to determine if a condition is new, improving, stable, or deteriorating.

Transfers and Returning Inmates

Health screening is much less elaborate when the inmate is a transfer from another facility that is within the same correctional system and intake screening has already been done, as long as the health record is transferred. If this is the case, the nurse only needs to review the record and make arrangements, as necessary, for continuation of the person's health care at the new facility. If the inmate is a transfer from another correctional jurisdiction (i.e., from prison in another state or from a state-operated prison to a county-operated jail), receiving screening needs to be done but it may be less detailed if the person's health information is also transferred.

Sometimes nursing staff will be very familiar with an inmate because they have been received many times at the facility. However, if the inmate has spent any amount of time in the community, initial health screening is still necessary upon admission. The nurse needs to gather the diagnostic and observational data, however if the prior record is available, the interview only needs to inquire about recent episodes of

- Trauma
- Communicable and chronic diseases
- Drug/alcohol use

- Symptoms of mental illness
- Suicidal ideation
- Hospitalizations
- Pregnancy

Closure of the Screening Encounter

Initial health screening may be the only contact a detainee will have with any health care personnel, or it may be the first of many contacts. The nurse is in a position to positively impact the individual and perhaps their family or the community as a result of this interaction. During the closure phase the nurse gives verbal and written instructions about how to access health care attention at the facility. The nurse also tells the patient what they can expect at the next health care encounter and provides any additional instructions needed about their health care (medications, assistive devices, etc.). If the detainee is likely to stay only a short time, a list of resources in the community should also be provided so that they can follow up on the results of screening or seek care as necessary. Case Example 14.1 provides the opportunity to apply the material reviewed in this section.

CASE EXAMPLE 14.1

On Saturday at 3:00 am, a 17-year-old man is booked into the juvenile detention facility. The young man is cooperative but appears intoxicated during the interview. Although he is brief in answering questions, he gives a history of taking medication for seizures, a recent psychiatric hospitalization, and moderate use of alcohol. He indicates that he has not been to jail before. Vital signs are normal, and on physical inspection he is noted to have a rash over his upper torso.

Discussion Questions:

1. What disposition decisions does the nurse make about this individual's health care?
2. What instruction does the nurse give the young man at the conclusion of receiving screening?

Mental Health Screening

The purpose of mental health screening is to prevent suicide and to identify inmates who are likely to require mental health services during incarceration (Spiers et al., 2006). Many people admitted to correctional facilities have a history of mental illness and the circumstances surrounding arrest and incarceration are correlated with increased risk of suicide or crisis. Urgent mental health needs can be identified at the time of receiving health screening and so questions related to history as well as signs and symptoms of mental illness and suicidality should be included in the receiving screening tool (Anno, 2001).

Role of the Nurse

A patient's mental health needs are assessed again at the time of the initial health assessment. The initial health assessment is a more complete history and examination than the minimum amount of information collected at intake. This assessment may be done at intake and replace receiving screening or it may take place several days to two weeks later. During the initial assessment, nurses may interview patients to amplify the health history, perform the physical exam, and collect lab or other diagnostic information (ACA, 2002; NCCHC, 2008a, 2008b, 2011). In some systems, mental health screening is also completed at this encounter, and can be done by a nurse as long as they received instruction and supervision in identifying and interacting with persons who may need mental health services (NCCHC, 2008a, 2008b, 2011; Spiers et al., 2006).

The key concepts of mental health screening are that it is completed by trained staff, a standardized form or process is used, and there is a low threshold for referral to mental health. Nurses should expect to interview inmates who are reluctant or unable to provide complete and accurate information about their mental health history or current symptoms. Ensuring patient privacy, conducting the encounter professionally, and giving information that addresses the patents' concerns will facilitate cooperation among persons who may be suspicious, confused, or frightened (Spiers et al., 2006).

Nurses should be familiar with all aspects of the initial mental health screening process as well as the forms used to document the results. An important clinical distinction is to accurately identify and describe symptoms of altered mental status so that medical emergencies like delirium or acute intoxication are treated appropriately and persons who are mentally ill are referred promptly so that their condition does not deteriorate during incarceration. Nurses need to be familiar with the terms and description of behaviors that distinguish psychotic symptoms, disorders of thinking, communication, or mood. Effective communication with mental health providers is achieved by thorough and accurate description of behavior indicative of mental illness more so than the use of diagnostic labels. Refer to Chapter 12 Mental Health for this information.

Triage and Referral

Patients identified by screening as likely to require mental health services need to be referred for a more complete mental health evaluation. Nurses should be provided with written guidelines or instructions for referral to mental health that include the timeframe for the follow-up encounter to take place (Anno, 2001; Spiers et al., 2006). Nurses need to know who to refer the patient to, how the referral is documented, and when the patient will be seen. Nurses use this information to arrange for the patient's safety and ongoing care (ANA, 2007). The nurse should also have the patient sign consent for release of information and take steps to obtain records from previous mental health providers so that this information can be incorporated into treatment planning early (Spiers et al., 2006). Guidelines provided in Table 14.3 include referral timeframes for the types of mental health concerns that may be identified during initial mental health screening.

All inmates, even those who are not identified as needing mental health services, must receive an explanation of how to request mental health services before release from the intake area. There are many aspects of detention or incarceration that stress mental well-being and contribute to development of emotional crisis or deterioration of a person's mental condition. The nurse should include an explanation of how to request attention for a mental health concern at the same time that instructions on how to access health care are given. The nurse's attitude and demeanor during mental health screening and the explanation about how to request services can greatly influence an inmate's inclination to request subsequent services, so it is important to avoid judgmental or stigmatizing behaviors (Burrow et al., 2006).

Screening for Work Assignment

Correctional systems often require a health screening when an inmate is going to be assigned to a specific type of work or program. The content of health screening should correspond to the purpose of the clearance requested. For example, someone being considered for work on a forestry or fire crew needs to be screened differently than someone being considered for placement in a residential alcohol and drug abuse treatment program. The nurse should be clear about the purpose of each type of health screening performed, familiar with the content of each screening tool, and know how to conduct the screening as well as the criteria for deciding the outcome of the clearance.

Food Service Worker Screening

The purpose of screening inmates for assignment to the kitchen is to prevent transmission of food-borne illnesses. There are federal, state, and county requirements for food safety, and health screening of food service workers may be required. In addition, correctional administrators sometimes voice concern that an inmate with an infectious disease might purposefully contaminate food and ask that inmates with these diseases be screened out.

Kitchen clearance at a minimum consists of checking that the inmate does not have an infectious disease that can be transmitted via casual contact and the person can understand and follow direction. More specifically, inmates who have open skin sores on arms or hands, respiratory infection, jaundice, vomiting, or diarrhea should be excluded from food service assignment until cleared medically. Prevention of food-borne illness also requires that workers rigorously follow procedures for food handling and hygiene. Individuals who are unreliable in their ability to follow direction because of a mental or cognitive disorder should also be excluded from food service assignments (Bick, 2006).

Screening for food service assignment may be accomplished by review of the record or as an encounter with the inmate. If it is a face-to-face encounter, the nurse can reinforce the importance of the inmate reporting to their supervisor if they are sick, have any open sores or skin infection, and to follow instruction on kitchen hygiene to prevent disease transmission.

Screening for Remote and Arduous Work Assignments

Another type of screening for work clearance is when the inmate will be housed at a remote location without health care or will be assigned particularly arduous work. Examples are forestry work, fire, or road crew. The purpose of screening for these assignments is so that inmates are assigned work they are physically capable of doing. The screening method, tool, or process used needs to be relevant to the type of work the person will be doing. If more than one type of assignment is possible, then the clearance criteria need to assume the most rigorous assignment. Screening will include consideration of ability to lift and carry weight, walk on uneven ground, coordination, and so on. The standard health screening may not include sufficient information to determine whether an inmate has the strength, agility, and other characteristics to perform specific, more rigorous, or specialized work. If it does not, then an appointment needs to be made to see the inmate and gather this additional information before a decision is made.

When the types and numbers of job assignments do not match the characteristics of the population being screened, not enough people are cleared to fill all the work slots. Nurses may be pressured about the clearance decisions they make if not enough inmates are available to perform the work. Nurses in this situation can suggest that the criteria for clearance be adjusted or modified but should not ignore clearance criteria or change a decision because of pressure. Screening for job assignment should err against assigning an inmate to work who has a condition that puts them at risk of injury or further harm. For example, an inmate on medication that causes drowsiness should not be assigned to drive a threshing machine on the farm or run a saw in the meat shop.

Sometimes, more caution is exercised in making clearance decisions than may be necessary. This could be because the description of the work clearance is inaccurate, the screening criteria may be too broad or set too high, or it may be simple miscommunication. Visiting the work location and observing the work being done may identify a gap between the description of the job and the actual criteria for clearance, which could then be clarified or defined more narrowly. It may also be that the work location is using criteria for hard labor when it actually has less strenuous jobs that inmates could be cleared for. When nursing leaders invest time collaborating with correctional personnel to facilitate health screening and clearances for job and program assignment, nursing staff are less pressured about the clearance decisions they are expected to make.

Screening for Treatment or Program Participation

Residential treatment, boot camp, or school may require health screening before enrollment or program participation. The process and content of the screening must be relevant to the reason for the clearance. As an example, some residential substance abuse treatment programs require that inmates be screened for tuberculosis. This is because the incidence of active tuberculosis is high among addicts and many programs do not have health care staff on site. In an effort to prevent tuberculosis outbreak among program participants, prospective inmates are screened out for active disease and, if they have infection, must have completed preventive treatment before admission to the program.

Physical and mental conditioning is a major emphasis of boot camp programs. Health screening may be required to ensure that potential enrollees are physically and mentally capable of participation (Wilson, MacKenzie, & Mitchell, 2003). This kind of screening may be accomplished by review of the record. If the initial health assessment was not be specific enough for boot camp clearance, an appointment needs to be made to see the inmate, and additional information gathered before a decision is made.

Documentation and Communication for Work and Program Assignment

The results of work or program screening need to be documented in the inmate's health record. If the inmate was not cleared, the reason should also be documented in the health record. Since review of the health record is often the primary part of many types of screening, the results of any prior screenings need to be considered in making decisions. The results of health screening for work or program assignment are also communicated to custody and program staff in writing. Communication to custody and program staff should be in relation to the assignment and not include confidential health information. This communication may be as simple as adding a notation to a list or a simple form.

Correctional facilities that do not have information about health status already available will notify the health care program that clearance is needed. For efficient operation of the correctional facility, getting these clearances has an urgency that is sometimes not shared by the health care program and this can be a source of conflict. Assigning inmates to work and programming is a complex process involving in addition to the inmate's health status, their classification, time left to serve, gang affiliation, needs and abilities matched to a finite set of jobs, and program slots that each has criteria for filling. Some correctional facilities have staff whose time is completely devoted to making these assignments. Having the wrong inmate in the wrong place at the wrong time because of an error in making assignments may result in an avoidable escape, injury, or death.

Other Types of Screening

The registered nurse in correctional health care must be prepared to address a wide spectrum of needs. Correctional nurses have experience and knowledge in the areas of public health, psychiatry, emergency, disease management, and chronic care (ANA, 2007). Screening inmates for contraindications for use of restraint, use of force, and placement in segregation or other type of isolated housing is a unique aspect of correctional nursing. Assessment, critical thinking, and professionalism are essential features of this nursing role.

Placement in Segregated Housing

Over the years, correctional systems have developed or adopted many different terms for the types of housing used for punishment and to contain those inmates who require higher degrees of custody supervision. These areas may be termed segregation, administrative isolation, protective custody, lockdown, supermax, death row, special housing units, and so on. These locations are distinguished from the general population by the fact that inmates are more isolated from contact with others and receive services separately (ACA, 2002; NCCHC, 2008a, 2008b, 2011).

Accreditation standards require that an inmate placed in segregation be screened so that if such a setting is contraindicated by a medical or mental health condition, an alternative placement is made. Screening also ensures that arrangements are made to continue necessary health care while the inmate is housed in the segregated setting (ACA, 2002; NCCHC, 2008a, 2008b, 2011). When nurses are notified of placement in one of these settings, they conduct the screening, indicate if there are any contraindications, and make arrangements for ongoing care.

Contraindications for placement in segregation are medical or psychiatric conditions that are more appropriately cared for in a clinical setting such as an infirmary, inpatient unit, or hospital (e.g., intoxication, diminished consciousness, suicide history or behavior, respiratory distress, etc.). Nurses who conduct this screening should do so using a list of contraindicating conditions developed by medical and

1.	Inmate's Name:		
2.	ID #:		
3.	INSTITUTION:		
4.	Date: _____ Admitted to: DSU____ IMU____ ADSEG____		
5.	Health Classification:		
6.	Verbal instructions given on inmate access to health care while in segregated housing	YES	NO
7.	Any existing medical contraindications to segregated placement? If yes, report to _____ or designee.	YES	NO
8.	Current medications?	YES	NO
9.	Was the inmate involved in an altercation?	YES	NO
10.	Does patient report any injuries? If yes, please detail in narrative form in progress notes.	YES	NO
11.	Does patient express or exhibit any intent for self-harm? If yes, please complete Suicide Risk Assessment.	YES	NO
12.	Does patient have history of self-harm?	YES	NO
13.	Does patient have history of suicide attempts? If yes: Co. Jail___, DSU___, IMU___, MHI___, GP___, Other____	YES	NO
14.	Does patient have a history of previous MH inpatient admission or treatment?	YES	NO
15.	Is the patient receiving involuntary medications?	YES	NO
16.	Yes to any of items 11 -15 requires immediate MH notification. Notification made to:		
17.	Patient is under MH care currently? MH referral sent to:	YES	NO
18.	Chart review completed by:		
19.	Printed name:		
20.	Time:		

FIGURE 14.1   Screening for contraindications to placement in segregation.

Source: From Oregon Department of Corrections (2010).

psychiatric clinicians. This list should be developed considering the conditions experienced by inmates in each of these settings as well as the availability of health care assistance. The nurse should ask about the inmate's current mental and physical state as well as the circumstances preceding the decision to place the inmate in segregation. Next, the nurse should review the health record and determine if a face-to-face evaluation should also be completed. If, for example, the inmate has been in an altercation, an assessment for possible head injury or other trauma is indicated. The results of screening are documented in the health record and may be narrative or on a form specific to the purpose of the screening. An example of a form used to guide screening for contraindications to placement in segregation, referral for ongoing care, and to document findings is provided in Figure 14.1.

Nurses need to be clear about their professional role in clearance for placement in segregated settings because there is potential for an ethical violation to occur. The purpose of screening is to identify anyone who has a condition that contraindicates placement in segregation, not to provide medical clearance or approval to proceed with punishment (Anno, 2001). The same is true in making arrangements for ongoing care; segregation should not result in denial of medically necessary care. There may be some types of procedures or appointments that can be scheduled electively and can take place when the person has been released from segregation (e.g., routine oral hygiene). These are decisions to be made by the responsible clinician after notification by the nurse. The responsible clinician may provide guidelines for the level of care provided while in segregation; if so, these should be written and formalized in protocol or policy and procedure. The decision to modify or delay scheduled services can only be made as a result of a review and consideration of individual's need for health care and not as a result of policy alone. The nurse is to advocate for a patient's health and well-being. If the nurse's assessment indicates that the patient's condition warrants additional consideration or intervention, the nurse must obtain needed clinical services (ANA, 2007). Accreditation standards are clear that health care providers determine the setting and timeframe appropriate for clinical care regardless of the inmate's custody status (ACA, 2002; NCCHC, 2008a, 2008b, 2011).

Use of Force and Custody Restraint

Many of the methods and tools used by correctional personnel to manage inmate behavior and maintain safety and security are also associated with some risk for injury, disability, or death. These include use of force, physical control, restraints, electric shock, irritating chemicals, and smoke. In an effort to reduce preventable adverse events, health care staff may be asked to screen and identify inmates with health conditions that contraindicate use of these devices.

Custody restraint is the tool most often employed to maintain inmates. One of the contraindications for use of custody restraint is pregnant and postpartum women. The NCCHC (2010) adopted a position statement that discourages use of restraints, especially in the third trimester. The ACA (2010) has adopted a similar accreditation standard. Other contraindications for limiting use of custody restraint are inmates with certain orthopedic, motion, or balance problems. Contraindications for use of the Taser or Oleoresin Capsicum (OC) or pepper spray include inmates with respiratory or cardiac disease. Symptoms of post-traumatic stress disorder may be exacerbated by use of force, so a plan of care should be developed by mental health staff to include early intervention to minimize use of force.

The purpose of screening inmates for conditions that may contraindicate use of force or restraint is to protect the inmate from injury. This is another area where erosion of the nurse's professional role is possible. This screening is not to approve use of force, restraint, or other forms of control, but to notify correctional personnel that there is additional risk of harm in the use of these methods with specific individuals (Anno, 2001).

This screening should be done in advance of need so that alternatives can be developed by correctional personnel to manage the inmate. The nurse should have a screening tool or written guidelines that describe what is to be evaluated and the criteria for decision making. These guidelines should be developed or approved by physician leadership at the facility. The notice that the inmate has a contraindicating condition needs to be communicated to corrections personnel in a way that does not violate medical confidentiality. The evaluation and resulting notification also should be documented in the health record.

SUMMARY

Nurses use many screening techniques and tools in the correctional setting to examine, identify, and act upon certain clinical conditions or needs that inmates have for health care and safety. The key concepts of screening are that it can be done quickly and that it identifies those conditions or needs for which it was intended to screen and that it makes efficient use of resources. When screening tools and processes are standardized, the same outcome is likely to be achieved, no matter who conducts screening. Many levels of personnel can be used to perform health screening; however, nurses are especially efficient and effective because of their ability to gain rapport with the patient, recognize abnormal conditions, prioritize, and then organize provision of subsequent treatment and care.

DISCUSSION QUESTIONS

1. What are the factors that challenge getting good interview information during receiving screening at your facility?
2. How do you respond to an assignment officer who challenges your screening decision to deny clearance of an inmate for food service assignment?
3. What are the contraindications for placement in segregation at your facility?
4. What instructions would you give to the officers transporting a woman who is 30 weeks pregnant to a prenatal appointment?

REFERENCES

American Correctional Association. (2002). *Performance based standards for correctional health care in adult correctional institutions.* Alexandria, VA: Author.

American Correctional Association. (2010). *2010 Standards supplement.* Alexandria, VA: Author.

American Nurses Association. (2007). *Corrections nursing: Scope & standards of practice.* Silver Spring, MD: Author.

Anno, B. (2001). Health care delivery system model. In B. Anno (Ed.), *Correctional health care: Guidelines for the management of an adequate delivery system* (pp. 172–174). Chicago: National Commission on Correctional Health Care.

Bick, J. (2006). Infectional control in the correctional setting. In M. Puisis (Ed.), *Clinical practice in correctional medicine* (pp. 234–235). Philadelphia: Moseby Elsevier.

Burrow, G., Knox, C., & Villanueva, H. (2006). Nursing in the primary care setting. In M. Puisis (Ed.), *Clinical practice in correctional medicine* (2nd ed., pp. 426–459). Philadelphia, PA: Mosby Elsevier.

Hammett, T. (2006). Epidemeolgy of HIV/AIDS and other infectious diseases in correctional facilities. In M. Puisis (Ed.), *Clinical practice in correctional medicine* (pp. 167–174). Philadelphia: Mosby/Elsevier.

Kistler, J., & Chavez, S. (2011, Winter). Spotlight on the standards: E-02 Receiving Screening. *CorrectCare* (pp. 7–8). Chicago, Illinois: National Commission on Correctional Health Care.

Knox, C. (2010, Fall). Correctional nursing practice: What you need to know (Part 4) screening, sick call and triage. *CorrectCare* (pp. 16–17).

Maruschak, L. (2008, April 22). *Medical problems of prisoners.* Retrieved October 17, 2011, from Bureau of Justice Statistics, Office of Justice Programs, U.S. Department of Justice: http://bjs.ojp.usdoj.gov/index.cfm?ty=pbdetail&iid=1097

National Commission on Correctional Health Care (NCCHC). (2008a). *Standards for health services in prisons.* Chicago, IL: Author.

National Commission on Correctional Health Care (NCCHC). (2008b). *Standards for health services in jails*. Chicago, IL: Author.

National Commission on Correctional Health Care. (2010, October 10). *Position statements: Restraint of pregnant inmates*. Retrieved August 18, 2011, from National Commission on Correctional Health Care: http://www.ncchc.org/resources/statements/restraint_pregnant_inmates.html

National Commission on Correctional Health Care (NCCHC). (2011). *Standards for health services in juvenile detention and confinement facilities*. Chicago, IL: Author.

Oregon Department of Corrections. (2010, October). *DOC health services, policies and procedures, P-E-09 segregated inmates*. Retrieved November 9, 2011, from Oregon Department of Corrections: http://www.oregon.gov/DOC/OPS/HESVC/docs/policies_procedures/Section_E/PE09.pdf

Raba, J. (2006). Intake screening and periodic health evaluations. In M. Puisis (Ed.), *Clinical practice in correctional medicine* (pp. 41–49). Philadelphia: Mosby Elsevier.

Raffle, A. (2011). *Further resources to interactive learning module: Screening*. Retrieved August 20, 2011, from HealthKnowledge: http://www.healthknowledge.org.uk/sites/default/files/documents/interactivel/screening/screening_resources.pdf?op=Resources

Spiers, E., Pitt, S., & Dvoskin, J. (2006). Psychiatric intake screening. In M. Puisis (Ed.), *Clinical practice in correctional medicine* (2nd ed.), (pp. 285–291). Philadelphia: Mosby Elsevier.

Wilper, A. P., Woolhandler, S., Boyd, J. W., Lasser, K.E., McCormick, D., Bor, D.H., & Himmelstein, D.U. (2009). The health and health care of US prisoners: Results of a nationwide survey. *American Journal of Public Health, 99*(4), 666–672.

Wilson, D., MacKenzie, D., & Mitchell, F. (2003). Effects of correctional boot camps. *Campbell Systematic Reviews, 1*, 1–42.

FIFTEEN

Nursing Sick Call

Sue Smith

D ue to the level of security required in correctional facilities, inmates must rely on the institution medical staff for assistance with common health problems and for access to the most mundane types of treatment, like nonprescription remedies for colds, headaches, muscle strains, and the like (Knox & Shelton, 2006; Smith, 2009). In 1976, the U.S. Supreme Court established that inmates have a constitutional right to a level of health care that protects them from unnecessary medical suffering. The Supreme Court mandate established a constitutional level of care that includes a functioning sick call system using properly trained medical staff, a priority system to ensure that those who need care most receive it first, and a system for staff training and ongoing quality control (Rold, 2006). The term "sick call" evolved from the military lineup of soldiers seeking medical attention, but the process is now used in correctional settings to describe their method of addressing access to health care for inmates. The term is well suited to correctional systems, as it provides an orderly process important to facility security (Knox & Shelton, 2006).

Sick call provides an important first level of health care services and a gatekeeper function in which nurses assess inmate patients and determine the level of care needed. This ensures that health care resources are not wasted, so that inmates with more serious illnesses are not competing with those who have minor complaints for advanced provider services (Knox & Shelton, 2006). Nursing sick call enhances the professional autonomy of nurses and is one of the signature practices that sets correctional nursing apart as a specialty. It allows nurses to *independently* assess patients, develop a nursing diagnosis and a treatment plan, and is an important opportunity to provide inmates with patient education and self-care information. So it is important for the nursing sick call process to be based on clinically sound principles that meet legal and professional standards of care.

UNDERLYING PRINCIPLES OF SICK CALL

Principles are fundamental standards or rules, upon which all other rules or standards rest (Agnes & Laird, 1996). The fundamental principles that underlie sick call are (1) unimpeded access to health care that is available to inmates daily and (2) that health care provided to patients will be safe.

Daily Access to Care

Access to care is one of the three basic rights guaranteed to prisoners in 1976 by the U.S. Supreme Court in *Estelle v. Gamble* (NCCHC, 2008). Unimpeded access to care means that the access is determined by qualified health care staff or health-trained staff and cannot be denied or delayed by security staff (Anno, 2001; Knox & Shelton, 2006). Although lay staff may convey sick call requests by providing sick call request forms or contacting health care staff about inmate health concerns, they may not decide whether inmates will receive medical attention (Anno, 2001). Following the decision by the U.S. Supreme Court, the right of access to care further evolved into access that is available daily. This standard of care is supported by the major correctional accrediting organizations, the American Correctional Association and the National Commission on Correctional Health Care, in mandatory or essential standards that require "daily access to care" (ACA, 2003; NCCHC, 2008).

Because nurses are very often the only health care providers consistently onsite in correctional facilities, sick call is one of the major ways in which the standards for access to care are met. The access to care standards further require that inmates must be fully informed about the health services that are available and how to access the services. The standards go on to require that information about health care services must be presented to inmates verbally and in writing and in a manner that they understand (ACA, 2003; Knox & Shelton, 2006; NCCHC, 2008). These standards are best met by providing information about sick call services in multiple formats and in multiple places throughout the facility (Anno, 2001; Knox & Shelton, 2006).

Professional Clinical Judgment

Adequate sick call operations require professional clinical judgment by health care personnel trained and licensed to carry out sick call procedures. Nurses engaged in sick call must be trained in the patient evaluation, triage, and treatment procedures required by sick call procedures. The nurses must also be appropriately licensed to carry out all procedures required by sick call practice (Knox & Shelton, 2006; Rold, 2006). Because sick call involves a high-level assessment and clinical decision making, the provisions in this chapter generally pertain to registered nursing practice. To determine what involvement licensed practical or vocational nurses (LPNs or LVNs) may have in sick call assessment and interventions, it is wise to review state nurse practice acts to determine what nursing actions practical or vocational nurses are permitted (Knox & Shelton, 2006; Smith, 2009).

Safe Patient Care

Following the publication of *To Err Is Human: Building a Safer Health System* by the Institute of Medicine (IOM), patient safety has been established as the right of all patients and the obligation of all health care workers (Kohn, Corrigan, & Donaldson, 2000). In 2008, the National Commission on Correctional Health Care acknowledged the importance of patient safety in correctional facilities by adopting a standard that directly addresses this issue; this standard requires the responsible health authority to promote a "patient safety culture that encourages staff to identify opportunities to reduce harm or potential harm to patients" (p. 26).

Subsequent study into patient safety has acknowledged that nurses are on the "sharp end" of patient care delivery because nurses often have the most direct contact with patients (Benner et al., 2006; Page, 2004). Nurses preserve patient safety by objectively measuring signs and symptoms, by evaluating changes in patient signs and symptoms, by executing nursing interventions, by maintaining respect for their patients, and by remaining vigilant to patient health status (Benner et al., 2006).

ESSENTIAL SKILLS FOR NURSING SICK CALL
Health Assessment Skills

Health assessment is fundamental to nursing practice; virtually all nursing clinical decisions are based on the subjective and objective data collected from patients during assessment. The purpose of health assessment is to gather information about the patient and use that information to describe the patient's health status and to determine any actual or potential health problems (LaMarre, 2006). In particular, correctional nurses must have strong assessment skills based on an in-depth knowledge of anatomy, physiology, and pathophysiology. Inmate patients come to sick call with a variety of health issues—some complaints are minor ones that would be self-treated in community settings, some are complex and life threatening, yet other complaints are self-serving and made to manipulate the prisoner's environment (Burrow, Knox, & Villanueva, 2006). It takes a skilled, observant, and knowledgeable

From the Experts ...

"In a correctional health care setting, Nurses' Sick Call represents the foundation of access to health care—a constitutional right of inmate patients. In addition to the provision of nursing care during a sick call encounter, referrals to advanced level providers, dental, optometry, podiatry, and mental health services are generated when the patient's need transcends a nurses' scope of practice. As a patient population, inmates present with diverse health concerns that span continuums of both age and acuity. For these reasons, well-developed assessment skills are critical in correctional health care, and are the most important tool a nurse can utilize to ensure that patients' needs are appropriately identified, triaged, and treated."

Jennifer Clayton, BA, RN, CCHP
Columbus, OH

nurse to thoroughly assess an inmate's complaint and collect adequate objective data to make a rational decision based on valid and reliable information.

Clinical Decision-Making Skills

Clinical decision making refers to the process that nurses use to reach judgments or conclusions about a patient's needs or health problems. It is based on the clinical reasoning that nurses use to interpret patients' signs and symptoms, to evaluate their responses to therapies, and to evaluate the relevance of any changes in patients' condition (Benner et al., 2006). It is a deliberate process of generating solutions and alternatives, weighing them, and choosing the best solution to the patient's problem. Good clinical decision making is complex and requires understanding of pathophysiology and the diagnostic aspects of the patient's clinical presentation (Tanner, 2006). During the clinical decision-making process, competent nurses use good communication and technical skills to obtain valid and reliable health information from patients . This complex set of data is then processed to make appropriate decisions and to develop responsive care plans (Lunney, 2010; Rogal & Young, 2008). In other words, nurses need to know what questions to ask and what assessments to conduct, then quickly and accurately analyze and process all of the data collected and, finally, compare that knowledge with an what they already know about health conditions to determine the correct diagnosis and plan appropriate interventions (Harjai & Tiwari, 2009).

Patient Education

Patient education is a major component of nursing care and nurses are frontline providers of patient education (Ignativicius, 2006; Kerns & Pinney, 2006). Sick call provides excellent, and frequent, opportunities for health promotion, self-care, and disease-specific patient education. Inmates have typically received little health education throughout their lives and often lack knowledge about healthy lifestyles or how to manage disease processes that might affect them; additionally, many have poor reading ability (Kerns & Pinney, 2006). Care must be taken to ensure that patient education is given in a manner that the patient will understand, so it is advisable for training materials to be simply stated and include little medical jargon; many find that materials containing pictures to be helpful.

All nursing protocols should assess the patient's knowledge about their health status and provide patient education specific to the disease addressed by the protocol. Many larger correctional systems have developed patient education programs and training materials specific to the correctional population, and many of these programs are willing to share their materials without cost. Smaller systems, including county jails, have obtained patient education materials in a variety of formats and languages from their county health departments. Additionally, there are many governmental and nonprofit organizations such as the Federal Bureau of Prisons (FBOP), the Centers for Disease Control and Prevention (CDC), the American Diabetes Association, and many others that will provide free patient education materials (Kerns & Pinney, 2006). A note of caution—while the FBOP and CDC provide corrections-specific patient education, material from noncorrectional organizations should be reviewed to ensure that it is appropriate for use within the correctional setting.

SICK CALL SUPPORT
The Sick Call Environment

Nursing sick call should take place in a room dedicated for this purpose. The room provided should be appropriate for clinical encounters, meaning that the room provides visual and/or auditory privacy and is of ample size to accommodate the nurse, the patient, a desk, chairs for both, an examination table, and equipment sufficient to do a thorough assessment of patient complaints. Handwashing facilities are essential. Suggested equipment for a sick call room includes

- Thermometers
- Stethoscope
- Blood pressure cuffs in appropriate sizes to fit small and large patients
- A calibrated weight scale
- A handheld light
- Oto-ophthalmoscope
- Q-tips
- Tongue depressors
- Exam gloves
- Dressing supplies
- Germicidal solution
- Reference materials, including any approved nursing protocols and patient education materials

Correctional nurses need to be aware that that, except in emergencies or other life-threatening situations, it is *not* appropriate to evaluate patients in cells, on tiers, in hallways, or other nonclinical settings (Anno, 2001; Knox & Shelton, 2006).

Nursing Protocols

Nursing protocols are written guidelines for nurses to use when assessing patients, making judgments about patients' clinical conditions, and implementing treatment plans (NCCHC, 2008). They should reflect strong collaboration between physicians and nurses because they allow nurses to initiate treatment for common nonurgent health complaints with physician oversight. Most nursing protocols address a wide range of health concerns, from minor complaints like sore throat, cold symptoms, or fungal skin infections, to more serious symptoms like chest pain or shortness of breath. Each nursing protocol should define the entire assessment and all interventions indicated for each complaint, including any indicated referrals, follow-up, and patient instructions (NCCHC, 2008).

Nurses and advanced providers who create nursing protocols may consider using handbooks developed for use by advanced practice nurses. The content of these handbooks includes many of the minor health complaints seen in sick call and is often presented in the logical step-wise fashion familiar to nurses. However, care must be taken to remove assessments and interventions that are not within scope of practice for registered nurses. Generally, effective nursing protocols contain information that includes

- Definition of the problem or complaint and its etiology.
- The minimum subjective and objective assessment that must be completed for each complaint.

- Appropriate nursing diagnoses; this should include alternative problems that need to be considered, including a worst-case scenario.
- Criteria for referrals to advanced providers, including specific time frames for appointments.
- A range of interventions that is appropriate for nurses to initiate.
- Patient education and instructions for evaluation and follow-up (Knox & Shelton, 2006; Smith, 2009).

It should be noted that while nursing protocols need to contain sufficient direction to guide the nurse's assessment and subsequent actions, they are not meant to restrict the nurse's assessment of patients. Nurses must be capable of critical thinking and drawing on expert knowledge to determine if different or additional information is needed. For instance, if a patient is seen for a complaint of a sinus problem, but presents with an elevated blood pressure, the nurse must be prepared to include additional assessment data, consider different nursing diagnoses, and develop a plan of care that addresses the problem of elevated blood pressure as well.

The format used for nursing protocols can vary greatly; however, most nursing protocols address one complaint and contain all assessments and assessment data related to that complaint. Some correctional systems, like those in Georgia and Texas, combined nursing protocols with assessment forms to form a complaint-specific form that prompts nurses through an assessment and treatment plan. Other systems utilize complaint-specific protocols without an assessment form so that sick call nurses document the encounters in the patient's medical record (Knox & Shelton, 2006). The Ohio Department of Rehabilitation and Correction (ODRC) developed complaint-specific protocols using a design similar to an algorithm or flow sheet. Separate assessment forms that addressed body systems were developed that provide prompts for adequate assessment of complaints involving that system, but allow the nurse to address more than one complaint on the form. Examples of the ODRC Nursing Protocols and Assessment forms are found in Figures 15.1 and 15.2.

The National Commission on Correctional Health Care has addressed development and use of nursing protocols in an "important" standard intended to ensure that nurses who participate in sick call do so under very specific guidelines and that the nurses are properly trained to use the protocols. The NCCHC standard, E-11, Nursing Assessment Protocols requires that

- Nursing protocols are developed and reviewed by nursing administration and the responsible physician.
- All new correctional nurses are trained in the use of nursing protocols.
- Nursing protocols do not include use of prescription medications except in the case of emergencies and other life-threatening situations (NCCHC, 2008).

Education and Training

When considering training, it is important to remember that (1) nursing sick call is not found in most mainstream nursing care settings and (2) nursing preparation can vary widely and it cannot be assumed that all nurses are proficient with all the assessment techniques included in most nursing protocols (LaMarre, 2006). Specific training in the sick call process and in the use of nursing protocols is needed and is required by the NCCHC standard for Nursing Assessment Protocols. Sick call training should be developed by experienced correctional nurse experts and correctional

Respiratory Complaints – Acute Bronchitis (Lower Respiratory Infections)

Definition: An acute infectious disease involving the bronchi and characterized by increased production of mucous and an inflammatory exudates of mucous and white blood cells.

Etiology: Most commonly caused by viruses; may also be caused by *Streptococcus pneumonia* and *H. Influenzae.*

Subjective: Patient History
Patient Complaint: "I've got a bad cold"
Gradual onset of symptoms over 2-3 days
<u>Generalized symptoms</u>
Malaise
Generally denies shaking chills
History of smoking
	<u>Respiratory symptoms:</u>
	• Productive cough
	  - Viral bronchitis produces small amounts (< 60 cc) of purulent sputum
	  - Bacterial bronchitis produces larger amounts (≥ 60 cc) of purulent sputum
	• Wheezing, slight dyspnea
	• May c/o dull substernal chest pain

Objective: Physical Assessment <u>Vital Signs:</u> T: afebrile or low grade fever Pulse/Respiratory rate: within normal limits BP: within normal limits <u>Neck:</u> Supple; mild or no cervical lymphadenopathy <u>Throat:</u> Within normal limits	<u>Eyes:</u> Within normal limits <u>Ears:</u> Normal <u>Nasal mucosa:</u> Within normal limits <u>Chest:</u> • Rhonchi and/or wheezing present; may also note scattered crackles
Nursing Assessment: • Ineffective airway clearance R/T tracheobronchial secretions **Differential Diagnoses:** (See appropriate nursing assessment guidelines) • Ineffective airway clearance R/T upper respiratory infection	**Differential Diagnoses:** (Referral to advanced care) • Pneumonia • Tuberculosis • Bronchial asthma • Congestive heart failure
Nursing Care Plan: <u>Refer to advanced provider immediately if:</u> ✓ Temperature ≥ 101° ✓ Pt. is unable to swallow or complains of neck rigidity ✓ Signs & symptoms of severe respiratory distress ✓ Pulse oximeter reading of < 95% <u>Routine referral to advanced provider:</u> ✓ All cases of suspected bronchitis require referral to an advanced provider <u>Nursing Actions:</u> ✓ Acetaminophen or Aspirin 325 mg/ 1–2 tabs every 4 hrs. as needed for low grade fever >100° and aching ✓ 1–3 day medical lay-in for severe malaise, fever <u>Patient Education</u> • Medication side effects; importance of completing full antibiotic regimen • Encourage rest • Increase fluid intake • Instruct in proper handwashing, cough etiquette and disposal of soiled tissues • Pt. to return to sick call if symptoms do not improve in 72 hours Adapted from: Hoole, A., Picard, C.G., Ouimette, R., Lohr, J. & Powell, W. (1999). Patient Care Guidelines for Nurse Practitioners.	

FIGURE 15.1   Nursing assessment guidelines.

Source: Adapted from the Ohio Department of Rehabilitation and Correction, Nursing Assessment Guidelines. Used with permission.

Respiratory Complaints

Name:	Number:	DOB:
Institution:	Date:	Time:

Subjective Data:
Patient Complains of:_____
_____
_____

Significant Medical History:

	Y	N	Comment		Y	N	Comment
Documented weight loss	□	□	_____	Diabetes	□	□	_____
Tobacco use	□	□	_____	Cardiac disease	□	□	_____
Asthma/COPD	□	□	_____	HIV disease/splenectomy	□	□	_____
History of TB infection	□	□	_____	Allergic rhinitis	□	□	_____
				Other:	□	□	_____

Objective Data:
1. T___ P___ R___ B/P___ Weight_____   4. Lungs:_____
   Pulse ox: _____ Peak flow rate: _____   _____
2. Appearance: _____   5. Cardiovascular:_____
3. EENT Assessment: _____
   □ Eyes:_____   6. Abdominal:_____
   □ Ears:_____
   □ Nasal Mucosa:_____   7. Extremities:_____
   □ Throat:_____
   □ Tonsils:_____   8. Skin:_____
   □ Neck:_____   _____

Nursing Assessment (see appropriate nursing assessment guideline)
Consistent with patient signs and symptoms: Ineffective Airway Clearance R/T
□_____   □_____
□_____   □_____
□_____   □_____

Nursing Care Plan:
Refer to advance health provider immediately if:

□ Temp. ≥ 101°   □ Purulent tonsils   □ PEF reading < 200
□ Unable to swallow   □ Neck rigidity/pain with flexions □ S/Sx of Influenza
□ Adventitious lung sounds □ Diminished breath sounds   □ R/O TB

Nursing Interventions (check medications ordered)
□_____   □_____
□_____   □_____

Patient Education: (check topics covered with patient)
□ Increase fluid intake   □ RTC if not better in 3 days
□ Medication side effects   □ Smoking cessation
□ Cough hygiene   □ Importance of hand washing & hygiene
□ Rest/avoid fatigue   □ Other:_____

Disposition: (check actions taken)
□ No restrictions on activity   □ Physician notified: ___/___/___ _____
□ Lay-in: Start:_____ Stop:_____   (date)   (time)
□ Admit to Infirmary
□ Transport to local hospital   □ Advance provider appointment:
□ Return to clinic if no improvement in ____ days.   ___/___/___ _____
                                                        (date)   (time)

Additional Notes: _____
_____

Nurse's Signature	
Name:	Number

FIGURE 15.2   Example nursing assessment/protocol.

Source: Adapted from the Ohio Department of Rehabilitation and Correction, Nursing Assessment Protocol. Used with permission.

physicians and then made available in a manner that ensures that all nurses are trained consistently. It is recommended that sick call training content include

- Design and content of the nursing protocols
- Review of health history assessment
- Review of physical examination techniques found in the protocols
- Practice in conducting an efficient and complete nursing sick call assessment
- Adequate sick call documentation
- Legal considerations (Smith, 2009).

Training in nursing sick call may be implemented in various ways, depending on the size of the facility or system. Larger systems may be able to conduct training in a classroom setting or as on-the-job training. Smaller facilities may need to make use of a detailed lesson plan delivered as independent study. Correctional health care professional organizations, such as the Academy of Correctional Health Care Professionals, the American Correctional Health Services Association, and the Health Professionals Interest Section of ACA, offer support in the form of educational conferences and professional mentoring that can be tailored to the needs of individual facilities.

For most nurses, hands-on experience contributes greatly to their ability to make appropriate decisions, so presenting training through the use of case studies, drills, and simulations may be helpful (Etheridge, 2007). When possible, health care administrators may consider assigning new correctional nurses to work with experienced nurses, as there is evidence that being able to observe the actions of experienced health care team members and sharing clinical judgments with them is helpful to newly hired nurses (Harjai & Tiwari, 2009). This method has yet another benefit, as there is increasing evidence that the use of nurse mentors helps novice nurses and nurses who are new to a specialty practice improve their clinical decision-making skills by sharing their clinical judgments with them and discussing how they arrived at that decision (Harjai & Tiwari, 2009).

Following training, nurses need to be evaluated for competency before conducting sick call, then regularly thereafter (Burrow et al., 2006; Smith, 2009). There are multiple ways in which this evaluation may take place. The Oregon Department of Corrections developed a checklist format that encompasses all examination components needed for a head-to-toe assessment for evaluating nursing competencies (Scott & Collatt, 2009). The Ohio Department of Rehabilitation and Correction took another approach by partnering with a commercial program to provide online competency evaluation for correctional nurses who are located in institutions that are geographically scattered throughout the state (J. Clayton, personal communication, November 29, 2011). Finally, peer review can be very helpful in evaluating nurses' competency in a manner that is more supportive and less intimidating than formal evaluations.

SICK CALL PROCESS
Common Complaints Seen in Sick Call

Sick call is intended for inmates with minor health complaints and to triage health complaints that need evaluation by advanced providers. While there are many minor health complaints, correctional systems have found there are a few complaints that are more commonly seen. Various correctional systems, including Georgia, Ohio, and Oregon, have surveyed their sick call operations and found that the most common health complaints include

- Pain—including back pain, muscle and joint pain, and headaches.
- Skin—rashes, including dry skin and fungal infections.
- HEENT complaints—including colds, sinus problems, and allergies (P. Garner, personal communication, November 16, 2011; Knox & Shelton, 2006).

Monitoring the common health complaints seen in sick call will help correctional health care administration in developing nursing protocols best suited to the needs of the facility or system (Knox & Shelton, 2006).

Triage and Disposition of Requests

Triage is defined as a system of determining the order in which acts of medical assistance are carried out (Agnes & Laird, 1996). Triage has most commonly been identified with emergency care, but can be used whenever priority of care must be determined. In the sick call process, triage refers to the review and prioritization of inmates' requests for health services. Because the volume of sick call requests can be very high and timeliness of response is important, triage ensures that response to requests is effective, timely, and clinically appropriate (Knox & Shelton, 2006). There are several ways in which sick call requests are triaged, but all methods are based on some common principles:

- When possible, all requests should be reviewed with the patient's medical record.
- All requests must be evaluated within 1 day of being made.
- Judgment about the disposition and urgency of each request is made by personnel trained and legally entitled to do so.
- Inmates are notified of the health care department's response.
- All requests and actions are documented (Anno, 2001; Knox & Shelton, 2006).

The triage process results in a disposition or decision about the actions that will be taken to address the request. The sick call procedure needs to define the dispositions available at each facility and may include the following:

- Emergent—the inmate is seen immediately.
- Routine—the inmate is scheduled for the next day's sick call.
- Routine dental complaints, excluding dental pain, are referred to Dental Clinic.
- Requests for medication refills are forwarded to the pharmacy, unless the medication is for a chronic disease, then the patient is seen by an advanced provider (ODRC, 2007).

Correctional accreditation standards allow for triage to be performed by trained health care staff or by other correctional personnel trained by the responsible physician (ACA, 2003; NCCHC, 2008). However, triage is most commonly completed by nurses who, by virtue of their education and with some additional training, are capable of conducting the entire sick call process, including initial assessment and evaluation, referral to advanced practitioners, and resolution of minor health complaints without referral. Health-trained correctional staff should not evaluate or treat clinical signs or symptoms independently (Knox & Shelton, 2006).

Assessment

Standard 1 of the Scope and Standards of Corrections Nursing Practice states that "[T]he corrections nurse collects comprehensive data pertinent to the patient's health and condition or the situation" (ANA, 2007, p. 19).

Assessment is the first step in the nursing process and involves the systematic, orderly collection of subjective and objective information about a patient's health status; it is the foundation on which nursing care is planned (Blair, 2002; Lee, Munger, Coxon, & Collins, 2004). In general, there are two types of assessment: comprehensive assessment and focused assessment. Comprehensive assessments are primarily performed to gather fundamental information on new patients. Focused assessments are used for established patients who are being seen for routine or urgent care visits; they address specific symptoms and usually only address the specific body systems related to the patient's concern (Bates & Szilagyi, 2009). Focused assessment is the format used for most patients seen in nursing sick call because these encounters are dictated by the patient's health concern. Well-constructed nursing protocols provide guidelines for gathering appropriate subjective and objective data. For efficiency and to ensure consistent and accurate information, the nurse needs to develop a systematic procedure; following a specific routine during assessments will help ensure the nurse does not miss anything (Bates & Szilagyi, 2009).

Subjective

Subjective assessment is the information that the patient tells the nurse; it includes health history information given by the patient about their health complaint, and may include information about the patient's past medical history, family history, and social history (Bates & Szilagyi, 2009). It may also be referred to as assessing the chief complaint or the history of the present illness. A thorough history is an essential component of a focused assessment, as it guides the objective assessment that follows. Unfortunately, it is the part of the focused assessment process that is most often neglected by nurses and other health care providers.

Subjective assessment begins by asking the patient to identify his or her health complaint or concern. When assessing a complaint, the nurse needs to elicit the seven attributes of a symptom (see Exhibit 15.1)—location, quality, quantity, or severity; timing, setting, remitting; or exacerbating factors and associated manifestations (Bates & Szilagyi, 2009). It is important to listen carefully to the patient's description of the health problem and try to document the patient's exact words. The nurse guides the interview by asking a series of open-ended or direct questions as indicated by the patient's responses. Open-ended questions elicit a lot of information in the patient's own words, but occasionally it is necessary to control the direction of the interview by using direct questions that ask for specific information. However, nurses do need to be cautious to avoid "putting words in the patient's mouth" by asking questions like "Are you coughing anything up? Is it green?" Observe the patient carefully for nonverbal clues about their stated problem, such as posture, facial expressions, and body movements throughout the interview. When the nurse has thoroughly assessed the patient's chief complaint, the nurse can begin to analyze the diagnostic clues obtained about the cause of the patient's symptoms and determine what physical assessment elements are needed to confirm or rule out a disease process.

EXHIBIT 15.1

Seven Attributes of a Symptom

1. Location—where is it, where does it radiate?
2. Quality—what does it feel like?
3. Quantity or severity—how bad is it? For pain, use a pain scale.
4. Timing—When did it start? How long does it last? How often does it happen?
5. Setting—What seems to make it happen? Consider environmental, emotional or activity related factors.
6. Relieving or exacerbating factors—what makes it better or worse?
7. Associated symptoms—does the patient notice any other symptom(s)?

Source: Adapted from Bates & Szilagyi (2009).

Objective

All objective, or physical, assessments should begin with assessment of vital signs and weight, as these measurements give valuable clues to the nature of the patient's specific complaint(s) and to the patient's overall well-being. Patients should be weighed with their shoes off on a calibrated scale. Vital signs include blood pressure, heart rate, respiratory rate, and body temperature. Vital signs need to be assessed using equipment that is accurate and in good working order, using correct assessment techniques (Bates & Szilagyi, 2009; Knox & Shelton, 2006). The nurse then proceeds to apply the techniques of inspection, palpation, auscultation, and percussion, as needed, to the body system(s) related to the complaint. Depending on the complaint, the physical assessment may involve one or more body systems so, here again, well-developed nursing protocols are essential to guide the nurse's actions.

Diagnosis

Standard 2 of the Scope and Standards of Corrections Nursing Practice states, "[T]he corrections nurse analyzes the assessment data to determine the diagnoses or issues" (ANA, 2007, p. 20). Nurses use nursing diagnoses when making judgments about a patient's condition. A nursing diagnosis is the nurse's clinical judgment made about patient responses to actual or potential illness and should be drawn from the North American Nursing Diagnosis Association (NANDA) approved list of nursing diagnoses (Ackley & Ladwig, 2011). Nursing diagnoses may be provided in a nursing protocol used for the assessment or may be devised by each nurse at the time of the assessment. If the nurse is using a self-developed nursing diagnosis, the nurse must include all of the components of a nursing diagnosis, which include the diagnostic label *and* the defining characteristics, related factors, or risk factors. For example, acute pain related to (specified) injury is an appropriate nursing diagnosis (Ackley & Ladwig, 2011); "altered comfort" is not.

Plan

Standard 4 of the Scope and Standards of Corrections Nursing Practice states, "[T]he corrections nurse develops a plan that prescribes strategies and alternatives to attain expected outcomes" (ANA, 2007, p. 22). When a nurse reaches a nursing diagnosis, the nurse determines the outcomes to be achieved and selects nursing interventions, or actions, that will result in the needed outcome (Ignatavicius & Workman, 2006; LaMarre, 2006). Here again, the use of nursing protocols is important to support the clinical decision making of correctional nurses as well-developed nursing protocols will contain the interventions that are approved by the facility medical director for nurses to use in sick call. After determining the appropriate plan of care, the sick call nurse needs to review the plan with the patient to ensure the patient understands and agrees, or consents, to the plan (LaMarre, 2006).

Implementation

Standard 5 of the Scope and Standards of Corrections Nursing Practice states, "[T]he corrections nursing implements the identified plan" (ANA, 2007, p. 24). When the nurse has completed the assessment, made the nursing diagnosis, selected the appropriate interventions, and reviewed the plan with the patient and obtained consent, it then is the nurse's responsibility to implement the plan of care in a safe and timely manner. This may involve providing interventions outlined in the nursing protocol or collaborating with other nurses, advanced providers, or other correctional personnel to ensure that the care plan is implemented (Ignatavicius & Workman, 2006; LaMarre, 2006).

Evaluation

Standard 6 of the Scope and Standards of Corrections Nursing Practice states, "[T]he corrections nurse evaluates progress towards attainment of outcomes" (ANA, 2007, p. 30). Evaluation is the final step of the nursing process. Correctional nurses need to have a plan that addresses the degree to which the patient's expected outcomes were achieved. This may involve one or a combination of the following outcomes:

- The patient's problem has resolved and no other nursing actions are needed.
- The patient's problem is still present; reassessment, a new plan of care or reevaluation is needed.
- The patient has a new problem that needs assessment and resolution (Ignatavicius & Workman, 2006).

This may be demonstrated in nursing sick call by instructing the patient to return to sick call within a given time frame if symptoms persist or worsen—without additional co-pay, if applicable—or by scheduling a return visit for the patient.

Clinical Backup

Nursing protocols are not designed to allow nurses to make medical decisions, nor can nurses be expected to make medical decisions that are beyond their scope of practice. Nursing protocols must be designed in a manner that ensures that nurses and advanced providers collaborate in managing care of patients, making appropriate referrals, and maintaining the chain of care (Knox & Shelton, 2006; LaMarre, 2006).

Criteria for Referrals

Nursing protocols need to address general reasons for referral to advanced level providers, which may include

- The nurse is unable to determine a nursing diagnosis after collecting subjective and objective data.
- Assessment findings are significantly out of normal, as defined in the nursing protocols.
- Additional diagnostic evaluation, beyond the nurses' scope, is needed.
- Treatment indicated is beyond the nurses' scope of practice.
- When the patient has come to sick call two or more times without resolution of the complaint (Knox & Shelton, 2006).

Referral Time Frames

In addition to addressing criteria for referral, it is important for nursing protocols to address the time frames in which referrals must take place. Generally, these time frames are:

- *Immediate*—the patient must been seen by an advanced provider immediately; usually reserved for potentially life-threatening conditions.
- *Urgent*—the patient needs to be evaluated by an advanced provider on the *same day*; used for patients with severe pain or health problems that may deteriorate if left untreated.
- *Routine*—the patient needs to have a scheduled appointment with an advanced provider; usually within 7 days (Knox & Shelton, 2006).

Failure to adequately address referral in sick call procedures and protocols may result in one of two primary problems—underreferral and overreferral. Underreferral means that a patient should have been referred to an advanced provider, but was not or was not referred timely. The outcome of this is that the patient may not be correctly treated or that needed treatment is delayed. Overreferral means that patients with complaints that could have been addressed by a nurse were sent to an advanced provider. Here again, the outcome is often that treatment for the patient is delayed, but also that advanced providers are burdened with unnecessary appointments that compete with the needs of patients with more serious health problems (Knox & Shelton, 2006).

Case Example 15.1 provides an opportunity to apply the material reviewed here using the nursing assessment guideline and protocol provided in Figures 15.1 and 15.2.

CASE EXAMPLE 15.1

A 57-year-old man presents to nursing sick call complaining of having a "heavy cold for a week." He is requesting cough medicine and an order for an extra pillow "so I can sleep better at night." Upon assessment, the patient states that he developed a "chest cold" about 14 days prior and that he often has cold symptoms "especially

(continued)

during the winter." He states that he coughs frequently and produces a large amount of yellowish mucus. He has smoked 1 1/2 packs of cigarettes daily for nearly 25 years.

The results of the physical assessment are: Vital signs—T 98°, P 88, R 18, BP 138/90, pulse ox 92%; General appearance—pale, moderately obese White male; HEENT—no redness, swelling or drainage noted in ears, nose, or throat; Neck—supple; no lymphadenopathy palpable; Cardiac—normal sinus rhythm; no extra sounds heard; Lungs—sounds diminished at bases bilaterally; coarse rhonchi heard in upper and middle lobes; no wheezing heard.

Discussion Questions:

Using the Nursing Assessment Guidelines and Protocol found in Figures 15.1 and 15.2, answer the following:

1. What is your nursing diagnosis?
2. What is your plan? What is the level of urgency?

SICK CALL OPERATIONS

If sick call is the "backbone" of correctional health care, then the sick call operations are the "legs" that carry the entire process. Having an efficient method of receiving and triaging inmates' requests for care and addressing the problems that arise will ensure that patients are seen within acceptable time frames, that nursing and other health care resources are not wasted, and inmate patients' concerns are addressed appropriately (Knox & Shelton, 2006).

Request Methods

Sign-Up/Show-Up Sheet

For this method, inmates put their names on a list designated for this purpose. Oftentimes, the sign-up sheet will be distributed to inmates either by security or by nursing staff the day prior to the scheduled encounter. All inmates on the list are scheduled by the health services staff for a face-to-face encounter with a qualified health care provider; a list of inmates scheduled is then sent to security staff so that inmate movement can be monitored. Triage for this method occurs when the inmate is seen by the nurse and includes assessment and evaluation of the presenting problem. An advantage of this system is that it does not rely on inmate literacy, except for the ability to sign their name. Disadvantages to this method are that the reason for the request may not be known until the inmate is seen, and there may be difficulty in determining needed staffing levels because volume can fluctuate (Burrow et al., 2006; Knox & Shelton, 2006).

Written Requests

This method requires inmates to write their health concerns on a specific health care request form or another institutional form, sometimes called a "kite." After completing the health care request, inmates are directed to place them in a box reserved for the purpose of collecting health care requests and accessible only by health care staff, or are conveyed to health care staff in some other confidential manner. This method allows health care staff to review the request with the inmate's health record present, direct it to the appropriate staff, and to prioritize the urgency of the request before seeing the inmate. The primary disadvantage is that it requires that the inmate have enough literacy to read the directions on the form and complete it (Burrow et al., 2006).

Telephone Triage

Telephone triage allows inmates, who may not be able to read or write on a request form, to discuss their health concern with nursing staff. It allows a nurse to ask clarifying questions and determine the disposition and priority of the request. It does not replace face-to-face encounters, which should be scheduled following the phone call. This method requires an adequate supply of telephones accessible to inmates and that nurses have strong interviewing and communication skills to adequately determine the nature of the patient's problem. Well-designed nursing protocols written specifically for telephone triage will assist nurses to gather all of the information needed to make decisions about the patient's needs without jumping to conclusions (Knox & Shelton, 2006; Mitchell, 2010).

Walk-In Clinics

This system allows inmates to come to Health Services at will during certain scheduled hours. Walk-in clinics allow inmates with low literacy to access health services in a confidential manner and are best used for health complaints that are easily addressed with patient education or self-care remedies. It eliminates the need for nurse time to triage health care request forms. However, this method makes it difficult to predetermine staffing needs and it is necessary to retrieve the inmate's health record for review after the inmate arrives at the clinic (Knox & Shelton, 2006).

Health Care Appointments

This method closely resembles the manner in which patients access care in the community; inmates decide who they need to see (i.e., physician, dentist, nurse, or mental health staff) and how urgently they need to be seen. No triage is necessary; the method requires a predetermined number of appointment slots sufficient for institutional need, an appointment scheduling method, and the patient's record. A variation of this method is to allow such appointments for patients considered to be medically fragile or have complicated conditions including chronic illnesses or mental illness (Knox & Shelton, 2006).

Segregated Settings

Segregation settings present particular problems to the sick call process. Because segregation inmates are confined to their cells for most of the day, American Correctional Association (ACA) and National Commission on Correctional Health Care (NCCHC) accreditation standards require that health care staff make face-to-face rounds on general segregation inmates at least 3 times per week, and daily on high-security inmates to ensure their health and mental status is not deteriorating because of confinement (ACA, 2003; NCCHC, 2008). Segregated inmates tend to request health services at higher rates than general population inmates because the increased confinement is more detrimental to their health and due to sheer boredom. Some correctional facilities have managed these problems by developing a dedicated segregation nurse assignment; the assigned segregation nurse makes rounds daily, checking on the health status of the inmates, collecting the names of inmates requesting health services, and often conducting sick call assessments in a room located in the Segregation Unit that is equipped for this purpose (Anno, 2001; Anno & Spencer, 2006; L. Bethel, personal communication, November 16, 2011).

Management of Problem Areas

Medicalization of Nonmedical Issues

Health care staff frequently come under pressure, from inmates and from security staff, to intervene in areas of inmate comfort and institutional operations. Such areas include requests for comfort items like low bunks, particular shoes or clothing, better bedding, or special diets; they can also include clearances for certain work details, determinations about shackling procedures, and prisoner searches. While it may be tempting and expedient to get involved in these types of decisions, the result may be an impossible burden of these types of demands that ultimately interferes with care directed at the real health care needs of inmate patients. Puerini and Shelton (2006) developed a model approach to addressing inmate's requests for care:

1. Find objective evidence of a serious medical problem. This involves meticulous subjective and objective assessment by correctional nurses and advanced providers.
2. Develop system-wide policies outlining therapeutic levels of care that address all levels of need from urgent to elective. Then, consistently follow these policies.
3. When there is no evidence-based intervention available, consider declining to order unproven remedies.
4. Provide consistent education to prisoners upon entry into the system and throughout their incarceration about the proper role of health care services with emphasis on what necessary medical care is, what is merely comfort care, and the therapeutic levels of care.

There are several ways to address medicalization issues described in the literature. Effective triage can direct requests for medication refills and routine dental or eye appointments to the appropriate services without the inmate being seen in sick call. Some correctional systems require inmates to obtain over-the-counter medications and self-care articles (dental floss, skin lotion, shoe inserts, etc.) at the inmate commissary or canteen. Finally, inmates requiring a different size or width of shoes or additional bedding or clothing may be referred to the facility quartermaster (Knox & Shelton, 2006).

No-Shows

Inmates who request sick call appointments, then do not show up for the appointment can be troubling for multiple reasons. There can be legitimate concern that the inmate is very ill and incapable of attending sick call and needs immediate attention. There are also security concerns that the inmate may be someplace other than where one is scheduled to be, which leads to escape and other concerns. Moreover, nurse staffing is often arranged based on the number of inmates scheduled for sick call; if there are a significant number of no-shows, nursing time and resources are wasted. For all of these reasons, it is important to encourage inmates to keep scheduled sick call appointments and discourage failure to attend an appointment. Continuous quality improvement (CQI) reviews can be particularly useful in determining the root causes of no-shows. All possible causes must be identified before they can be addressed. Since sick call passes are usually issued by security staff, addressing causes of no-shows requires cooperation between security and health care staff. As soon as it is known that an inmate has not reported for sick call, either a nurse or a corrections officer assigned to Health Services should contact the inmate's housing unit to determine the whereabouts of the inmate and why the inmate failed to report at sick call. If the inmate is located and determined to have no legitimate excuse for missing the appointment, some correctional systems will issue conduct reports to inmates who fail to report for scheduled appointments in order to hold them accountable for their actions (L. Bethel, personal communication, November 16, 2011). Another method of addressing no-shows is to insist that the inmate come to the Health Services area to refuse or cancel the appointment, as this allows the health care staff to know that the inmate voluntarily changed his or her mind without using staff time to research why the inmate did not appear (Anno, 2001).

Frequent Flyers

Every correctional facility or system reports experiences with frequent flyers—inmates who, for a variety of reasons, access sick call services very frequently, often every day. Some of the reasons may seem trivial, such as requests for comfort items or food that is more acceptable to the inmate. However, nursing administrators have found that there can be legitimate reasons for the inmate's frequent complaints. One example of this involved an inmate who continued to complain of severe abdominal pain at the site of a past surgical procedure for several months. After receiving many kites and complaints from the inmate, the Health Care Administrator prevailed upon the institution physician to reevaluate the inmate. Subsequent testing revealed that the inmate had some serious adhesions that required further surgery. The inmate's complaints stopped after the second surgical procedure (L. Bethel, personal communication, November 16, 2011). Another approach that has been successful is to schedule such inmates for routine appointments at brief intervals, then lengthening the time between appointments as the inmate's needs are addressed (C. Knox, personal communication, December 27, 2011).

Negative Behaviors

In a survey of correctional nurses, Flanaghan and Flanaghan (2001) reported that correctional nurses describe their patients as "difficult, manipulative, aggressive, and demanding" (p. 75). The study went on to note that many correctional nurses believe that inmate patients seek medical attention primarily to avoid work assignments and for secondary gain rather than for legitimate health reasons (Flanaghan & Flanaghan, 2001). Thus, it becomes important for correctional nurses to be trained in management of disruptive and manipulative patients.

Experienced correctional nurses often report that demonstrating consistent, considerate, and professional behaviors when interacting with inmates to be most successful. Rather than allowing a disruptive inmate to dictate the tone of the sick call encounter, nurses need to maintain a consistent and unshakeable professional demeanor, quietly insisting on respectful behavior. If particular inmates are known to frequently be disruptive or aggressive, the nurse may consider asking a correctional officer to remain nearby during the encounter to discourage such behavior.

Manipulative behavior is best managed by setting firm boundaries. Nurses need to be familiar with and consistently follow policy and procedure when providing care for inmate patients—every inmate patient, every time (L. Bethel, personal communication, November 16, 2011). It is also very important that there is consistency among the nursing staff when providing care for patients, as this will discourage inmates from playing staff against staff or nurse shopping (Burrow et al., 2006).

High Volume of Sick Call Requests

Anno (2001) noted that research on health care utilization by inmates does exceed utilization patterns in community settings; other correctional health care sources report that anywhere from 5% to 30% of the inmates in any given correctional facility will request health services on any given day (Knox & Shelton, 2006). Additionally, sick call requests can fluctuate seasonally due to viral illnesses like colds and influenza and due to injuries incurred in warm weather. Managing high sick call volume can be challenging, but there are many reports of successful solutions.

Offering sick call on a consistent and frequent schedule can lower the daily volume of sick call requests by reassuring inmates that they will be seen timely when needed (Dowdy, 2005). Appropriate and skilled triage of requests is also a highly effective method of managing sick call requests. Skilled triage of sick call requests allows nurses to prioritize care so that patients having the greatest need are seen first and allows nurses to refer inmates to other services, such as pharmacy services for routine medication refills, rather than being seen in sick call (Anno, 2001; Dowdy, 2005; Knox & Shelton, 2006). If sick call volume is extremely high, facility policy may allow routine requests to be deferred until a later nursing shift (L. Bethel, personal communication, November 16, 2011). If sick call volume continues to be very high, the health care staff should consider using the CQI measures to identify and resolve the problems leading to the high volume (Dowdy, 2005).

LEGAL AND ETHICAL ISSUES
Legal Issues

Given the high level of professional autonomy present in nursing sick call it can be very easy for correctional nurses to slip outside their professional boundaries. It is important for correctional nurses to be familiar with and practice in accordance with the standards of safe nursing practice as determined by their respective state laws and Board of Nursing regulations (LaMarre, 2006; Morris, 2007). It is further important that correctional nursing leadership provide administrative and clinical guidance in the form of policies and protocols that are consistent with the Board of Nursing regulations in their respective states (LaMarre, 2006).

The most common legal questions about nursing protocols involve the use of medications, over-the-counter preparations, and prescription medications, often found in the protocols and nursing scope of practice. Generally speaking, over-the-counter medications are regulated by the Food and Drug Administration via the Federal Food, Drug and Cosmetic Act (1938) and do not require prescription by a licensed provider (Morris, 2007). Moreover, as sick call interventions do require a high level of clinical assessment and decision making, it is prudent to have strong nursing protocols that include a properly authorized list of interventions developed in collaboration with the institution's licensed medical providers (Morris, 2007; Smith, 2009). There is considerable variance in state laws concerning the initiation of prescription drugs by registered nurses (RNs) for minor illnesses. Review of applicable state nursing laws is needed before considering these types of protocols. It is recommended that a physician or other advanced provider review any interventions involving prescription medications and confirm these orders by the next working day (Knox & Shelton, 2006).

Ethical Issues

Sick call practice places correctional nurses on the frontlines of correctional health care and brings certain ethical dilemmas to the forefront (Anno & Spencer, 2006). Correctional health care experts have noted that even excellent nurses can change their ethical perspectives when they walk through the gates of a correctional facility—developing punitive attitudes toward inmates, determining that their health care complaints are inflated or for secondary gain only, and believing that inmates are generally undeserving of quality health care (Brodie, 2001). Compounding this problem is the fact that nurses often feel isolated from mainstream nursing when they work in correctional settings, which reinforces the nurses' feelings that things are different in correctional settings (Brodie, 2001; Muse, 2009). This presents significant risk that such disrespect for inmate patients could impact the nurses' clinical decision making, potentially leading them to discount inmates' complaints as always being false or inflated and possibly delaying or even failing to respond to their requests for health care (Benner et al., 2006).

CONTINUOUS QUALITY IMPROVEMENT

The Continuous Quality Improvement (CQI) elements of monitoring, problem identification, and corrective action are integral to ensuring that sick call services meet the needs of the inmate population, while making the most efficient use of available health care resources (Knox & Shelton, 2006). During monitoring, problems are identified for study and quality measures are developed, generally using the requirements found in written sick call procedures and nursing protocols, but may also include requirements found in ACA and NCCHC accreditation standards pertinent to sick call. Finally, indicators are formulated that will measure the quality of the sick call services. An example of indicators developed for nursing sick call can be found in Exhibit 15.2.

There are a few examples of sick call quality measurement found in the literature. Dowdy (2005) described an out-of-control sick call process that had resulted in a very high volume of requests and delayed access to care. Using the CQI tools of problem identification, monitoring, and corrective actions, she was able to resolve the problems leading to the high volume and was able to bring her facility's process into compliance with NCCHC accreditation standards (Dowdy, 2005). Referral, or "pass-through," rate is yet another process area that has been monitored. Knox and Shelton (2006) reported that some correctional systems reported as much as 70% of patients seen in sick call were referred to advanced providers, while other correctional systems reported much lower rates of referral. The Ohio Department of Rehabilitation and Correction conferred with correctional health care authorities and reviewed Nurses' and Doctor's Sick Call records before setting a departmental target rate of 35%–50% of patients to be referred from nurse sick call to advance providers. Persistent monitoring tracked compliance with the standard, identified outliers, and the reasons behind the outliers (L. Bethel and P. Garner, personal communication, November 16, 2011).

EXHIBIT 15.2

Sick Call Continuous Quality Improvement Indicators

- Health Service Request was appropriately triaged and signed by a RN.
- Inmate was scheduled for sick call within the time frame dictated by protocol.
- Nursing assessment is complete and contains chief complaint, subjective, and objective data.
- Subjective assessment includes 3–4 descriptors of the History of Present Illness.
- Complete vital signs and weight were assessed and recorded.
- The nursing plan noted is consistent with the applicable nursing protocol and clinical guidelines.
- The treatment plan is appropriate for the assessment findings and includes patient education.
- Nursing notes are documented in SOAP format.
- Documentation includes date and time of encounter.
- Documentation includes legible signature and title of the writer.
- Documentation includes patient follow-up, referral to advanced care, or nursing plan.

Source: Adapted from the Ohio Department of Rehabilitation and Correction Continuous Quality Improvement form: Nursing Sick Call. Used with permission.

From the Experts . . .

"Since correctional nurses sometimes work alone and without a physician always present, strong physical exam/nursing assessment/triage skills and the ability to provide appropriate nursing interventions are essential for new nurses to run nursing sick call in the correctional setting. The nursing sick call process must provide appropriate treatment/interventions based on the need so that the inmate's health is not compromised. The ability of the nurse to accurately assess/treat the inmate results in fewer returns to nursing sick call and decreases demands on the advanced level providers in doctors' sick call.

Pam Garner, RN
Chillicothe, OH

SUMMARY

In secure correctional settings, inmates must rely on the institution medical department for access to OTCs and other types of self-care treatment that may not available to them. Sick call provides correctional systems with a mechanism to ensure inmates have access to health care services. Sick call further serves a gatekeeper function, allowing inmates to be evaluated and their needs met in a clinically appropriate manner at the appropriate level of care so that scarce health care resources are not wasted and so that inmates with more serious illnesses are not competing for physician time with inmates who have minor problems (Knox & Shelton, 2006). The fundamental principles of sick call practice are that unimpeded access to care is available to inmates daily, that care will be provided by properly trained and licensed staff, and that the care given in sick call will be safe.

Sick call is one of the signature practices that set correctional nursing apart as a nursing specialty. Properly executed, sick call can be a "thing of beauty," allowing nurses to practice at the fullest level of their knowledge and experience. Few other health care situations within nursing allow a nurse to independently assess, develop a nursing diagnosis and a treatment plan that may involve administering over-the-counter medications for a patient without direct oversight from an advanced provider. The high level of autonomy inherent in nursing sick call requires collaboration between nurses and advanced health care providers and meticulous attention to state laws concerning nursing scope of practice. Development of strong protocols that support and direct the nurses' actions and clinical decision making is necessary for legally and clinically appropriate sick call practice.

DISCUSSION QUESTIONS

1. What aspects of nursing assessment are you most and least comfortable with?
2. Sick call was described as a "thing of beauty" in this chapter. How would you describe a sick call process that operates at this level of excellence?
3. What resources are used to develop nursing assessment and treatment protocols at your facilities?
4. Inmate PJ presents at nursing sick call with complaints of "migraine headaches." What subjective and objective assessment should the nurse perform? What is a potential nursing diagnosis for inmate PJ?
5. What are some approaches to reducing high volume sick call? What CQI tools would you suggest using?
6. What problems are seen at sick call that could be addressed in another way at your facility?

REFERENCES

Ackley, B. J., & Ladwig, B. G. (2011). *Nursing diagnosis handbook* (9th ed.). St. Louis, MO: Mosby-Elsevier.

Agnes, M., & Laird, C. (Eds.). (1996). *Webster's new world dictionary and thesaurus*. New York: Hungry Minds, Inc.

American Correctional Association. (2003). *Standards for adult correctional institutions* (4th ed.). Alexandria, VA: Author.

American Nurses Association. (2007). *Corrections nursing: Scope and standards of practice*. Silver Spring, MD: Author.

Anno, B. J. (2001). *Correctional health care: Guidelines for management of an adequate delivery system*. Chicago: NCCHC.

Anno, B. J., & Spencer, S. S. (2006). Medical ethics and correctional health care. In M. Puisis (Ed.), *Clinical practice in correctional medicine* (2nd ed.). Philadelphia: Mosby Elsevier.

Bates, L. S., & Szilagyi, P. G. (2009). *Bates' pocket guide to physical examination and history taking* (6th ed.). Philadelphia: Wolters Kluwer Health/Lippincott, Williams & Wilkins.

Benner, P., Malloch, K., Sheets, V., Bitz, K., Emrich, L., Thomas, M. B. et al. (2006). TERCAP: Creating a national database on nursing errors. *Harvard Policy Review, 7*(1), 48–73. Retrieved November 14, 2011, from http://www.hcs.harvard.edu/~hhpr/publications/previous/06s/Benner_et_al.pdf

Blair, P. (2002). Corrections nursing: What's wrong with this picture? *CorrectCare, 16*(4), 8.

Brodie, J. S. (2001). Caring: The essence of correctional nursing. *Tennessee Nurse, 64*(2), 10–12.

Burrow, G. F., Knox, C. M., & Villanueva, H. (2006) Chapter 29: Nursing in the primary care setting. In M. Puisis (Ed.), *Clinical practice in correctional medicine* (2nd ed.). Philadelphia: Mosby Elsevier.

Dowdy, M. (2005). Sick call out of control? This jail nurse tamed the beast. *CorrectCare, 19*(4), 10.

Etheridge, S. A. (2007). Learning to think like a nurse: Stories from new nurse graduates. *The Journal of Continuing Education in Nursing, 38*(1), 24–30.

Federal Food, Drug and Cosmetic Act (21 U.S.C. § 301 et seq). Retrieved from http://www.fda.gov/RegulatoryInformation/Legislation/FederalFoodDrugandCosmeticActFDCAct/default.htm on 11/6/11.

Flanaghan, N. A., & Flanaghan, T. J. (2001). Correctional nurses perceptions of their role, training requirements, and prisoner health care needs. *Journal of Correctional Health Care, 8*(1), 67–85.

Harjai, P. K., & Tiwari, R. (2009). Model of critical diagnostic reasoning: Achieving expert clinician performance. *Nursing Education Perspectives, 30*(5), 305–311.

Ignatavicius, D. D., & Workman, M. L. (2006). *Medical-surgical nursing: Critical thinking for collaborative care* (5th ed.). St. Louis, MO: Mosby-Elsevier.

Kerns, J., & Pinney, B. (2006). Promoting systems for continuity of care. In M. Puisis (Ed.), *Clinical practice in correctional medicine* (2nd ed.). Philadelphia: Mosby Elsevier.

Kohn, L. T., Corrigan, J. M., & Donaldson, M. S. (Eds.). (2000). *IOM: To err is human: Building a safer health system.* Retrieved November 6, 2011, from http://www.nap.edu/catalog/9728.html

Knox, C., & Shelton, S. (2006). Sick call. In M. Puisis (Ed.), *Clinical practice in correctional medicine* (2nd ed.). Philadelphia: Mosby Elsevier.

LaMarre, M. (2006). Chapter 28: Nursing role and practice in correctional facilities. In M. Puisis (Ed.), *Clinical practice in correctional medicine* (2nd ed.). Philadelphia: Mosby Elsevier.

Lee, C. A., Munger, C. D., Coxon, V., & Collins, E. (2004). In G. B. Altman (Ed.), *Delmar's fundamental and advanced nursing skills* (2nd ed.). Clifton Park, NY: Delmar Learning.

Lunney, M. (2010). Use of critical thinking in the diagnostic process. *International Journal of Nursing Terminologies and Classifications, 21*(2), 82–88.

Mitchell, J. K. (2010). Telephone triage: Your job is on the line. *ONS Connect, 25*(9), 8–11.

Morris, K. (2007). Issues and answers: Occupational health nurses and OTC's. *Ohio Nurses Review, 82*(3), 10.

Muse, M. V. (2009). Correctional nursing: The evolution of a specialty. *CorrectCare, 23*(1), 3–4.

National Commission on Correctional Health Care. (2008). *Standards for health services in prisons.* Chicago, IL: Author.

Ohio Department of Rehabilitation & Correction. (2007). *ODRC Medical Services Protocol Manual: Nurse's Sick Call Access.* (Rev. 2007).

Page, A. (Ed.). (2004). *Keeping patients safe: Transforming the work environment for nurses and patient safety.* Retrieved November 6, 2011, from http://nap.edu//catalog/10851.html

Puerini, M., & Shelton, S. (2006). Doc, I gotta have that pillow: When requests for "comfort" and care collide. *Correct Care, 20*(1), 1, 16.

Rogal, S. M., & Young, J. (2008). Exploring critical thinking in critical care nursing: A pilot study. *The Journal of Continuing Education in Nursing, 39*(1), 26–33.

Rold, W. J. (2006). Legal considerations in the delivery of health care services in prisons and jails. In M. Puisis (Ed.), *Clinical practice in correctional medicine* (2nd ed.). Philadelphia: Mosby Elsevier.

Scott, B., & Collatt, M. (2009, October). Assuring nursing skills through competency development. In *NCCHC National Conference,* Orlando, FL.

Smith, S. (2009). The nurse is in: Designing effective nursing sick call guidelines. *CorrectCare, 23*(3), 14–15.

Tanner, C. A. (2006). Thinking like a nurse: A research-based model of clinical judgment in nursing. *Journal of Nursing Education, 45*(8), 204–211.

SIXTEEN

Emergency Care Delivery

Margaret M. Collatt

All correctional nurses are expected to respond to medical emergencies including psychiatric emergencies. Nursing assessment and treatment intervention in the correctional environment is similar to prehospital emergency medical response and emergency department care in the community. This chapter describes emergency preparation, including organization, response strategies, and approaches for nursing assessment in the field. The sequencing and interventions used in emergency life support, along with the nurse's command role with correctional staff during the emergency, are discussed. Finally, how to prepare for and debrief an emergency medical response are described.

STANDARDS AND EXPECTATIONS FOR EMERGENCY RESPONSE
Access to Care

Provision of emergency care is a fundamental expectation of any correctional facility. Emergency care includes 24-hour availability of basic first aid and CPR, evacuation and emergency transport, and services of a hospital emergency department or equivalent (Anno, 2001). The capacity to cope with inmate emergencies and access to specialists and/or inpatient hospital treatment when warranted by the patient's condition applies to all correctional institutions, regardless of size (Rold, 2006). The obligation to provide emergency services is the same even if there are no regular health care services provided on-site. Both the American Correctional Association (ACA) and the National Commission on Correctional Health Care (NCCHC) have established standards that detail expectations for responding to emergencies (ACA,

2002; NCCHC, 2008a, 2008b, 2011). Correctional nurses are expected to respond to emergencies and, as the first medical responder, to take charge, directing the response and arranging for definitive care. Correctional officers retain responsibility for safety and security in a medical emergency; the additional emphasis in these situations is that definitive, timely care and treatment must be delivered and to do so the nurse must be organized, decisive, and communicative. Medical emergencies can take place at any location in the facility or on grounds. In addition to inmates, the subject of a medical emergency may be a staff member or visitor (American Nurses Association [ANA], 2007).

From the Experts ...

"Typically, emergency situations are extremely chaotic and people don't always stop and think first before doing things in an organized fashion. I've seen it over and over, and being in that type of situation you need someone who stops, thinks and takes control—nurses are great at it."

Karen Schmedeke, RN, BSN, CCHP
Denver, CO

Medical emergencies provide a unique perspective on the adequacy of the health care program in particular and, more generally, the safety and security of the operation of the facility. If inmates are unable to access primary care services or are dissatisfied with the quality of care, often the number and severity of medical emergencies will increase. Access to items considered contraband in a correctional facility increases the likelihood of incidents that result in trauma, assault, or overdose. If inmates are assigned work that is unsafe, occupational injuries may occur. While skilled and responsive emergency services save lives, each emergency should be evaluated to determine if there is a trend or problem area in the delivery of other services or the operation of the facility, that if addressed may prevent another emergency.

Right to a Clinical Judgment

In a medical emergency, inmates are entitled to a professional medical judgment (Rold, 2006). Since correctional nurses are most likely the first medical professional to respond to the medical emergency, they are therefore expected to also exercise their clinical judgment about the patient's immediate care. As a colleague pointed out, two thirds of the day at a typical jail, there is no doctor on-site and it will be the nurse who manages the emergency response (Laffan, 2010).

The nurse has two obligations; one is to be knowledgeable and competent to provide basic emergency care and the other is to exercise clinical judgment in the emergency. Clinical judgment or problem solving using the nursing process (assessment, nursing diagnosis, plan, implementation, and evaluation) that is consistent with guidelines established by the facility for emergency care will facilitate decision making and timely transfer of the patient if necessary.

Training and Competency

It is imperative that the correctional nurse has expertise in clinical assessment and a strong grasp of underlying pathophysiology. These skills and knowledge improve the nurse's decision making and problem solving, resulting in better patient outcomes (Laffan, 2010). Correctional nurses must be capable of providing emergency care anywhere on the site of the correctional facility and under many different kinds of conditions. The techniques to stabilize the patient at the scene and prepare for rapid transport are also part of the correctional nurse's skill set. These include opening and protection of the airway, respiratory support by Ambu, Bagmask, or through intubation (if trained), perfusion support, including cardiopulmonary resuscitation (CPR), initiation and maintenance of an intravenous (IV), recognition of soft tissue damage and fracture with manual stabilization, immobilization of the spine, control of hemorrhage, and delivery of a newborn.

In emergency response, correctional nurses carry O_2 tanks and change regulators to administer oxygen, employ various transfer techniques and equipment, apply cervical collars and other possible fracture stabilization supplies, control bleeding through dressings and other techniques, start IV fluids and administer medications in adverse conditions, recognize and manage cardiac and neurological compromise, and treat other conditions that may be unique for each facility.

In most correctional settings, the level of training and proficiency expected of nurses is that of Basic Life Support (BLS). Nurses should also be taught how to prepare specialty medications that a practitioner who is ACLS trained may request during a life-threatening emergency. Sometimes, a facility will establish certification in Advanced Cardiac Life Support (ACLS) as the expectation for emergency response. This decision is based upon the medical status and needs of the population housed at the correctional facility, ambulance response times, and the ability to retain staff proficiency at the ACLS level. Even nurses who have prior expertise and knowledge of emergency care must be trained to the specific policies, procedures, guidelines, and equipment used at the correctional facility. This training includes where equipment is kept, how to arrange for transport, guidance for clinical decisions, and documentation. Emergency response requires coordination by the nurse with the facility, the physician and health care program, ambulance, and hospital emergency room.

Response Times and Skill Levels

Responding to medical emergencies within the correctional facility is complex and cannot be performed solely by the correctional nurse. The safety of each team member as well as the health of the patient requires that staff work as a team for the best possible outcome. Correctional officers are critical members of the team; often, they are the first responder, they secure and clear the area, direct traffic, carry equipment, escort EMS, and facilitate off-site transport.

Each facility should have an emergency response plan that defines how individual medical emergencies are handled as well as a more elaborate plan to respond to larger-scale emergencies or disasters. The ACA (2002) has defined 4 minutes as the acceptable amount of time for the first person to respond to an emergency, and many facilities have adopted this standard. This time frame takes into consideration the delays that are inherent in correctional facilities, such as locked equipment and doors that are controlled by others.

From the Experts

"During an emergency, take care of the patient as best you can. Deal with the emergency in the most effective way possible and remember you are not there by yourself. Ask anybody who is there by you to help and tell them what you need. Remember, this is a population of people that probably need our care the most."

Susan Laffan, RN, CCHP-RN, CCHP-A
Toms River, NJ

Meeting the 4-minute standard requires that correctional officers be trained in basic first aid and BLS because they will most often be the first to respond. ACA and NCCHC require training of correctional officers to include in addition to first aid and CPR, recognition of life-threatening conditions, intoxication and withdrawal, mental illness, and suicide intervention (ACA, 2002; NCCHC, 2008a, 2008b, 2011). Some correctional officers may have EMT and/or paramedic training and experience as well. Correctional staff also will have been trained in the facility's procedures to refer or obtain assistance from health care staff, notification of the emergency medical system, and transfer to off-site medical facilities.

The correctional nurse will determine if the patient's condition is beyond the capabilities of the staff, equipment, and supplies that are readily available at the facility and arrange for the transfer of the patient. Both ACA and NCCHC require that arrangements for ambulance services, hospitals, and specialists are established in advance of need so that transport to a community-based health care facility takes place when medically necessary (ACA, 2002; NCCHC, 2008a, 2008b, 2011). Some correctional facilities work very closely with EMS in the community to standardize equipment and procedures and may practice emergency response drills together. Correctional nurses should be familiar with the local EMS system and be prepared to stabilize the patient if the ambulance is delayed. This may necessitate moving the patient to the health care area at the correctional facility until transport is available.

INITIAL RESPONSE TO EMERGENCY
Notification

Notification of an emergency may come by word of mouth, over the telephone, or via radio communication. The nurse receiving notification needs to get sufficient information to determine what supplies and equipment will be necessary to respond to the needs of the patient. Information to be communicated includes

■ Name of the requester and the phone number they are calling from (if applicable) in case additional information is needed.
■ Exact location where health care staff is to respond.
■ Information about the person with the emergency (bleeding, severe pain, or unconscious).
■ Any other factors that staff should be aware of, such as a disturbance or other security issue.

■ Instruct the reporting individual what assistance to provide to the patient until health care staff respond.

Sometimes, correctional staff will move the emergent patient to another area or bring them directly to the health services area. This may be an immediate means to protect the inmate or staff from injury or deescalate a situation. The nurse may also determine during the initial notification that the patient can be brought to the clinic for assessment or should be transported to the emergency department because their need for care exceeds the facility's capabilities. A nurse should not determine on the basis of telephone or radio contact alone that an emergency does *not* exist. A face-to-face assessment and evaluation by the nurse must take place whenever staff or an inmate thinks that there is a medical emergency.

Facilities that have more than one nurse on duty at the same time will typically designate one or more positions as responsible for emergency response. Some health care programs may also designate specific positions responding to mental health emergencies. These nurses wear a pager, radio, or other device to receive emergency notifications. Most of the time, these nurses have other responsibilities, such as managing the outpatient clinic, which can be stopped long enough to respond to the emergency. The emergency response nurse is also responsible for ensuring that the equipment and supplies are available and in working order. It is preferable to rotate this assignment so that all nurses retain their proficiency in emergency response.

Scene Survey and Safety

Safety is a top priority, and collaboration between the nurse and custody staff will reduce the possibility of staff injury. An emergency may be falsified; serve as a diversion for other prohibited activity, or be used to observe how the emergency team responds in planning a future disturbance. The nurse must be observant when entering the area where the emergency is taking place. If the scene is not safe, it may be detrimental to the response effort and to the response team. For instance, the responding nurse may be unaware of a potential hostage situation or that an inmate has a weapon. It is the responsibility of the custody staff to secure the scene for safety, and to notify the medical response team. The nurse is not obligated to enter the scene until it is safe and should have an exit strategy if the scene becomes unsafe. Most important is to have a means of communication and remain aware of other events taking place in the environment surrounding the emergency.

Once the scene is safe, the nurse determines the nature of the medical emergency, how it took place, whether there were precipitating factors, and how many people are involved. If the emergency is an injury, the nurse needs to estimate the extent of trauma. If it is an illness, the nurse needs to assess the person's health status immediately preceding the emergency. Additional information to be gathered includes whether the individual has any preexisting medical or psychiatric conditions, if the person has allergies or is taking a high alert medication, and when they last consumed food or fluid. This information is gathered by observation of the area, asking questions of the person involved, and others who witnessed the event. From this information the nurse determines the urgency or priority of care and if additional resources are needed. Next, the nurse assesses the patient's condition using a systematic approach to identify and treat or stabilize the patient until transport for definitive care, either to the medical unit or to a hospital setting.

Primary and Secondary Assessment

The primary assessment consists of a quick visual inspection of the patient to assess and correct any immediately life-threatening conditions. Primary assessment begins with the patient's general appearance and respiratory status, cardiac perfusion, and mental status. The cervical spine is stabilized as the airway is established. Mental status is a measure of neurological ability or disability, the patient's level of consciousness, and cognitive ability. If respiration and/or circulation are compromised, resuscitative measures are initiated before any further assessment. This primary assessment should take no more than 30–60 seconds, followed by a secondary assessment.

The secondary assessment is a quick head-to-toe assessment. The nurse uses this information to determine how to manage the patient medically without doing further harm. The secondary assessment includes a full set of vital signs; an inspection of the body for obvious injuries and foreign bodies; a relevant health history, including immunization, medications, assistive devices; and a more thorough assessment of neurological function if there is a possibility of head injury. The secondary assessment should take no more than 2–3 minutes.

Triage

The quick primary and secondary assessments allow the nurse to decide and communicate with others the priority and urgency for treatment. Clearly defined criteria should be established to use in determining when the patient's condition cannot be handled on-site. These criteria will depend upon the medical capability at the facility, numbers and skills of nurses, physicians and other health care providers, the equipment and supplies maintained at the facility, and the distance to off-site services. The emergency plan will also identify the triage categories and provide definitions for the use of each category. Many correctional facilities have adopted the same code system used by EMS in the local community. After triage occurs, the patient is treated and may be moved to the health care area and/or is stabilized for transfer to EMS and transport to the hospital.

Treatment

Treatment, also known as tertiary assessment or stabilization, should take place in the health care area. The nurse monitors and reassesses the patient until the emergency is resolved or the patient's care transferred to EMS. During this time, the patient should be protected from hypothermia and an IV started if fluid replacement and medications are to be anticipated. The nurse will be providing treatment according to established protocols and/or implementing direct or telephone orders from the provider.

Emergency guidelines or written protocols should be developed by the nursing director in collaboration with the medical director at the facility to address the types of medical emergencies that are life threatening. These protocols should outline the requisite subjective and objective findings for each type of condition, the steps the nurse should take to stabilize the patient, and when and how to transfer the patient for additional care. The NCCHC standards anticipate that nurses use assessment protocols, which may include directions to use prescription medication to treat emergent, life-threatening conditions (NCCHC, 2008a, 2008b, 2011). When the clinician is contacted the emergency response is reviewed, including use of any

TABLE 16.1 Example of Content Areas Addressed by Emergency Protocol

Anaphylaxis	Diabetic ketoacidosis
Angina	Hypoglycemia
Asthma	Myocardial infarction
Cardiac arrest	Poisoning
Cerebral vascular accident	Puncture wound
Chest wound	Shock
Childbirth	Suicide

Source: Adapted from Oregon Department of Corrections, Health Services (n.d.).

prescription medication, then adjustments or additions may be made to the patient's care as necessary. Examples of medical conditions considered life threatening that should be addressed in emergency protocols are listed in Table 16.1.

Emergencies can be the result of a medical condition such as asthma, diabetic crisis, or pregnancy; an intentional or unintentional injury such as suicide or rape; or an accident at the work site such as a laceration, amputation, or other musculoskeletal injury. Nurses need to be prepared to respond to the variety and range of emergencies that may take place in the facility. Preparation includes being competent and knowledgeable of the treatment protocols for life-threatening emergencies so that the response is not delayed because of the need to consult the reference. Assessment protocols need to be simple and main points enunciated to aid memorization. Some facilities have developed flash cards, drills, and mnemonics with frequent review and sign off to assist nurses in committing the emergency protocols to memory. See Figure 16.1 for an example of an emergency assessment protocol; note the summary at the top of the first page.

The nurse who responds to a "man down" may arrive to discover that the event is much larger than reported. When an emergency is declared that overwhelms the staffing, equipment, or supplies available, the role of nurses will still be that of medical care; the focus changes to managing multiple casualties and directing treatment efforts to inmates and staff that can be saved. The National Institute of Corrections (NIC) has maintained a substantial focus on emergency preparedness since the 1980s by providing resources and technical assistance to correctional facilities. The events of 9/11 and Hurricane Katrina emphasized the need for correctional facilities to be prepared for large-scale disasters both natural and manmade, and to coordinate the response with the community (Schwartz & Barry, 2009). Common large-scale emergencies include fire, explosions, hostage situations, riots, hurricanes, earthquakes, and storms.

COMMUNICATION AND INFORMATION SHARING

Communication during an emergency is one of the most important aspects of a coordinated response. Nurses are in communication with correctional staff, physicians, and other health care providers, and off-site medical personnel. The nurse who has responsibility for emergency response maintains an awareness of events within the facility that could result in an emergency or complicate the response (Laffan, 2010).

30 Second Review: Possible MI/Intractable Angina

1) Continue NTG 0.4mg SL. q 5-10 min. if pain is persistent and vitals stable (SBP>90).
2) O₂ by nasal cannula or mask at 4-8 L/min.
3) ASA 325mg chewable if no allergy.
4) The following steps are to occur concurrently:
   a. Call 911. Prepare patient for transport
   b. While waiting, start normal saline lock or IV TKO
   c. Notify Practitioner (do not delay transport)
   d. 12 lead EKG as last step while waiting

DEFINITION: Increased cardiac discomfort, refractory to treatment and/or physically disabling. Chest pain and systemic signs consistent with ongoing myocardial ischemia and/or myocardial compromise. Not relieved by oxygen, rest and sublingual nitroglycerin tablets.

Lack of sufficient oxygenation of myocardial tissue to meet current cardiac demands, with impending myocardial tissue damage.

Clinically it is often difficult in this situation to be sure if the chest pain is related to a heart attack or not. If you, as a nurse, think this _may be_ an MI, act completely as if it is (i.e., once started go all the way.)

If chest pain is relieved by NTG, and patient's vitals are stable, see Angina Protocol.

DATA BASE:

Subjective: Intense substernal chest pain or pressure. Pain to left jaw, shoulder or arm. Vague but intense chest heaviness, shortness of breath, weakness, nausea, diaphoresis, "I don't know what it is but I've never felt like this before." OR "It feels like it did when I had my other Heart Attack." Bilateral jaw pain is frequently myocardial in etiology.

Objective: Patient looks bad. Any combination of the following: Diaphoretic with grey, ashen complexion, ↑ HR, ↑ or ↓ BP, cool, clammy, anxious, abnormal respirations. Signs and symptoms not relieved by sublingual NTG, rest and Oxygen. Many people having a myocardial infarction have a normal physical exam.

Assessment: Possible Myocardial Infarction

Plan:
1. Prepare patient for transport. While waiting, continue to use NTG 0.4mg sublingual q 5-10 minutes if pain is unrelieved and if SBP is at least 90.
2. O₂ by nasal prongs or mask, low to medium flow at 2-8 LPM. Use ambu-bag (15L) if patient is obtunded.
3. ASA 325mg chewed if no allergy.
4. Monitor Vitals at least every 5 min. while awaiting transport.
5. Start IV TKO or heparin/saline lock.
6. May do Stat 12 lead EKG while waiting for emergency transport.
7. Notify the practitioner. Do not delay transport.

FIGURE 16.1   Myocardial infarction, possible (intractable angina).

Source: Adapted from Oregon Department of Corrections, Health Services, Emergency Protocols, January 2009. Used with permission.

An example would be an emergency that takes place on the control room floor at the time of a scheduled inmate movement will require officers to direct traffic and clear the area. Another example would be a severe flood that may delay ambulance response times or crowd the emergency room. In both examples, the nurse needs to anticipate and prepare for additional contingencies to address potential delays.

Communication that is clear, concise, and in a common language facilitates a timely response and smooth transition as responsibility for patient care is transferred because everyone is working from the same information. Plain language should be used in all instruction, both verbal and written, and tested during drills and exercises (Safecom Program, 2009). The use of plain language does not prohibit the use of in-house emergency codes to communicate with facility staff. When communicating with entities outside the facility, however, plain language should be used in place of internal terminology or facility-specific emergency codes (Federal Emergency Management Agency [FEMA], 2006). For example, rather than requesting "Ambulance crew report to DSU," the plain language version is "Escort the ambulance crew to the emergency site in the Disciplinary Segregation Unit".

Facility procedures will specify the channels of communication and any particular codes that are to be used when requesting assistance, reporting findings, and giving direction. The nurse must be practiced and familiar with numbers and language used to communicate effectively during the emergency.

Activating the Emergency Medical System and Transport

Activating the emergency medical system (EMS) to transport the patient is usually as easy as memorizing a number and waiting for assistance to arrive. An accurate report of the patient's condition, using the agreed-upon code, ensures that EMS responds with the necessary equipment to initiate treatment. In many procedures, the nurse notifies the Commander or Officer-in-Charge of the facility that EMS is needed, what level or code the emergency is, and where the patient will be located. The Commander or Officer-in-Charge contacts EMS so that access to the facility and escort, if required, is made available. Timeliness in response means that EMS needs to know exactly where to go to respond to the patient (Laffan, 2010).

Security measures must be continually enforced; eliminating variation in these practices reduces opportunity to develop an escape plan using a medical emergency as a ploy. Security measures include positive identification of the patient, the necessary security restraints and the number of security personnel needed to provide security and protection. The nurse needs to reassess the patient and communicate with security staff if the patient's condition will become or is compromised by restraints or positioning used to maintain security.

Handoff to EMS

While waiting, the nurse prepares information (verbal and written, if possible) to be provided to EMS. This information includes

- The immediate history of the emergent condition
- Treatment interventions
- Current assessment with most recent vital signs
- Suspected diagnosis
- Any allergies or critical medications

When EMS first arrives on the scene, the nurse provides a briefing of the situation and condition of the patient(s) as described above.

DOCUMENTATION AND RECORDKEEPING

Usually there are several types of documentation that are required during and after the response to an emergency. First, the condition and care of the patient during and after the emergency must be documented in the health record. A report of the incident is also completed, which is not part of the health record but is a record of the emergency, who was involved, and how the response took place. Some correctional facilities also use video recording during an incident that is retained as a record and may be used for review purposes also. Finally, there may also be a verbal and/or written critique of the clinical aspects of the emergency response used to improve future performance by eliminating barriers or improving capacity to respond.

Health Record

Recording health information during an emergency can be very challenging because saving the patient's life is the focus of care, not documentation. Some correctional systems have identified a position to serve as a recorder. The person with this assignment accompanies the emergency response nurse to the site. This person can be a member of the clerical staff or any other staff person as long as they have been trained on how to record the information. Recording can be done in narrative format and, if so, the nurse calls out what the findings are to be recorded. Some correctional facilities use a form with check boxes to record positive findings or interventions, much like forms used by EMS or by emergency rooms.

In a mass-casualty emergency, recording may be limited to the triage decision and very brief information about the patient's condition and what treatment was initiated. Once again, many correctional facilities have adopted the tagging and documentation system used by the emergency response system in the local community because it facilitates transfer of information and accuracy in communicating important information about the patient's condition and interventions that took place before EMS arrived. Regardless of the selected format for sharing general information, the method must be easy to obtain and use.

In addition to contemporaneous documentation of the emergency, the health care program may require a summary progress note be made in the patient's record that documents in more detail the patient's condition, treatment provided, and response to intervention.

Incident Report

The nurse may also complete an incident report after the emergency response. Usually, incident report forms are completed by each of the staff members who respond. This form may be a simple template as in Figure 16.2. Once these are compiled from all responding individuals, they may be used to audit the health care team's response or to study the facility's combined response to identify possible improvements. If treatment protocols were used to initiate life-saving measures, post-event clinical review is required by NCCHC (2008a, 2008b, 2011). This involves, at a minimum, review of the patient's health record and the incident report.

Clinical Review

Since so much of the emergency response relies upon practiced application of skill and knowledge, the nurse may also be expected to reflect upon their own performance to identify opportunities for clinical enhancement or systems issues that would benefit from resolution. An example of a clinical review form for BLS response is provided in Figure 16.3. This more detailed summary of the response is useful to describe common or reoccurring themes that are in need of correction or would improve the response. Another purpose is to report possible improvements,

DATE: _____

WHO: (List name of C.O./staff initiating call) _____

WHAT: (State mechanism of injury or emergency) _____

_____

WHERE: Cell #: _____ Tier #: _____ Block #: _____ Other: _____
(Indicate *specific* site/location of incident)

WHEN: _____ to _____
(Note precise time when call initiated; synchronize with caller)

Responding Staff present (Record ALL staff) _____

_____

HOW/WHY: (Precipitating events; signs & symptoms; complaints) _____

_____

EQUIPMENT: (Taken to area, and other equipment used during event) _____

_____

FOLLOW-UP: (Disposition of victim; transfer, etc.) _____

RESPONDING TEAM REVIEW: _____

_____

(Analysis of Emergency Medical Response & Interventions)

RECOMMENDATIONS: _____

_____   _____
Signature: Health Services Personnel/E.M.R. Team Leader   Date

Note: The purpose of this tool is to support the staff involved, review the full situation, and to propose any modifications.

FIGURE 16.2 Emergency medical response incident debrief form.

From Oregon Department of Corrections (2008). Used with permission.

suggested support, and recognition/commendation of those who contributed to a good response and/or positive outcomes. This format allows the health care team to review responses quickly, identify training needs of the staff, learn from trends in emergency response, determine additional equipment and supplies needed, and demonstrate the workload of staff in responding to medical emergencies.

EQUIPMENT FOR RESPONDING TO EMERGENCIES

The responding nurse must bring the necessary equipment and supplies to the scene, similar to EMS in the community. These should be portable and standardized so that time is not lost locating supplies and transporting equipment to the scene. Emergency equipment and supplies should not be part of the day-to-day clinical operation, but located in multiple places that are easy to access and ready for use immediately upon notification. In establishing the equipment and supplies that should be available for an emergency response kit, the nurse can use samples of emergencies that took place at the facility or adopt a list from another facility that is similar in size, mission, and location. The equipment and supplies selected also need to be commensurate with the level of health care and staffing at the facility as well as the distance from emergency services in the community (NCCHC, 2008a, 2008b, 2011).

It is not possible to anticipate every type of medical emergency scenario. Also, the more equipment and supplies, the heavier it is to carry and the harder it is to find

Responding Personnel _____
(From all Functional Units)

Date: _____Time:_____

Site: _____
(Level, Tier, Cell; Other – specify)

Reason for Stopping: _____

Circulation restored: _____

Respirations restored: _____

Procedure unsuccessful (i.e., pt. expired): _____

Treatment Rendered:_____

Adequate Personnel Available: Yes_____ No _____

Comments: _____

_____

Performance of Personnel Responding:

Strengths: _____

Areas for Improvement: _____

Equipment and Supplies Available & Working Properly: Yes _____ No _____

Comments: _____

Documentation Review

Comments: _____

Suggestions/Recommendations

Comments: _____

FIGURE 16.3   Basic Life Support (BLS) critique form.

From Oregon Department of Corrections (2008). Used with permission.

things within the kit quickly. It is important to keep these two variables (weight and simplicity) in mind and select material that can be used in multiple ways, is going to be needed in most responses, and is lightweight and easy to carry. The correctional nurse must be flexible and creative, and in that way can be responsive to anything that may present as an emergent situation (Laffan, 2010).

Minimum Requirements

At a minimum, emergency equipment should include personal protective equipment (PPE), along with face masks or face shields, a bag valve mask, and oxygen to provide respiratory support, supplies to control bleeding, and an Automatic External Defibrillator (AED) to provide essential care. IV equipment and supplies should also be included in the initial response kit. Additional health care equipment may include electrocardiogram (EKG), suction, nebulizer, and rescue medication commensurate to the training of the health care staff and patient needs. Figures 16.4 and 16.5 are examples from the Oregon Department of Corrections of a standardized emergency response kit and medications that are taken with the AED on an initial response to the site of an emergency (Health Services Section Policy and Procedure #P-A-07, 2008).

QTY.	DESCRIPTION	EXP.DATES		QTY.	DESCRIPTION	EXP.DATES
	OUTSIDE POCKET			10 ea	Sanidex sanitizer wipes	exp.
1 ea	Ace Perfit Cervical Collar			1 ea	Digital Thermometer w/covers	exp.
1 ea	CPR Mask Laerdal (yellow)			1 pr	Utility Scissors	
1 ea	Ambu. Bag, Disposable			1 ea	Airway small	
1 ea	Burn Sheet, sterile, 60x96, Disposable			1 ea	Airway medium	
2 ea	Underpads (blue chux)			1 ea	Airway large	
1 ea	Sharps Disp.Container,1.5qt. BD#305487			4 ea	Tongue Blades	
				1 ea	Flashlight w/batteries	exp.
	COMPARTMENT 1 / INSIDE POCKET			1 ea	Penlight	
1 ea	Splints, air, full arm			2 ea	Face Masks, Ear Loop	
1 ea	Splints, air, full leg					
					COMPARTMENT 5	
	COMPARTMENT 2				**ziplock bag/yellow zipper bag**	
2 pkg	Burn Dressing, 5x9, Xeroform	exp.		1 ea	Irrigation Solution Nacl. 500ml	exp.
2 ea	Combine Dressing 8x10 / 5x9			1 ea	Eye Wash Solution 4oz.	exp.
10 ea	Dressing 4x4 Pads, sterile			2 ea	Safety goggles plastic,clear	
2 ea	Kerlix Dressing / Gauze 4"			4 pkgs	Eye Pads sterile - 1 per package	
2 ea	Gauze Roll 4", sterile					
					ziplock bag/orange zipper bag	
	COMPARTMENT 3			5 pr	Exam Gloves N/S Small	
12 ea	Alcohol Prep Pads	exp.		5 pr	Exam Gloves N/S Medium	
1 ea	AssurePro Glucometer & test strips	exp.		5 pr	Exam Gloves N/S Large	
1 ea	AssurePro control solutions 1&2	#1 exp.	#2 exp.			
2 ea	AAA batteries	exp.			**ziplock bag/blue zipper bag**	
5 ea	Safety Lancets			1 ea	Blood Pressure Cuff	
2 ea	Betadine/Povidine Swab Sticks	exp.		2 ea	Bio-Hazard Bags Red	
2 rl	Coban self adhesive roll 4"			1 ea	Stethoscope	
1 rl ea	Tape, cloth 1" & 2" roll					
1 ea	Triangular bandage				**ATTACH TO OUTSIDE OF BAG**	
1 ea	Ace Wrap bandage 4"			1 ea	List of items in Bag	
4 ea	Cotton Tip Applicators, 6" sterile			1 ea	Black notebook and pen	
1 ea	Cold Pack					
1 ea	Rescue Blanket					
		**after using bag, circle what has been used or what is needed				
	Bag Location:_____					
	Refilled by:				**Date refilled/checked:**	

FIGURE 16.4   Contents of emergency man-down kit.

From Oregon Department of Corrections (2008). Used with permission.

Qty.		Medication & Misc. with expiration dates	Exp. Date	Initial	Qty.		Sharps & Supplies		Sharps Sign-Out			
1	EA	Ventolin HFA (albuterol) inhaler			1	EA	SYRINGE, STANDARD	20CC				1
8	TAB	ASPIRIN 81 mg Chewable U/D (4/dose)			1	EA	SYRINGE, SAFETY	12CC				1
1	EA	ATROPINE (0.1 mg/ml) 10ml INJ			2	EA	SYRINGES, SAFETY	6CC			2	1
1	EA	DEXTROSE 50% IV INJ 25gm			3	EA	SYRINGES, SAFETY	3CC	3		2	1
1	EA	DIAZEPAM INJ 5mg/ml 2ml (Valium)			2	EA	NEEDLES green filter	18Gx1.5			2	1
4	caps	DIPHENHYDRAMINE 50mg (Benadryl) U/D			2	EA	NEEDLES green	18Gx1.5			2	1
1	EA	DIPHENHYDRAMINE INJ (50mg/ml) 1ml (Benadryl)			8	EA	NEEDLES purple	21Gx1.5	8	7	6	5
							(continued count)	21Gx1.5	4	3	2	1
2	EA	epinephrine (Adrenaline) 1:1000 1mg/ml 1ml SDV			4	EA	NEEDLES red	25Gx1	4	3	2	1
3	EA	FUROSEMIDE INJ 10mg/ml 40mg (Lasix)			4	EA	NEEDLE,SAFETY VACUTAINER	21Gx1	4	3	2	1
2	EA	GLUCAGON IM KIT			1	EA	NEEDLE,SAFETY VAC.BUTTERFLY	23Gx3/4				
2	bags	LACTATED RINGERS 500ml IV SOLN			2	EA	IV CATHETER, SAFETY	18Gx1.25			2	1
2	EA	LIDOCAINE INJ 2% (20mg/ml) 5ml			2	EA	IV CATHETER, SAFETY	20Gx1			2	1
1	EA	NALOXONE INJ 1mg/ml 2mg (Narcan)			2	EA	IV CATHETER, SAFETY	22Gx1			2	1
					2	EA	IV TUBING, PRIMARY SET	10D/ML			2	1
1	BT	NITROGLYCERIN Sublingual 0.4mg 25 tbs			1	EA	SCALPELS, SAFETY	#11				
6	TAB	ORAL GLUCOSE TABS			1	EA	SCALPELS, SAFETY	#10				1
1	EA	ORAL GLUCOSE GEL 15gm			2	EA	TRACHEA NEEDLES	14Gx1.5			2	1
9	EA	ALCOHOL WIPES			1	RL	TAPE, CLOTH 1"					
5	EA	BETADYNE WIPES or SWABSTICKS			1	RL	TAPE, CLOTH 2"					
5	EA	SANIDEX WIPES (replaced hibistat wipes)			1	RL	TAPE, PAPER 1"					
2	EA	TUBES RED			2	EA	TOURNIQUETS					
2	EA	TUBES BLUE (changed from gray)			4	EA	TUBE/NEEDLE HOLDER, STANDARD					
2	EA	TUBES PURPLE			10	EA	BAND AIDS ASSORTED					
1	EA	CARPUJECT INJECTOR	N/A		1	BG	GLOVES, 5 PAIR/1bag	SMALL				
1	EA	TUBEX INJECTOR	N/A		1	BG	GLOVES, 5 PAIR/1bag	MEDIUM				
					1	BG	GLOVES, 5 PAIR/1bag	LARGE				
First Item to expire _____ date _____												
Refilled or checked by _____ date _____					**Please note: Please account for sharps after emergency.							

FIGURE 16.5   Contents of emergency medication box.

From Oregon Department of Corrections (2008). Used with permission.

Backup Requirements

Backup equipment and supplies should be stored strategically throughout the facility. This provides a means to access equipment and supplies if it is timelier than transport from the clinic or warehouse or the route to the clinic is blocked. Additional or backup equipment and supplies may also be needed for stabilization while waiting to transport the patient off-site for further treatment. This equipment should include a gurney, back board, basket, or other device that can easily navigate stairs if they exist within the facility. A wheelchair may be used if the patient has the ability to sit upright.

The health care staff must have knowledge of and access to all locations where emergency equipment and supplies are stored to prevent delay in response or transfer of the patient. Correctional officers should also have access to backup supply and can carry it to the scene if directed to by the responding nurse. Figure 16.6 is an example of a form attached to an emergency response plan used to indicate where emergency equipment is located at one of the correctional facilities operated by the Oregon Department of Corrections (2008). It is provided as an example of the number of locations and types of equipment that are maintained for emergency medical response at a typical correctional facility.

MANDOWN KIT LOCATIONS	
1 – Minimum	
1 – Room behind the clinic nurse's desk	
1 – Segregation	
1 – Clinic area Intake Unit A/B	
1 – Medium Medication Room	
OB KIT LOCATIONS	
1 – Minimum	1 – Trauma Room
1 – Room behind the clinic nurse's desk	1 – Gatehouse
1 – Segregation	1 – Special Procedures Room
1 – Clinic area Intake Unit A/B	1 – Medium Medication Room
1 – Medium Medication Room	1 – Infirmary
MEDICATION KIT LOCATIONS	
1 – Minimum	1 – Clinic area Intake Unit A/B
1 – Room behind the clinic nurse's desk	1 – Medium medication room
STRETCHER LOCATIONS	
1 – Minimum Clinic	2 – Medium Trauma Room
WHEELCHAIR LOCATIONS	
2 – Minimum	
1 – Segregation	
5 – Medium Clinic	
AED LOCATIONS	
1 – Medium Clinic Nurse Station	1 – Administration Control Sally Port
1 – Minimum Medication Room	1 – Minimum Control Sally Port
O2 LOCATIONS	
1 – Minimum	1 – Segregation
1 – Room behind the clinic nurse's desk	1 – Clinic area Intake Unit A/B
DISASTER KIT LOCATIONS	
1 – Minimum	1 – Gatehouse
1 – Room behind the clinic nurse's desk	1 – Records building
1 – Clinic area Intake A/B	

FIGURE 16.6   Example of emergency equipment locations at a 1692-bed women's correctional facility.

Adapted from Oregon Department of Corrections (2008). Used with permission.

Large-Scale Response

The equipment and supplies for a large-scale emergency at a correctional facility are different than a standard emergency response, so simply increasing the amount is not necessarily sufficient. Establishing the equipment and supplies needed to respond to requirements to handle future large-scale emergencies should be based upon review of previous events. Since large-scale events at any one correctional facility are for the most part infrequent, planning for these is often accomplished by reviewing the experience of other facilities. This material can be obtained from the library or via one of many trainings and technical assistance offered by the NIC.

Common injuries and conditions that should be anticipated in a large-scale event include but are not limited to lacerations, burns, smoke inhalation, sprains/strains and fractures, chest pain related to anxiety, cardiac and muscle injury, gunshot wounds, stabbings, and impaled objects. Provision of emergency care to both staff and the inmates must be considered when determining amount and variety of supply needs. The ability to obtain additional supplies and equipment should be anticipated, and plans for obtaining and transporting patients should be established prior to need. Figure 16.7 provides an example from the Oregon Department of Corrections of the contents of a standardized disaster bag (Health Services Section Policy and Procedure #P-A-07, 2008).

QTY.	DESCRIPTION	EXP.DATES	QTY.	DESCRIPTION	EXP.DATES
6 ea	CPR Mask Laerdal (white)		1 ea	Eye Irrigation Solution	EXP
2 ea	Cervical Collar		2 ea	Antiseptic Scrub 4% 8oz	EXP
1 ea	Ambu bag		5 ea	N/S IV Fluids 500 ML	EXP
20 ea	Alcohol prep pads		4 ea	Xeroform (Burn dressing)	EXP
12 ea	Antibicrobial Wipes	EXP	1 ea	Burn sheet Sterile	
10 ea	Povidone-Iodine Wipes	EXP	3 ea	Coban 2"	
4 ea	Eye pads Sterile		3 ea	Coban 4"	
12 pkg	Sponge 4x4 Sterile 2/pkg		3 ea	Coban 6"	
1 pkg	Sponge 4x4 Non Sterile		2 ea	Elastic bandage 4"	
1 ea	Kerlix Dressing / Gauze 4"		2 pr	Gloves Sterile 7	
1 ea	Tape Paper 1"		2 pr	Gloves Sterile 8	
1 ea	Tape Cloth 1"		2 pr	Gloves Sterile 9	
1 ea	Tape Cloth 2"		2 bg/10	Gloves non Sterile Sm	
4 ea	IV Tubing W/ inj. Site		2 bg/10	Gloves non Sterile Med	
1 ea	Rescue Blanket		2 bg/10	Gloves non Sterile Lg	
2 ea	Bio-Hazard bags Red		2 bg/10	Gloves non Sterile X Lg	
1 ea	Sharps container Sm BD #305487		1 ea	Air splint arm	
			1 ea	Air splint leg	
	Fanny Pack			***Fanny Pack***	
2 ea	Tourniquets		1 ea	IV Tubing w/Inj Site	
1 ea	Penlight		2 ea	Needle 14g x 1.5" Tan	
1 ea	Flash light w/battery	EXP	2 ea	Needle 18g x 1.5" Green	
1 ea	Bandage scissors		2 ea	Needle 21g x 1.5" Purple	
1 ea	Utility scissors		2 ea	Needle 22g x 1" Blue	
1 ea	Stethoscope		2 ea	Needle 25g x 1" Red	
1 ea	Blood Pressure cuff		1 ea	Scalpels #10 SAFETY	
1 ea	Air way LG		2 ea	Butterfly 23g x 3/4" SAFETY	
1 ea	Air way med		2 ea	IV Cath 18g x 1 3/4" SAFETY	
1 ea	Kelly Forceps		2 ea	IV Cath 20g x 1 3/4" SAFETY	
			2 ea	IV Cath 22g x 1 3/4" SAFETY	
				OUT SIDE OF BAG	
10 ea	Post orders		1 ea	pen	
10 ea	Vests		1 ea	Note pad	
50 ea	Met tags		1 ea	List of Contents	
	Bag Location:_____				
	Expired Contents Checked or Refilled by:_____			**Date refilled/checked:**_____	

FIGURE 16.7   Contents of disaster bag.

Maintaining Readiness

No nurse wants to arrive at an emergency and find there is not enough oxygen in the tank or there are no gloves. In an emergency, no nurse wants to further jeopardize the patient by making a medication error because the epinephrine is where the atropine was supposed to be. Correctional nurses prevent this by monitoring and maintaining emergency equipment and supplies so that they are immediately ready for use.

Every shift, the emergency equipment should be checked to verify that it is available and in proper working order. An entire inventory of the contents of the emergency kit does not need to be completed if the emergency equipment has not been used. Some facilities use a numbered breakaway lock as a way to verify that the material and supply contained within is in the same condition as last inventoried. The date of the first item in the kit to expire should be listed on the outside of the emergency kit and the nurse should replace the outdated item as necessary. Items that will expire in the next few months should be rotated out of the emergency kit so that it can be used in the normal course of care delivery before it outdates. The AED battery, EKG, and oxygen supply should also be checked each shift. The need to check availability and readiness applies to every emergency kit maintained at the facility, not just the equipment and supplies kept in the clinic.

The emergency equipment and supplies should also be restocked after every emergency is resolved and prepared immediately for next use. If this cannot be accomplished at the time, the emergency kit should be removed from the area and a backup put in its place. In no case should nursing staff use an emergency kit multiple times during a shift of duty and not replenish its stock.

Periodically, the entire contents of the emergency kit should be inventoried to ensure that all items are accounted for and stored in the proper location. Many facilities conduct this inventory monthly. Periodic inventory is also recommended as a way for nursing staff to remember where things are kept and how the equipment is used. If only one or a few nurses respond to the majority of emergencies, other nursing staff will not be familiar or used to working with the emergency kit. Having nurses who have not had recent experience with the emergency kit complete the inventory is a way to maintain their knowledge and skill.

CHALLENGES

There are a number of standard challenges during the day-to-day operations of a correctional facility that become more challenging in an emergency or disaster, adding confusion to an already tense environment. The proficient and competent services of both health care and security are vital to a safe outcome in an emergency; this increases the importance of a collaborative and respectful appreciation of the responsibilities of each team member.

Nonurgent Health Care Requests in the Guise of an Emergency

The challenge most correctional staff, including nurses, will bring up first is that emergencies are called that, upon arrival and assessment, are clearly not emergent. An inmate may declare that they are having an emergency for many reasons that are not emergent. It may be lack of knowledge or anxiety, it may be a diversion so staff are distracted from an assault or escape attempt, it may be to observe the response and look for breaks in the system for future use, or it may be boredom or an assurance that assistance will be provided when requested.

Misuse of emergency response is not a problem unique to inmates or correctional facilities. Inappropriate use of ambulance and emergency department services is a problem in the community as well; a recent review of 39 articles published concerning nonurgent patients in the emergency department concluded that a median of 32% of emergency encounters were nonurgent (Durand et al., 2011). In emergency medicine, there is a struggle to reduce nonurgent use of emergency services as a way of managing overcrowded emergency departments and prevent ambulance diversion (Durand et al., 2011; Olshaker, 2009; Vardy, Mansbridge, & Ireland, 2009).

When a nurse responds to an emergency and discovers a nonemergent condition, the nurse has the opportunity to talk with the patient about what constitutes an emergency. This conversation may reveal other concerns about the adequacy or competency of health care provided at the facility. The nurse may be able to clarify important information or follow up on concerns. A word of caution: respond to every emergent call as if it is a life-threatening emergency. Just because a previously reported "emergency" was deemed nonemergent does not mean that the next call will follow suit. Every emergency requires that health care staff assesses the patient and decides what clinical care is medically necessary (Anno, 2001).

Working With Correctional Officers

An effective emergency response begins with an effective team leader. In a normal scenario, the correctional setting is controlled by security staff with regimented schedules, secure doors, and other barriers that control inmate movement. The security staff is trained to take control and command in all situations, and this is true in an emergency as well. If the nurse does not immediately take charge and manage the emergency *medical* response, control of the clinical response will quickly be taken over by security. The responding nurse must determine the type of care, time frames, and the transfer or transport needs of the patient; while the security staff determines the type of restraint, egress from the area and staffing to maintain safety and security. Safety and security remain paramount during medical emergencies.

Correctional officers bring to the team both assets and perhaps liabilities that the nurse should be attentive to in managing the emergency response. Some may have emergency medicine experience and may offer suggestions that could be misinterpreted as telling the nurse how to practice nursing. Some correctional staff may not be as comfortable during emergent situations or in a disaster and are distracted by concerns about their own safety or become hyperaware of their need to provide a secure environment. Nurses should take comments, suggestions, and ideas from team members without internalizing the message as wrongdoing or feeling that they are being chastised by their coworker or peers.

EVALUATION AND IMPROVEMENT

Emergency preparedness includes training and professional development, review of procedures and treatment protocol, practice working with other responding members of staff, and familiarity with the equipment and materials used. The

ACA and NCCHC have set explicit standards for training of health care and correctional staff in emergency response, drills of both small-scale "man-down" emergencies and mass-casualty disasters (ACA, 2002; NCCHC, 2008a, 2008b, 2011). Practicing a variety of scenarios, using established assessment protocols and explicit criteria for response times and methods allows all staff the opportunity to gain experience from one another and learn to work as a team in responding to emergencies. Every emergency response is also an opportunity to learn and improve; this is one of the reasons that every response should be debriefed and critiqued.

Debriefing

A debriefing is normally done within 72 hours of the incident. This gives the individual responder or group of responders the opportunity to talk about their experience, and how it has affected them, and to return to regular duty and operation as soon as possible. Principles used in debriefing emergency and disaster response include

- Ensure a supportive learning environment.
- Encourage attention to teamwork processes.
- Ensure that team members feel comfortable during debriefs.
- Focus on a few critical performance issues during the debriefing process.
- Describe specific teamwork interactions and processes that were involved in the team's performance.
- Support feedback with objective indicators of performance.
- Provide feedback on process measures first and more thoroughly; feedback on outcome comes last.
- Provide both individual and team-oriented feedback, but know when each is most appropriate.
- Record conclusions made and goals set during the debriefing to facilitate feedback during future debriefings (Salas et al., 2008).

Incident Review

An incident review is a recap of what happened during the emergency situation as a whole and not necessarily each individual response to the event. The review is a basis for improvement, future planning, and training opportunities. Once the health care program has completed an incident review, a corrective action report should be created. The action plan should address each of the following points for each issue identified for correction:

- The identified action to correct the issue or deficiency
- The responsible person or group of people to implement the action
- The due date for completion of the action
- The resulting corrective action that should be incorporated into plans and procedures once completed (FEMA, 2006).

SUMMARY

The correctional nurse has a responsibility to respond to medical emergencies of all types and scope. The nurse also has a responsibility to provide competent, responsive nursing care in an emergency. Emergency response requires knowledge, skill, and ability to assess and apply clinical interventions in the "field" according to established criteria and protocols. Correctional nurses must be trained and competent in the delivery of emergency care. Case Example 16.1 provides an opportunity to review and apply the material from this chapter.

CASE EXAMPLE 16.1

An emergency call is received by the clinic nurse on Sunday evening at 5:35 pm from the Intensive Management Unit. The officers report that the inmate has not eaten his dinner and is unresponsive. The nurse arrives on the unit and at the cell calls the inmate by name, bangs on the door, and raises her voice calling his name out. The inmate does not respond. He is lying on his side on the bunk, facing away from the door. The nurse knows the inmate takes medication for depression and hypertension. She informs the officers to open the door so she can examine the inmate. At 5:45 pm, staff enters the cell. When the inmate is turned over there is dried blood around his nose and mouth and on the front of his shirt. He is breathing on his own but not responsive to verbal commands. Vital signs are T: 98, P: 76 carotid, thready, BP: 90/57, O_2: 80%.

Discussion Questions:

1. Identify within this description when the scene survey, primary assessment, and secondary assessment were completed.
2. As a responder with BLS training, what are the next immediate steps you will take?
3. In debriefing this response, what processes might be considered for improvement?

DISCUSSION QUESTIONS

1. In an emergency at your facility, what triage categories do nurses use to communicate the patient's priority and urgency for treatment
2. What aspect of emergency response are you most comfortable with? What aspect are you least comfortable with? What steps can you take to increase your comfort in this area of emergency response?
3. Are the supplies and equipment at your facility adequate to effectively respond to a medical emergency? Are they adequate for a mass-casualty situation? What is the basis for your opinion?
4. Multiple patients reported to sick call with GI complaints. This may be the beginning of a facility-wide epidemic, or diversion to escape or riot. Identify the stakeholders that need to be notified and who you will contact for assistance.

REFERENCES

American Correctional Association. (2002). *Performance based standards for correctional health care in adult correctional institutions.* Alexandria, VA: Author.

American Nurses Association. (2007). *Corrections nursing: Scope & standards of practice.* Silver Spring, MD: Author.

Anno, B. (2001). *Health care delivery system model*. Chicago: National Commission on Correctional Health Care.

Durand, A., Gentile, S., Devictor, B., Palazzolo, S., Vignally, P., Gerbaux, P. et al. (2011). ED patients: How nonurgent are they? Systematic review of the emergency medicine literature. *The American Journal of Emergency Medicine, 29*, 333–345.

Federal Emergency Management Agency (FEMA). (2006, September 12). *NIMS implementation activities for hospitals and healthcare systems implementation*. Retrieved January 5, 2012, from http://www.fema.gov/pdf/emergency/nims/imp_hos.pdf

Laffan, S. (2010, February 9). Medical emergencies. *Correctional Nursing Today*. (L. Schoenly, Interviewer).

National Commission on Correctional Health Care (NCCHC). (2008a). *Standards for health services in prisons*. Chicago, IL: Author.

National Commission on Correctional Health Care (NCCHC). (2008b). *Standards for health services in jails*. Chicago, IL: Author.

National Commission on Correctional Health Care (NCCHC). (2011). *Standards for health services in juvenile detention and confinement facilities*. Chicago, IL: Author.

Olshaker, J. (2009). Managing emergency department overcrowding. *Emergency Medicine Clinics of North America, 27*, 593–603.

Oregon Department of Corrections. (2008, October). *Health services section policy and procedure #P-A-07*. Retrieved January 5, 2012, from Oregon Department of Corrections: http://www.oregon.gov/DOC/OPS/HESVC/docs/policies_procedures/Section_A/PA07.pdf

Oregon Department of Corrections, Health Services. (n.d.). *Nursing treatment protocols, emergency protocols*. Retrieved January 5, 2012, from Oregon Department of Corrections: http://www.oregon.gov/DOC/OPS/HESVC/protocol.shtml

Rold, W. (2006). Legal considerations in the delivery of health care services in prisons and jails. In M. E. Puisis (Ed.), *Clinical practice in correctional medicine* (pp. 520–528). Philadelphia: Elsevier.

Safecom Program. (2009, October). *Tools supporting communications interoperability aligned to National Emergency Commuinications (NECP) initiatives*. Retrieved January 5, 2012, from Homeland Security: http://www.safecomprogram.gov/library/Lists/Library/DispForm.aspx?ID=271

Salas, E., Klein, C., King, H., Salisbury, M., Augenstein, J. S., Bimbach, D. J. et al. (2008, September). Debriefing medical teams: 12 evidence-based best practices and tips. *The Joint Commission Journal on Quality and Patient Safety, 34/9*, 518–527.

Schwartz, J., & Barry, C. (2009). *A guide to preparing for and responding to jail emergencies: Self-audit checklists, resource materials, case studies*. Washington, DC: U.S. Department of Justice, National Institute of Corrections.

Vardy, J., Mansbridge, C., & Ireland, A. (2009, March). Are emergency department staff's perceptions about the inappropriate use of ambulances, alcohol intoxification, verbal abuse, and violance accurate? *Emergency Medicine Journal, 26*(3), 164–168.

SEVENTEEN

Management and Leadership

Lorry Schoenly

B asic management and leadership skills are necessary for nurses in all levels of the organization. Correctional nurses practice in settings which may have few leadership positions or in large facilities with an organized nursing structure similar to a hospital setting. Providing health care in a secure setting involves collaboration within the health care team as well as with corrections staff. Conflict resolution skills can be particularly helpful. Correctional nurses may be called upon to supervise other health care staff, volunteers, or inmate workers. Correctional nurses working as health services administrators, directors of nursing, shift supervisors, or charge nurses also need an understanding of organizational change principles.

DEFINING AND DIFFERENTIATING LEADERSHIP AND MANAGEMENT
Leadership

Leadership is a key standard of correctional nursing practice as defined by the American Nurses Association (2007). This leadership is expected, not only in the practice setting, but also within the profession. Nurses use leadership skills at all levels in an organization. Leadership principles are used by staff nurses to motivate team members to meet positive patient goals. Charge nurses lead shifts of staff to accomplish care processes efficiently. Nurse directors and administrators use leadership concepts to encourage support for health care outcomes at warden meetings.

Kouzes and Posner (2007) extensively researched transforming leaders and discovered five key leadership practices (Table 17.1). These practices can provide guidance for nurses to improve their leadership abilities. By role modeling desirable behaviors and inspiring a shared vision, nurse managers can lead staff by example. In addition, staff nurses need encouragement to challenge the status quo and

From the Experts ...

"I have observed nurses in the correctional setting go through rapid professional and personal growth. As a result, management skills are most important in the selection of staff. The nurse must function as leader/caregiver; training and managing nursing and correctional staff, while caring for a difficult, needy, and underserved patient population. In addition to managing others, the correctional nurse is in a vulnerable position and must manage the "need to be needed" that sometimes drives nurses. I have found that there is a fine line to be walked, and that in order to be successful the correctional provider of care must be able to manage on many levels: self, other staff, correctional personnel, and, most importantly, the patients that they serve. This is not easy for many nurses, but those who endure and grow with the field, and who continuously hone their management ability, have the most success in this growing specialty."

Johnnie R. Lambert, RN, CLNC, CCHP, LHRM
Miami, FL

advocate for improvements in the health care system. Nurse managers are in an ideal position to enable others to act on behalf of patients. In a system that can be harsh or uncaring, correctional nurse leaders have an opportunity to encourage and recognize true acts of compassion. Put into practice, these five leadership practices can positively affect correctional nursing practice.

Management

Management is also an important skill for correctional nurses. Management and leadership are often paired and differentiated as if nurses must choose which "camp" they will advocate. However, today's nurses must have both leadership and management skills to successfully navigate patients safely through the complex health care

TABLE 17.1   Key Leadership Practices

PRACTICE	DESCRIPTION
Model the way	Effectively model behaviors desired in other team members
Inspire a shared vision	Create a vision of the future that engages the entire team and inspires all to participate in making it happen
Challenge the process	Taking the risk to create positive change by establishing a climate for change and encouraging experimentation
Enable others to act	Enabling change through fostering collaboration and building trust
Encourage the heart	Genuine acts of compassion and encouragement, including recognizing contributions and celebrating victories

Source: Adapted from Kouzes and Posner (2007).

From the Experts . . .

"Health care managers in corrections must possess all the skills of a manager in any health care facility, but with much more finesse, creativity, and critical thinking."

JoRene Kerns, BSN, RN, CCHP
Nashville, TN

system. Management has been described as controlling (Owen, 1990), however, the control is most effectively focused on systems, processes, and environments of care. Other important areas of control include controlling costs and resource utilization including health care staff. By successfully managing the mechanisms of care delivery, nurses are freed to creatively solve patient problems and deliver effective patient care.

The correctional health care delivery system is composed of a variety of simple to complex processes that require management attention. "Effective management depends on knowing, adhering to, and improving processes for efficiency and effectiveness." (Bleich, 2011, p. 18). Nine key management tasks have been proposed to guide nurses in a management role (Exhibit 17.1).

The hustle and bustle of a busy unit may look chaotic and unorganized. Invisible systems and processes are at work in the midst of the activity. Nurses must

EXHIBIT 17.1
Bleich's Tasks of Management

1. Identify systems and processes that require responsibility and accountability, and specify who owns the process.
2. Verify minimum and optimum standards/specifications, and identify roles and individuals responsible to adhere to them.
3. Validate the knowledge, skills, and abilities of available staff engaged in the process; capitalize on strengths; and strengthen areas in need of development.
4. Devise and communicate a comprehensive 'big picture' plan for the division of work, honoring the complexity and variety of assignments made at an individual level.
5. Eliminate barriers/obstacles to work effectiveness.
6. Measure the equity of workload, and use data to support judgments about efficiency and effectiveness. Offer rewards and recognition to individuals and teams.
7. Recommend ways to improve systems and processes.
8. Use a social network to engage others in decision making and for feedback, when appropriate or relevant.

Source: From Bleich (2011 Box 1–3, p. 19), used with permission.

understand the full continuum of each process and how they work together as a system of care in order to effectively manage care delivery. Those in a management role must also assure that each element of a care process is understood as a responsibility of staff members. Correctional nurse managers can create post duty lists that identify the specific responsibilities of a staff member on a particular shift and day of the week. For example, a day shift registered nurse may be assigned to perform sick call. The post duties for day shift sick call may also include transcribing orders and reviewing transfer charts. A written list of duties for each staff role on each shift assists in clarifying accountability and responsibility. Nursing management also involves establishing written policies and procedures to guide care delivery. Policies can be based on the best practices provided by accrediting bodies and current nursing literature. Policies also improve the transparency of the care delivery system and assist new staff in quickly acquiring the systems knowledge to function effectively (Croll, 2008). When creating policies, reference the best practice in writing on the policy to assist when reviewed or revised.

Effective management also involves systems for recruiting, orienting, and developing the abilities of staff members. Efforts to make visible systems and processes can speed new staff on-boarding and standardize care delivery. In addition, practical job descriptions allow for clarity of roles and act as an effective recruitment and evaluation tool for ongoing staff development (Price, 2008).

Post duties, policies, and orientation programs assist nurses in managing care delivery in a health care unit. Nurse managers can use these tools to help team members understand the big picture of care delivery and their role in delivering that care. With this big picture in mind, staff members can play a part in the management of health care by providing continuous feedback on system operations. Nurse managers create this feedback loop by establishing a social network among staff members where positive change is encouraged and recommendations sought (Bleich, 2011). Manager–staff communication is vital to an effective clinical system.

Another important concept of managing nursing care is eliminating barriers and obstacles to effective practice. Nurse managers have a position in the organizational structure that allows for negotiation among other entities to reduce obstacles staff members may be facing in accomplishing care delivery. For example, changes in other service delivery in the facility may hamper effectiveness of a clinical process. Or, staff reporting through another organizational leader may not be fulfilling responsibilities of their job description which affect timeliness of care delivery.

Finally, nurse managers have the ability to monitor workload equity among staff members and make alterations to improve efficiency and effectiveness of the health care program. In addition, monitoring and acting on workload inequities improves staff satisfaction and decreases friction among team members. By attending to the various tasks of management, nurses can make a difference for staff and patients alike.

SUPERVISING OTHERS

Many correctional nurses supervise others in their daily activities. Understanding basic supervisory principles can reduce conflict and improve team efforts toward care delivery. Nurses working in defined management positions such as Nurse Executives, Chief Nursing Officers, Directors of Nursing and Administrators must also understand human resource principles and labor law to manage employees.

For example, recruiting and interviewing new staff members must be accomplished within the boundaries of equal opportunity and disability legal aspects.

Charge nurses and shift supervisors have time-determined supervisory roles with responsibility to effectively accomplish shift processes by engaging the resources and staff available for the time period. Nurse managers and unit administrators have additional responsibilities for determining adequate staffing and scheduling. Nurses in formal management roles also have responsibilities for selecting, developing, and evaluating staff.

Staff Members

When supervising other staff members, it is important to have both the big picture and the individual experience in mind. With the patient as the central focus, nurses supervise others to accomplish necessary care processes efficiently. Supervising others requires skill in communicating and engaging others in the goal of care. Unhelpful clinical and interpersonal behaviors by staff under supervision must be addressed quickly to avoid derailing clinical goals (Cully, 2008). Delegation skills and effective conflict resolution principles are discussed later in the chapter.

Nurses supervising other care providers may need to reevaluate and reassign responsibilities when care factors change. Patient and staff emergencies may require workload shifting and reprioritizing of care goals. Those supervising others have a responsibility to remain in contact with team members to guide activities and change priorities in real time. Correctional nursing care delivery is rarely accomplished in an ideal setting with ideal staffing. Continuous evaluation and reevaluation of progress toward short- and long-term patient care goals helps to maximize goal accomplishment.

Volunteers

Some correctional health care units may have community volunteers involved in care tasks. Connecting inmates with community health services can assist with successful reentry following release. Community volunteers should have a thorough orientation to facility safety procedures. As with other unlicensed individuals in the care area, nurses must be careful to limit delegation to nonnursing functions after competency evaluation. Volunteers may provide clerical and coordination assistance such as assembling charts or creating rosters.

Inmate Workers

Although a more ideal situation is for security staff to supervise inmate workers, correctional nurses may have regular contact with inmates working as porters or other service positions in the institution. Be sure to understand and follow any facility policies about interaction with inmate workers. Care should be taken to be aware of inmate activity in the health care unit to maintain patient confidentiality and staff safety. Consider patient privacy when giving tasks to inmate workers, as confidentiality must be continuously protected. For example, all patient record information should be shredded by health care staff before inmate workers dispose of papers. Inmate workers should be regularly rotated out of positions in the unit, as familiarity with staff and medical schedules can prove a security risk.

Delegation Principles

As a licensed health care professional, nurses have a legal as well as ethical responsibility to appropriately delegate tasks within the health care team. The National Council of State Boards of Nursing (NCSBN) and the American Nurses Association (ANA) publish guidelines to assist nurses in making safe delegation decisions (ANA, NCSBN, 2006). These guidelines are supported by nursing boards in various states and are often used as a basis for further state-level interpretation. Correctional nurses are encouraged to seek specific state application of these national guidelines.

Although tasks and components of the nursing process may be delegated to unlicensed staff, the assessment, planning, and evaluation of care is always the responsibility of the registered nurse, who remains accountable for the outcome (ANA, NCSBN, 2006). Indeed, professional nurses retain accountability for the entire nursing process. Not every component of the nursing process is appropriate for delegation. Observations by others can be considered in a nursing assessment, and particular interventions of the plan of care can be delegated (Table 17.2).

Care should be taken in the delegation process to evaluate various components of the situation to determine appropriateness. Nurses must consider their scope of practice, their own authority to delegate, and the qualifications of the staff member to which they are delegating a task or component of nursing care (NCSBN, n.d.). Although an employer may structure the care team on a shift to take into consideration the delegation of set functions to unlicensed staff, licensed nurses are still responsible to evaluate the context of the current nursing needs and staff competency before each delegation episode.

Nurses must consider several areas when delegating to other staff members. "The RN assigns or delegates tasks based on the needs and condition of the patient, potential for harm, stability of the patient's condition, complexity of the task, predictability of the outcome, and abilities of the staff to whom the task is delegated" (ANA, NCSBN, 2006, p. 2.). The overarching concern of delegation decisions is the health and safety of the patient (ANA, 2005).

The five rights of delegation can be used as a framework for delegation decisions (NCSBN, n.d.). By considering the task, circumstances, person, communication, and supervision in a delegation situation, correctional nurses can make sound judgments about the appropriateness for delegating (Table 17.3). The correctional setting has contextual issues that affect delegation decisions. When health care is delivered at

TABLE 17.2   Elements of the Nursing Process Appropriate for Delegation

NURSING PROCESS ELEMENT	APPROPRIATENESS FOR DELEGATION
Assessment	No, input can be solicited
Planning	No, input can be solicited
Intervention	Yes, with supervision
Evaluation	No, input can be solicited

Source: Adapted from ANA (2005).

TABLE 17.3 Five Rights of Delegation

DELEGATION CONSIDERATION	DESCRIPTION
Right task	One that is delegable for a specific patient
Right circumstances	Appropriate patient setting, available resources, and other relevant factors considered
Right person	Right person is delegating the right task to the right person to be performed on the right person
Right direction/communication	Clear, concise description of the task, including its objective, limits, and expectations
Right supervision	Appropriate monitoring, evaluation, intervention, as needed, and feedback

Source: Adapted from NCSBN (1997).

several sites within a facility, nurses may be asked to delegate to staff members in a different location. In these situations, the availability of resources and the competency of the staff member to know when there is need for higher-level evaluation become particular concerns.

Clear communication is of utmost importance when delegating nursing functions. Ambiguity and assumption have no place in the delegation process. Communication of delegated expectations should include direction for when the delegating nurse should be contacted for assistance, what information to report and record, and any specific patient concerns. Have the staff member affirm understanding by communicating back the delegated assignment. This will confirm full communication of expectations (ANA, NCSBN, 2006).

The delegation process has not concluded once a delegation assignment is made. Professional nurses retain accountability for care provided and therefore need to monitor the delegated tasks. Evaluation of care provided is also necessary. While the purpose of evaluation is to measure the patient's status in relation to the goals for care, the nurse also is attending to how well the staff member performed the delegated task. The nurse uses this evaluation of staff performance to provide feedback, coach, and suggest additional training in the interest of improving the staff member's ability to provide patient care. Elements to consider in the evaluation process include level of outcomes achieved, communication effectiveness, concerns to be addressed, and any need for staff skill development (ANA, NCSBN, 2006). Case Example 17.1 provides opportunity to apply delegation principles.

CASE EXAMPLE 17.1

The charge nurse during an evening shift at a large state penitentiary is making delegation assignments for the shift. He is working with another RN, an LPN, and two nursing assistants certified to pass medications. There is a 2-hour medication pass on this shift and an evening sick call. In addition, they have four patients in the six-bed infirmary and two inmates on suicide watch. Using the delegation principles from this chapter, discuss considerations the charge nurse should make when determining staff assignments. Suggest an assignment plan based on this information and your understanding of possible other post duties for the evening (e.g., emergency response, order transcription, shift reports).

Scope of Practice Issues

Licensed health care professionals are governed by legal statutes regarding the boundaries of the care that can be provided. Nurses in supervisory positions must have a clear understanding of the scope of their own practice and the practice of others on the health care team. Scope of practice is governed by the jurisdiction of the licensure, usually the state. Practice in a correctional setting can be complicated by a lack of understanding on the part of correctional authorities of the legal scope of practice issues. Nurses may be asked to practice outside the bounds of licensure. It is important for correctional nurses to communicate scope of practice concerns when they arise. For example, a correctional nurse might be expected to intervene and make diagnostic decisions without a medical professional present. Processes should be in place for accessing a medical professional when needed to determine care and treatment. This may involve transport to an acute care facility or contacting a physician or nurse practitioner who is on-call for consultation.

Nurses enjoy an expanded level of autonomy in the correctional setting and are often the first health care staff member to see an inmate for a medical condition. Self-evaluation of competency to perform nursing care is also important for ethical and legal practice. Nurses are responsible to maintain competence to practice at the level of expectation for their position and seek out education where needed. A clear understanding and communication of legal licensure boundaries can reduce the potential for patient harm.

BEST PRACTICES IN HEALTH CARE MANAGEMENT

Correctional nurse managers can find best practice information to model health care processes and standards from several sources. The National Commission on Correctional Health Care (NCCHC) and the American Correctional Association (ACA) publish standards of practice that have been shown to support quality patient outcomes in corrections. In addition, some accreditation standards from traditional settings such as the Joint Commission standards have application to a correctional setting. Discovering best practices is discussed in Chapter 18.

American Correctional Association (ACA)

The ACA accreditation program is a voluntary accreditation process evaluating the entire service delivery of a correctional facility. Eighty percent of U.S. correctional facilities are involved in ACA accreditation (ACA, n.d.). Specific health care standards were developed in 1989. These standards evaluate key components of inmate health care delivery, including systems, processes, and staff credentialing (ACA, 2002, 2010). ACA standards are revised annually and both the basic manual and latest standards supplement should be reviewed to determine current practice requirements.

National Commission on Correctional Health Care (NCCHC)

NCCHC standards are widely recognized as a basis for effective health service delivery in the correctional setting. This association emerged from the American Medical Association's work to improve prison health care in the late 1970s. Standards are published for prisons, jails, and juvenile facilities (NCCHC, 2008a, 2008b, 2011) and cover the health care processes of care and treatment, health records, administration, personnel, and medical–legal issues. NCCHC suggests that correctional health care systems guided by their standards "help facilities improve the health of inmates, staff, and the communities to which inmates return; increase the efficiency of their health services delivery; strengthen their organizational effectiveness; and reduce their risk of adverse legal judgments" (p. 1) (NCCHC, n.d.). Although a facility may not choose to seek accreditation through NCCHC, the standards provide a guide to best practices in correctional health care and can be used to create systems and processes in all key areas of health care delivery.

The Joint Commission (TJC)

The health care programs operated by Federal Bureau of Prisons (FBOP) have been accredited under the ambulatory health care standards of TJC (FBOP, 2005). TJC standards, provide very applicable best practices for correctional units and should be considered as a guide for practice. For example, TJC National Patient Safety Goals (NPSGs) provide the basis for a solid patient safety program in the correctional setting and are discussed in greater detail in Chapter 4, Safety for the Nurse and the Patient.

COLLECTIVE BARGAINING IN HEALTH CARE

Collective bargaining units, also called unions, have been declining steadily in the U.S. workforce but have been increasing in health care (Malvey, 2010a). Collective bargaining units represent the interests of employees to management regarding the terms and conditions of work, such as wages and hours of work (Gromley, 2011). Many reasons have been cited for increased union activity among nursing groups (Exhibit 17.2). Nurses may turn to unionization when they feel powerless to make positive change or to eliminate risk in their work environment.

Unions allow employees to negotiate workplace issues with management and have been successful in increasing job satisfaction regarding wages. However, nonbargaining unit nurses were found to have greater satisfaction with the image of nursing, professional relationships, and patient care in a comparison study among unionized and nonunionized nurses (Pittman, 2007). Regardless the environment, unionized or nonunionized, nurse managers must work together with staff members to accomplish patient care.

Relationship building among management and staff is an important component of good management. Nurses resort to unionization when they feel disconnected

---

EXHIBIT 17.2
Issues Leading to Increased Union Activity

- Lack of professional autonomy and professional practice models
- Inadequate staffing and unqualified caregivers
- The absence of procedures for the reporting of unsafe work environments and poor quality care
- Mandatory overtime and work overload
- Low wages and poor benefits

Source: Adapted from Gromley (2011).

from organizational management and perceive that they have no voice in the way their work is structured (Malvey, 2010b). Clear and consistent communication is needed to engage staff appropriately.

Fairness of treatment is another major management issue that can affect staff nurse desire to unionize. Nurse managers, of course, should always treat staff members fairly in employment dealings. However, much of fair employee treatment is invisible at the staff level. Nurses in management who make visible the equity principles used in dealing with staff matters communicate a strong message to employees.

Perceived lack of involvement in decision making has been cited as a cause of unionization among nurses (Gromley, 2011). Recently devised and supported participatory management structures such as shared governance involve staff in decision-making and accountability as an alternative to the need for collective bargaining. Participatory management structures have been linked to improved clinical outcomes, as well. Involvement of staff in management decision-making processes has been linked to decreased medication errors and increased customer service indicators in addition to reduced staff turnover and burnout (Angermeier, Dunford, Boss, & Boss, 2009).

Correctional nurses can effectively manage in unionized and nonunionized environments by applying principles of open communication, fair staff treatment, and shared decision making. Professional nurses ultimately desire work environments that allow safe and effective patient care (Gromley, 2011). Applying modern principles of participatory management in the correctional setting can improve nurse manager effectiveness.

COLLABORATION TO ACCOMPLISH GOALS

The complexity of health care delivery in any setting, including corrections, requires a team of care providers. Healthy collaboration among care team members and with correctional peers is required to successfully navigate a patient through the system and accomplish a positive health outcome. The ANA confirms the importance of collaboration to correctional nursing practice and identifies the responsibility of nurses to collaborate with patient, family, health care providers, and corrections staff (ANA, 2007).

Fostering Collaborative Relationships

Providing effective correctional health care requires strong collaborative relationships among care providers, corrections staff, the patient, and sometimes even family members. Effective collaboration requires truthfulness, directness of communication, and the willingness to listen to the point of view of others (Stalbaum & Valadez, 2011). Merely communicating information to another care provider or security staff does not constitute collaboration. Communication imparts information while collaboration consists of cooperative involvement and shared decision-making to create and implement patient care (O'Daniel & Rosenstein, 2008). Therefore, collaboration is a component of effective teamwork and critical to meeting patient goals.

Collaboration among members of the care team allows for a coordinated plan of care with integrated actions and goals. All members of the care team know and understand the interventions of others as well as how their actions affect progression to the goal. A cohesive team approach through collaborative efforts also provides a united front to the patient, adding confidence and lessening frustration (O'Daniel & Rosenstein, 2008).

Care team collaboration extends to the specialty consults and outside services required for care delivery in a correctional setting. Nurses can more effectively manage care outcomes when relationships are built with off-site medical specialty offices, emergency services, and outpatient surgical units. Manager-to-manager relationships across these services improve the collaborative interface and flow of information.

Correctional nurses have the added responsibility to collaborate with correctional staff in order to meet patient goals. Security officers become a part of care delivery as they monitor inmate movement and escort inmates outside the security perimeter. In addition, housing officers must initiate emergency treatment and may monitor inmates with chronic illness in the living quarters for symptoms that need to be brought to the attention of nursing staff. Additional challenges exist in collaborating with custody staff. Correctional nurses and corrections professionals can have differing priorities and goals in inmate management. Relationship development and open lines of communication are of particular importance here for successful outcomes.

Many barriers exist to effective collaboration (Exhibit 17.3). Nurses in management roles have opportunity to reduce these barriers and improve the collaborative environment. When blocks to collaboration are noted, a review of possible barriers may help in resolving conflict.

Conflict Resolution

Conflict is merely the presence of differences (Porter-O'Grady & Malloch, 2011). Although it is desirable to avoid conflict, it is present in any work setting. Indeed, conflict can be detrimental, but discussion and resolution of conflicting views can be a catalyst for necessary change and can lead to the generation of creative options

---

EXHIBIT 17.3
Common Barriers to Interprofessional Communication and Collaboration

- Personal values and expectations
- Personality differences
- Hierarchy
- Disruptive behavior
- Culture and ethnicity
- Generational differences
- Gender
- Historical interprofessional and intraprofessional rivalries
- Differences in language and jargon
- Differences in schedules and professional routines
- Varying levels of preparation, qualifications, and status
- Differences in requirements, regulations, and norms of professional education
- Fears of diluting professional identity
- Differences in accountability, payment, and rewards
- Concerns regarding clinical responsibility
- Complexity of care
- Emphasis on rapid decision making

Source: From O'Daniel and Rosenstein (2008, p. 4), used with permission.

(Folse, 2011). In addition, conflict can actually deepen and develop relationships in the care team. Therefore, conflict can produce personal and professional growth (Sportsman, 2007). Positive conflict resolution in the correctional health care setting is important for effective care provision and team cohesion.

TABLE 17.4   Conflict Management Styles

STYLE	COMPETITIVE STANCE	DESCRIPTION	POSITIVE USES
Avoiding	Lose-lose	• Withdrawing rather than dealing with disagreement • Postponing conflict leading to escalation of friction	• To await a better time or place for dealing with the conflict • To allow for personal reflection when immediate resolution is unnecessary
Accommodating	Lose-win	• Unassertive cooperation or capitulation to another • Self-sacrificing obedience	• When personal reflection indicates the other's option is understandable, although not ideal • If the issue is more important to the other individual • To preserve harmony when this is more important than conflicting issue
Competing	Win-lose	• Pursuing personal needs at the expense of others. • Use of cruelty, manipulation, or aggression to reach goal	• When speed is needed in an emergency decision • To right a wrong • If an unpopular decision must be made by leadership
Compromising	No win-no lose	• Each party relinquishes something in the resolution • Each side is appeased but neither totally wins	• Both sides are powerful and have mutually exclusive goals • Time pressures require an expedited resolution • If collaboration fails
Collaborating	Win-win	• More time-consuming problem solving approach requiring cooperative analysis of issues and goals • Collective decision making taking into account important issues from all perspectives	• Time available to creatively merge differing viewpoints • High need for significant and long-lasting resolution of differences

Source: Adapted from Folse (2011) and Sportsman (2007).

An understanding of personal preferred conflict management style is helpful in developing skills in resolving conflict. Table 17.4 reviews common conflict management stances. Each style can be effective when used in an appropriate context. Therefore, it is most desirable to actively evaluate each conflict and intentionally apply a particular management style.

A collaborative management style is most frequently the style of choice for positive conflict resolution, as it results in the greatest benefit to all and preserves relationship among the conflict participants (Sportsman, 2007). However, nurses most often use a compromising style of conflict resolution while unlicensed and allied health staff are more likely to avoid conflict (Sportsman & Hamilton, 2007). Developing skill in collaborative conflict resolution is necessary for the satisfying resolution of personal and clinical conflict in the correctional setting.

Collaborative conflict resolution uses problem-solving principles to engage the conflicting parties in the resolution process. A collaborative framework starts with acknowledgement that all parties have both diverse and common interests that need to be considered. Both common and competing interests are explored and understood by all participants. Important during this phase is the establishment and maintenance of trust and communication among all parties to the conflict (Porter-O'Grady & Malloch, 2011). This can be extremely challenging but crucial to an effective and sustainable outcome.

Once full understanding is reached, participants move to gathering and analyzing data to determine the best solutions to the conflict. This information is used to creatively generate possible solutions. Many solution-generating techniques are available such as brainstorming and root cause analysis structures like a fish-bone diagram (Welch, 2011). It is important for all participants to maintain an open-minded, resolution-focused perspective during this phase of the process.

Once a solution that honors the concerns of all participants is selected, implementation is planned. This phase of conflict resolution may be very short or take a considerable amount of effort, depending on the initial conflict. As with any implementation, an evaluation of the outcome is then initiated with any ensuing changes based on evaluation results (Welch, 2011).

PROFESSIONAL DEVELOPMENT

A hallmark of professional practice is the continuing need to maintain and improve knowledge, skills, and abilities. Correctional nursing practice is ever evolving and there is need to revise practice using the newest information and evidence-based findings.

A professional staff development program provides educational experiences during initial entry into a position and continues through ongoing renewal and refreshment of basic practice information. Learning experiences are also needed whenever there is a change in practice or a change in roles within the care team. Education is important whenever a gap in knowledge is revealed, such as when clinical errors emerge or a performance evaluation indicates deficiencies. In addition, health care accrediting bodies have annual staff education requirements. NCCHC requires 12 hours of continuing education for each staff member, while ACA requires 40 hours of training (ACA, 2010; NCCHC, 2008a, 2008b). Several components make up an effective clinical unit professional development program.

Orientation

New staff are introduced to the organization's mission, policies, procedures, and their role expectations during an orientation process (ANCC, 2009). In addition, orientation allows the new staff member to meet the rest of the care team and learn the work environment. In correctional practice, this includes an understanding of security services and the communication processes among custody, service, and health care staff.

A well-organized orientation program speeds the acclimation of new staff and prevents early turnover (Twedell, 2011). A comprehensive plan includes all elements of the job description, clinical processes, policies and procedures, and applicable regulations. Although this will involve reading material, a skill-based clinical orientation is vital. New staff members should have an opportunity to have a protected time of performing all areas of the job description before placed into the staffing mix.

Preceptorships are a popular and successful method for staff orientation. Preceptors are experienced staff who guide the new staff member through the various learning experiences necessary to assimilate into the role (Moore, 2008). When possible, preceptors should obtain additional training in clinical teaching and voluntarily assume the role.

Competency Evaluation

An important component of a professional development plan is evaluation and improvement of staff competence. Competency is "the application of knowledge, skills, and behaviors that are needed to fulfill organizational, departmental, and work setting requirements under the varied circumstances of the real world" (Wright, 2005, p. 8). Competence evaluation can serve many purposes (Exhibit 17.4) and should be an ongoing process. Competency evaluation begins during the hiring process and continues throughout employment.

The most frequently used method for competency evaluation is a skills checklist (Kowalski, 2011). Care should be given to the selection of skills to be evaluated. The most important skills for effective and safe patient care should be prioritized. Too much detail in a competency evaluation can make the process cumbersome, time-consuming, and ineffective. The position description and post duties should be considered in determining a competency evaluation checklist. Priority safety skills such as cardiopulmonary resuscitation, responding to emergencies, intravenous administration, and wound management can be considered (Harman, 2007). In addition, an initial competency evaluation should be considered any time a new procedure or piece of equipment is introduced into the care setting.

EXHIBIT 17.4
Purposes of Competency Evaluation

- Evaluate individual performance
- Evaluate group performance
- Meet standards set by a regulatory agency
- Address problematic issues within the organization
- Enhance or replace performance review

Source: Adapted from Wright (2005).

Although creating a skills checklist for various staff positions is a good start, inserting the competency evaluation process into the nurse manager's pattern of activities can be problematic. Consider ways to incorporate staff competency evaluation into other management structures. Staff competency can be assessed as a part of quality improvement activities, documentation reviews, and as preparation for annual performance evaluations. The nurse manager may increase participation by using self-evaluation and peer evaluation processes.

When staff competence is determined to be below standard, a time-limited written remediation plan is recommended (Kowalski, 2011). Sometimes called a written contract, the plan should include specific remediation steps along with the method of reevaluation.

Inservice Education

Nurses and other staff members have a continuing need for education about policies, procedures, and processes specific to their job duties and description. Inservice education is specific to the performance of assigned functions for a particular agency or institution (ANCC, 2009). Inservice education also includes skill development with treatment equipment. Any new policy or procedure should initiate inservice education activities to assure that all staff members understand their role in the new procedure.

Nurse managers are responsible for providing necessary education for staff members to properly perform their job functions. The need for inservice education can come from performance evaluations, continuous quality improvement reports, mortality and morbidity data, and clinical error reports. It can be helpful to create an annual calendar of inservice activities to guide the planning of educational experiences. Some inservice efforts may be a part of the monthly meeting process. For example, nurse managers may review a particular policy with staff based on some monthly clinical data. Regular inservice topics can come from seasonal needs, such as treatment of heat-related injury in summer or infectious disease protocols during influenza season.

Inservice materials can come from many sources and in flexible formats. Managers can acquire videos from pharmaceutical and equipment companies. Many educational resources are available for download from the Internet. Even when Internet access is limited onsite, materials can be printed for use in a self-study format. Senior staff can be asked to provide simple policy overviews or demonstrate rarely used skills during staff sessions. Members of other units can be asked to address staff about important elements of care provision such as the mental health staff reviewing the concepts of suicide risk.

Continuing Education

Unlike inservice education, which is specific to the performance of a role within an organization, continuing education focuses on professional knowledge, skills, and attitudes necessary for general nursing practice (ANCC, 2009). Continuing education experiences build on basic licensure education and can be applied broadly to many work settings. For example, a program on nursing ethics can be applied in a current work setting as well as future professional endeavors.

Many state boards of nursing require nursing continuing education credits for relicensure. Nurses certified in a specialty practice may also need continuing education credits to maintain certification. Nursing continuing education is measured in hours and can include fractions of hours. The national standard in the United States for nursing contact hours is the American Nurses Credentialing Center (ANCC) accreditation. Certificates of completion for programs accredited through ANCC are accepted by all state boards of nursing and nursing certification boards. ANCC accreditation establishes that quality standards have been used to create the program and that the program is free of bias in presentation of treatment options (ANCC, 2009).

Although the accreditation process can be cost prohibitive for an individual facility, nurse managers can make accredited nursing continuing education available to staff members through journal self-study programs, online courses, and professional conferences. Both the National Commission on Correctional Health Care and the American Correctional Association offer ANCC accredited nursing continuing education through their conferences. NCCHC also provides nursing continuing education through the Journal of Correctional Health Care.

Professional Development for Nonclinical staff

Nurse managers must also consider the ongoing professional development of nonclinical staff under their direction. Clerical, medical records, and pharmacy supply staff perform vital functions to support clinical processes. In addition, security staff may be regularly assigned to the clinical area and require inclusion in educational experiences. Professional development activities specific to these roles should be a part of the overall clinical program.

Special care in competency evaluation should be given to those support roles closest to clinical care processes, such as medication technicians and nursing assistants. Consider and include the role of nonclinical staff in any unit orientation, competency evaluation, inservice, and continuing education activity. Accreditation standards also require orientation and ongoing appropriate training for volunteers, interns, students, and inmate workers in the clinical area (ACA, 2002; NCCHC, 2008a, b).

Management of Education Records

Records of staff involvement in education are an important component of employee files. These records establish levels of staff participation for accreditation purposes. More important to the nurse manager, staff education records verify the maintenance of staff competency and affirm staff ability to perform specific clinical functions within the care setting. With the advent of computerized documentation, a staff spreadsheet can be maintained. This speeds the organization of annual credentialing processes, such as CPR, first aid, or institution-required skill validation. Some institutions have staff members complete post tests for each education program and use the post-test as validation of critical learning. Post tests are signed and dated, providing a record of staff accountability for the new information or skill.

ORGANIZATIONAL CHANGE

The saying that "change is not the unusual but the normal" is true in all health care settings, including corrections. Paired with the corollary that "the only person who likes change is a wet baby," and a continuing need for skills in managing organizational change and the human factors attached to it is evident. Nurse managers must act as effective change agents by coordinating and balancing competing priorities within the organization and among the various staff members. The plan and process for change may appear organized and systematic on paper. The actual implementation of change, depending on the magnitude, can, instead, seem chaotic, uncertain, and imprecise. Nurse managers must be flexible and able to alter the course mid-progress while remaining focused on the desired goal.

Guiding the Change Process

Consistency and attention are needed to successfully guide a change process. The nursing process (Assessment, Planning, Implementation, Evaluation) and the continuous quality improvement process (Plan, Do, Check, Act) can provide guidance in managing a change implementation. The IMPROVE model developed by Pennsylvania State University expands on the elements of the continuous quality improvement process and is a helpful guide for clinical change (Table 17.5).

When planning for clinical change, the first step seems obvious—identify and select the process for improvement. However, pausing to determine the order of a complicated change or the priority of change elements can speed the change process and avert disaster. Once the process has been identified, a map of the current process is created to make visible process steps and prepare for a description of how that process will be changed. Next, the current process is analyzed to obtain baseline data to establish the critical need for change and compare with the new process during the evaluation phase. At some point during the first phases of the change process, the nurse manager may be required to validate the need for a clinical change to garner support from other managers and organizational leaders. Indeed, data about the current process can assist with gaining staff support for change, as well.

The next phase involves researching and developing an alternative solution for the identified problem. Best-practice information can be obtained from accrediting bodies, other facilities within the system, federal guidelines, or research articles. Open up the discussion to staff members involved in the process. Many good ideas can be generated and evaluated for implementation.

Armed with this information, the nurse manager can organize and implement necessary improvements. This can be a lengthy and messy process as systems are moved from old to new. Expect alterations and adjustments in the midst of change implementation. Take as long as necessary to fully implement and habituate the new process.

Once a change is in place, verification and documentation is necessary to establish positive results. A thoughtful evaluation concludes the change process and allows comparison of new outcomes with the previous process performance data.

TABLE 17.5   Penn State's University IMPROVE Model

STAGE	DESCRIPTION
I	Identify and select the process for improvement
M	Map the critical process
P	Prepare analysis of process performance
R	Research and develop solutions
O	Organize and implement improvements
V	Verify and document results
E	Evaluate and plan for continuous improvement

Source: From Sherlock (2009), used with permission.

TABLE 17.6   Bridges Stages of Transition During Change

STAGE	CHARACTERISTICS
Endings	Letting go of the past to embrace the new
Neutral zone	Chaotic middle straddling old and new forms
Beginnings	Embracing the new and moving on

Source: Adapted from Bridges (2009).

Evaluation of the change should also include evaluation of the team's performance and the management of the various steps of the process.

The Human Side of Change

Reluctance and resistance can be a common staff response to change (Donohue, 2011). Encouraging acceptance, involvement, and ownership can speed transition and lead to lasting change. Understanding the change behavior patterns of various staff members can assist managers in speeding assimilation and implementation of new processes and staff requirements. Tailoring the response to the context and staff characteristics improves outcomes in managing a change process.

Bridges' (2009) model of change is helpful in understanding the impact of major organizational change on staff members (Table 17.6). Most change begins with the ending of an "old way" of doing or being in the work place. Sometimes it is helpful to acknowledge that ending and the meaning it has for team members. Depending on the magnitude of change initiated, staff may need a time of grieving. For example, changing a prison from male to female or eliminating long-held rituals may require a period of grief.

The neutral zone is a time of straddling old and new ways. It can be a time of chaos and confusion. Increasing communication with staff during this time period is recommended. Keeping staff informed of change progress and readjustments in the change path is important. Also important is role modeling the new desired behavior and taking suggestions from the staff in the implementation process.

The final phase of transition according to Bridges is the new beginning. At this phase staff members need to be reminded of the purpose of the change and visualize the picture of what the new process looks like. They need to see the plan and what their part is to play, or where they fit in the big picture (Bridges, 2009). By considering the human side of organizational change, nurse managers can speed transition and gain staff support. Case Example 17.2 provides an opportunity to apply these principles.

CASE EXAMPLE 17.2

After much evaluation and deliberation, facility management of a medium-size female prison has decided to change the nursing sick call process for general population inmates. Instead of using sick call slips to triage and assign visits by appointment, open sick call hours will be posted and inmates needing to see a nurse can report to the medical unit for evaluation during these hours. Discuss ways the nurse manager can involve staff in the change process and brainstorm methods for managing the project.

SUMMARY

Correctional nurses in all levels of the organization benefit from developing management and leadership skills. Understanding and complying with licensure requirements when delegating nursing functions is important. Collaboration, in particular, is necessary to meet patient care goals in a correctional environment where the health care team must coexist with security and service units. Conflict among staff requires additional resolution skills. Nurse managers can foster the continuing professional development of staff members through a structured staff development program involving orientation, competency assessment, inservice, and continuing education opportunities. Effecting organizational and clinical change through a structured process and attention to the human factors of change can move a clinical program forward, even in the challenging correctional environment.

From the Experts ...

"Mark Twain said, "If you don't where you are going, any road will get you there." It is critical for the correctional nurse leader to have a clear picture of what should be accomplished and have the leadership skills to get others to follow them on their journey to nursing excellence in the correctional setting."

Becky Pinney, MSN, CCHP-RN
Nashville, TN

DISCUSSION QUESTIONS

1. Can a nurse be both a leader and a manager? What are the characteristics of each?
2. Based on the information in this chapter, what goals do you have for improving your leadership or management skills?
3. Analyze an ongoing conflict in your work setting. What is blocking the effective resolution of the conflict? Are there opportunities for positive resolution based on information from this chapter?
4. What professional development resources are available to you in your work setting? Consider internet, print, conferences, and internal education opportunities. Make a list of all resources and create a monthly plan for staff professional development at your facility.

REFERENCES

American Correctional Association. (2002). *Performance-based standards for correctional health care in adult correctional institutions.* Alexandria, VA: Author.

American Correctional Association. (2010). *2010 Standards supplement.* Alexandria, VA: Author.

American Correctional Association (ACA). (n.d.) *Standards and accreditation.* Retrieved from http://www.aca.org/standards/agency.asp

American Nurses Association (ANA). (2005). *Principles of delegation.* Silver Spring, MD: Author. Retrieved from http://www.healthsystem.virginia.edu/internet/e-learning/principlesdelegation.pdf

American Nurses Association (ANA), National Council of State Boards of Nursing (NCSBN). (2006). *Joint statement on delegation.* Retrieved from https://www.ncsbn.org/1056.htm

American Nurses Association (ANA). (2007). *Corrections nursing: Scope & standards of practice.* Silver Spring, MD: Author.

American Nurses Credentialing Center (ANCC). (2009). *Application manual: Accreditation program.* Silver Spring, MD: Author.

Angermeier, I. A., Dunford, B. B., Boss, A. D., & Boss, R. W. (2009). The impact of participative management perceptions on customer service, medical errors, burnout, and turnover intentions. *Journal of Healthcare Management, 54*(2), 127–140.

Bleich, M. (2011). Leading, managing, and following. In P. S. Yoder-Wise (Ed.), *Leading and managing in nursing* (5th ed.), St. Louis, MO: Elsevier Mosby.

Bridges, W. (2009). *Managing transitions, making the most of change* (3rd ed.). Philadelphia: Da Capo Press.

Croll, N. (2008). Writing policies and procedures. In A. Crowther (Ed.), *Nurse managers: A guide to practice* (2nd ed.). Melbourne: Ausmed Publications.

Cully, M. (2008). Dealing with unhelpful nurses. In A. Crowther (Ed.), *Nurse managers: A guide to practice* (2nd ed.), Melbourne: Ausmed Publications.

Donohue, M. A. (2011). Leading change. In P. S. Yoder-Wise (Ed.), *Leading and managing in nursing* (5th ed.). St. Louis, MO: Elsevier Mosby.

Federal Bureau of Prisons. (2005). Program Statement P6010.02 Health Services Administration. Accessed 7/4/2012 at http://www.bop.gov/policy/progstat/6010_002.pdf.

Folse, V. N. (2011). Conflict: The cutting edge of change. In P. S. Yoder-Wise (Ed.), *Leading and managing in nursing* (5th ed.). St. Louis, MO: Elsevier Mosby.

Gromley, D. K. (2011). Collective action. In P. S. Yoder-Wise (Ed.), *Leading and managing in nursing* (5th ed.), St. Louis, MO: Elsevier Mosby.

Harman, E. (2007). Maximizing employee performance. In R. A. P. Jones (Ed.), *Nursing leadership and management: Theories, processes and practice.* Philadelphia: F. A. Davis.

Kouzes, J. M., & Posner, B. Z. (2007) *The leadership challenge* (4th ed.). San Francisco, CA: Jossey-Bass.

Kowalski, K. (2011). Managing personal/personnel problems. In P. S. Yoder-Wise (Ed.), *Leading and managing in nursing* (5th ed.). St. Louis, MO: Elsevier Mosby.

Malvey, D. (2010a). Unionization in healthcare: Background and trends. *Journal of Healthcare Management, 55*(3), 154–157.

Malvey, D. (2010b). Unionization in healthcare: strategies. *Journal of Healthcare Management, 55*(4), 236–240.

Moore, M. L. (2008). Preceptorships: Hidden benefits to the organization. *Journal for Nurses in Staff Development, 24*(1), E9–E15.

National Commission on Correctional Health Care (NCCHC). (2008a). *Standards for health services in prisons.* Chicago, IL: Author.

National Commission on Correctional Health Care (NCCHC). (2008b). *Standards for health services in jails.* Chicago, IL: Author.

National Commission on Correctional Health Care (NCCHC). (2011). *Standards for health services in juvenile detention and confinement facilities.* Chicago, IL: Author.

National Commission on Correctional Health Care (NCCHC). (n.d.) *Publications: NCCHC standards.* Retrieved from http://ncchc.org/pubs/index.html

National Council of State Boards of Nursing (NCSBN). (1997). *5 Rights of delegation.* Retrieved August 5, 2011, from https://www.ncsbn.org/fiverights.pdf

O'Daniel, M., & Rosenstein, A. H. (2008). Professional communication and team collaboration. In *Agency for healthcare research and qualtiy (AHRQ). Patient Safety and quality: An evidence-based handbook for nurses.* AHRQ Publication No. 08-0043. Agency for Healthcare Research and Quality, Rockville, MD. Retrieved from http://www.ahrq.gov/qual/nurseshdbk/docs/O%27DanielM_TWC.pdf

Owens, H. (1990). *Leadership is.* Maryland: Abbot Publishing.

Penn State University. (2003). *A structured approach to organizational improvement, Innovation Insights, 7.* Retrieved from http://www.psu.edu/president/cqi/innovation/improve7.pdf

Pittman, J. (2007).Registered nurse job satisfaction and collective bargaining unit membership status. *Journal of Nursing Administration, 37*(10), 471–476.

Porter-O'Grady, T., & Malloch, K. (2011). *Quantum leadership: Advancing innovation, transforming health care* (3rd ed.). Boston: Jones & Bartlett.

Price, G. (2008). Working with job descriptions. In A. Crowther (Ed.) *Nurse managers: A guide to practice* (2nd ed.). Melbourne: Ausmed Publications.

Sherlock, B. (2009). *Integrating planning, assessment, and improvement in higher education.* Washington, DC: National Association of College and University Business Officers.

Sportsman, S. (2007). Constructive conflict management. In R. A. P. Jones (Ed.), *Nursing leadership and management: Theories, processes and practice.* Philadelphia: F. A. Davis.

Sportsman, S., & Hamilton, P. (2007). Conflict management styles in nursing and allied health professionals. *Journal of Professional Nursing, 23*(3), 157–166.

Stalbaum, A. L., & Valadez, A. M. (2011). Developing the role of manager. In P. S. Yoder-Wise (Ed.), *Leading and managing in nursing* (5th ed.). St. Louis, MO: Elsevier Mosby.

Twedell, D. M. (2011). Selecting, developing, and evaluating staff. In P. S. Yoder-Wise (Ed.), *Leading and managing in nursing* (5th ed.). St. Louis, MO: Elsevier Mosby.

Welch, R. A. (2011). Making decisions and solving problems. In P. S. Yoder-Wise (Ed.), *Leading and managing in nursing* (5th ed.). St. Louis, MO: Elsevier Mosby.

Wright, D. (2005). *The ultimate guide to competency assessment in health care* (3rd ed.). Minniapolis, MN: Creative Heath Care Management, Inc.

EIGHTEEN

Research Participation and Evidence-Based Practice

Lorry Schoenly

Research is a foundation of correctional nursing practice (ANA, 2007). Nurses must understand how to integrate research findings into practice and, at a minimum, participate in research activities. In addition, the corrections environment can pose ethical situations requiring nurse actions to protect human subjects during research activities. The ANA Scope and Standards of Corrections Nursing Practice expect nurses to integrate research into their practice by participating in various research activities and using the best evidence to guide practice decisions (ANA, 2007). The Code of Ethics for Nurses (ANA, 2001) also directs nurses to participate in advancing the profession through, among other things, contributions to knowledge development in the field.

THE IMPORTANCE OF RESEARCH FOR NURSING PRACTICE
Scientific Basis of Practice

From the very start of the profession, nursing was based on science. The art and science of nursing is often mentioned, and with good reason. The nursing profession requires whole brain thinking with actions based on knowledge, skill, and appropriate attitude. Florence Nightingale, commonly held as the first nurse leader, used observation and statistics in the first attempts to quantify nursing practice. Her work is the basis of nursing research and evidence-based practice (EBP) today (Burckhardt, 2008).

Nursing, then, is a caring profession based on a scientific foundation of ever-expanding information. Knowledge about the best application of nursing practice is created through nursing research. Research, a basic scientific process, validates and refines existing knowledge while also creating new knowledge (Burns & Grove, 2009).

Since research is the scientific basis for practice (AACN, 2006), nurses in every specialty need to understand the research process and be able to apply research findings to their practice setting. Correctional nurses can apply general nursing research to the correctional patient population and environment to improve care outcomes. In addition, research specific to correctional nursing practice can provide a basis for nursing care delivery in the specialty setting.

Evidence-Based Practice

EBP expands upon research utilization to include clinical expertise and patient preference (Fawcett & Garity, 2009). Indeed, research application is a major component of EBP, however, consideration is also given to clinician expertise and patient characteristics (Figure 18.1). The search for solutions to clinical problems drives the EBP process (Zalon, 2011).

EBP is an organized process that begins with a spirit of inquiry about an area of clinical interest or concern (Melnyk & Fineout-Overholt, 2011). After an area of interest is selected, a clinical question is created that guides the search for evidence. All sources are used to locate evidence for evaluation. This evidence, once collected, is appraised for credibility and applicability then integrated with clinical expertise and patient preferences before being implemented. The final steps in the process are to evaluate and disseminate the outcome of the EBP application (Melnyk & Fineout-Overholt, 2011).

Best Practices Development

It would be fortunate to locate solid, research-based evidence on which to base all nursing practice, but this is not available in many cases. Much of nursing practice is based on clinical knowledge and past practices that have been effective in

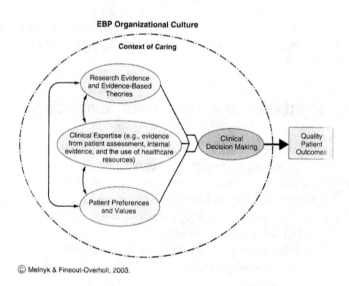

© Melnyk & Fineout-Overholt, 2003.

FIGURE 18.1   The components of EBP.

Source: From Melnyk and Fineout-Overholt (2011, p. 6). Used with permission.

From the Experts ...

"Evidence-based nursing is critical to incorporate in correctional nursing, as it draws on the experience and traditions of correctional nurses, and solidifies them through research. This validates the specialty and experience of correctional nurses."

Mark Ellsworth, MSN, RN
Salt Lake City, UT

dealing with the human response to disease and injury (Benner & Leonard, 2011). When research evidence is not available, nurses can, instead, rely on best practice guidelines and protocols to guide practice.

Best practice guidelines combine all available information on a particular practice to determine the best course of action. These guidelines may not be as rigorous as EBP guidelines and include a greater degree of expert opinion and anecdotal reports of success. Best practices still hold great value for improving nursing practice by applying expertise from the larger practicing community and therefore establishing greater credibility in clinical decision making.

Best-practice recommendations can come from a wide array of internal and external sources. Practitioners within the system may share practices from experiences in other settings. Clinical experts may share practice experiences from their clinical settings during conference presentations or in journal articles. Although not as strong an evidence source as research studies, information shared from expert clinicians and other settings provide best practice resources when stronger evidence is not available.

Quality Improvement Activities

EBP and best practice guidelines apply external sources of information to local clinical practice. For correctional nurses, external sources most often, of necessity, come from other clinical specialties and can require alteration for application to the correctional setting. Quality improvement activities provide an internal source of knowledge (Melnyk & Fineout-Overholt, 2011). Internal quality improvement projects can evaluate current nursing practices and lead to refinements that improve patient outcomes. Brown (2009) suggests a method for the integration of EBP with quality improvement activities that involves four steps. First, a system weakness can be identified and evaluated through QI activities to establish a baseline. Next, external sources of information can be researched to create a new practice model to replace the system weakness. The third step in the process is to strategically integrate the innovation into the existing clinical system. Finally, following implementation of the best practice or EBP, a post-implementation QI evaluation is performed. Modifications of the newly implemented practice can take place based on the evaluation outcome.

BASIC RESEARCH PRINCIPLES

An understanding of basic research principles can improve both the application of external evidence and the creation of reliable internal evidence through the quality improvement process. By using research principles in practice, correctional nurses can have greater confidence when changing clinical practice to improve patient outcomes.

Adequate Sample Size

A study of a nursing intervention needs to have a large enough sample to show the effect of the intervention. This can be challenging because the effects of a nursing intervention are often of moderate impact, meaning a fairly large sample size is needed to show significant change (Brown, 2009). Generally speaking, a large sample size is better than a small one. If the study under review has a small sample, search for similar studies to validate the results. Even better, search for credible reviews of the literature on the intervention in question. For example, meta-analyses and research review articles are often available. In addition, organizations such as the Agency for Health Research and Quality, Cochran Collaborative, and the Joanna Briggs Institute published reviews of the literature on specific health care interventions (Table 18.1). These sources are of particular help to nurses new to the research process.

Randomization

Randomization refers to the method for selecting and assigning subjects to groups (Fawcett & Garity, 2009). Each subject should have equal opportunity to be included or to be placed in any of the groups under study. For example, in an experimental study, subjects should not be given a choice as to the group they will be assigned. Subjects should represent the larger population under study and each group should be equivalent in the diverse characteristics of the population (Brown, 2009). When randomization is adequate among the test groups, a difference between the groups can more confidently be attributed to the intervention (DiCenso, Ciliska, & Guyatt, 2005). For example, a study of inmate response to a patient education intervention should not compare results between the administrative segregation population and the general population, as there is variability in the characteristics of these two groups, which might affect the results of the intervention.

In the case of an internal quality improvement study, care must be taken to be representative in the sample selection. Consideration should be given to the inclusion of all characteristics of the population or data under study. For example, a review of medication administration should include samples from each medication line, weekday and weekend shifts if characteristics are different. All levels of staff should be considered, such as both LPN and medication technician, if appropriate. By considering randomization in quality improvement activities, correctional nurses can be more assured that differences are a result of the intervention.

TABLE 18.1   Sources of Nursing Research Reviews

SOURCE	INTERNET LOCATION
Agency for Healthcare Research and Quality Cochrane Collaborative Joanna Briggs Institute	www.ahrq.gov www.cochrane.org www.joannabriggs.edu.au

Generalizability

Generalizability refers to the applicability of research findings to the larger population (Fawcett & Garity, 2009). Appropriate randomization, as described earlier, is a key component of generalizability. In addition, the subjects in the study should be similar to the target population. This is also called transferability. Since the body of nursing research in the corrections specialty is still developing, nurses must often consider the application of research from other specialties to the corrections setting. The difference in patient population and setting characteristics should be evaluated when making an application to correctional health care. When there is little risk of patient injury, questions of transferability are of less concern.

When an internal process or procedure is being evaluated, the results can be applied overall if data was collected among all variables. However, if sampling was limited to a particular time, group, or patient set, the results may not represent the process in general. For example, a quality improvement review of nursing sick call documentation performed using the first 10 visits of each month would not adequately represent the various staff and patient conditions. This study would not be generalizable to the full nursing sick call process in the facility.

Credibility

Credibility refers to the trustworthiness of the information and focuses on both the author's background and the design of the study (Powers, 2011). In other words, can this information be used with confidence in clinical practice? It is a common misconception that all published information is credible. While that is often the case, many published studies include bias or have faulty sampling and research design (Fawcett & Garity, 2009).

FINDING AND EVALUATING EVIDENCE

A major component of research utilization, EBP, and best-practice identification is finding and evaluating evidence about the area of health care under investigation. Without sufficient evidence, nurses may have difficulty determining the right course of action. Sometimes the difficulty is the amount of published information about the particular topic. However, sometimes the difficulty lies in an insufficiently formulated question.

Framing the Research Question

A poorly created research question will often lead to an ineffective information search (Fineout-Overholt & Stillwell, 2011). Time spent developing research questions is well spent and decreases the subsequent search time. The PICOT question development process leads to a systematic and consistent process for identifying elements of a clinical issue needed for a successful evidence search (Stillwell, Fineout-Overholt, Melnyk, & Williamson, 2010). By focusing on the five key elements of PICOT construction, as listed in Table 18.2, nurses can develop search strategies to more effectively uncover appropriate evidence.

Applying the PICOT process, correctional nurses at a female facility are interested in creating a support group for the growing number of inmates who are having bulimia symptoms. They wonder if this would really be worth the time and effort. Will there be a positive outcome? Their research question, then, might be: "Would a support group help female inmates reduce bulimic episodes if held over a 6-month period?" Armed

TABLE 18.2   Elements of the PICOT Research Development Process

ELEMENT	CHARACTERISTICS	SAMPLE SEARCH COMPONENTS
P	Patient population or disease	Young adult women
I	Intervention or issue of interest	Support group
C	Comparison intervention or issue of interest	Individual education
O	Outcome	Reduce bulimia activities
T	Timeframe (optional)	Over 6 months

Source: Adapted from Fineout-Overholt and Stillwell (2011).

with this specific question, the nurses are ready to search for information. Often the topic under question does not need to be time limited or does not yet have a comparison intervention. The search might be started by seeking all interventions for bulimia. In such a case, the PICOT process can be modified to fit the need. As an example, the nurses in this situation might have worded their question: "What interventions have been successful in dealing with bulimia in young adult females?"

Although the PICOT system of question generation is strongly advocated, it can be problematic for correctional nurses. There are so few studies of nursing interventions in the corrections population that little evidence will be found. When this is the case, consider a similar population for the evidence search. For example, if inquiring about bulimia, use a general population, such as young adults, or consider gender, such as female population, if that is appropriate. This will yield a greater amount of information that the correctional nurse can consider for application to the specialty setting.

The "I" component of a PICOT question can refer to an intervention, but also could be a diagnostic test, prognosis, etiology, or even the meaning of an illness or condition to the patient (Fineout-Overholt & Stillwell, 2011). When considering the intervention or issue of interest, start by using a common term. Once several information sources are located, review these for other key terms that might assist in gleaning appropriate information. For example, a search may start by using the term "eating disorders." Once several studies are located, key terms such as "bulimia" or "binge-purge eating" may emerge. Use of that term in the search field may then yield more applicable studies.

A comparison intervention may not be desirable at first. Often it is an effective strategy to start with a broader search without using a comparison to see what literature is available. Once early returns are reviewed, a comparison intervention may present itself and can be used for a more in-depth search. Adjust the search question accordingly.

The outcome component of a PICOT question may be obvious, such as a reduction of the condition or greater patient compliance with treatment. In the case of a subject with extensive published research, considering a specific outcome can narrow the findings to a few valuable results. A PICOT question can be revised and expanded during the search process.

Timeframe is the most often omitted element of a PICOT research question. However, timeframe for an intervention may be of importance to correctional nurses working in a setting with high inmate turnover such as a jail. Limiting the timing of an intervention can help in finding evidence for short-term treatment options. If a time limit greatly reduces the number of evidence options, try eliminating this requirement and evaluating the resulting literature for application on an individual basis.

Information Searching

Once a researchable question is developed, the search can begin for any published research and best practices to answer the question. The expansion of cost-free Internet sources of professional literature has been a boon to correctional nurses who do not always have access to medical libraries or librarian resources. Several other sources of searchable databases may be available and are listed in Exhibit 18.1. Some state nursing licensure boards provide medical library access through licensure fees. Nurses continuing their formal education have access to university library systems. Some public library systems link to the public university search systems and can allow both searching and obtaining copies of articles and books for loan. Both Google Scholar and PubMed are cost-free resources available on the internet, although they are less robust than medical library resources and often will only provide abstracts of appropriate articles.

EXHIBIT 18.1
Information Resources for Evidence Searching

- University library systems
- Public library
- State licensure access
- Internet sources
- Google Scholar—scholar.google.com
- PubMed—pubmed.gov

Evaluating Evidence

Not all information is credible or useable in the correctional setting. Even information published in a peer-reviewed journal needs to be evaluated for credibility and application. A three-component evaluation suggested by Brown (2009) can help nurses determine what research findings and best-practice recommendations to implement in clinical practice. Credibility, clinical significance, and applicability appraisal can guide correctional nurses reviewing search results.

Credibility

This concept was discussed earlier as one of the basic principles of conducting research. In evaluating evidence from the literature search, the nurse also considers credibility. First, determine if the organization or persons performing the study have the credentials to do so (Brown, 2009). Nationally recognized research clearinghouses such as previously mentioned AHRQ, Cochran Collaborative, and Joanna Briggs Institute provide credibility for the findings. In fact, using systematic reviews and practice guidelines created by such credible sources is an excellent first step for correctional nurses eager to incorporate evidence into practice but unsure of their research evaluation skills.

A second area of credibility evaluation is the determination of any undue bias or influence upon the research and interpretation of results. Very basic potential bias may emerge from the research funding source. Interpretation of study results may be skewed based on the support perspective. For example, care should be taken when considering research findings on medication efficacy when efforts have been funded by the pharmaceutical company producing the medication in question (Mathuna, Finehout-Overholt, & Johnston, 2011).

In addition to evaluating author credibility and bias, nurse reviewers should consider the study format to determine credibility. There are many systems for determining the strength of evidence of a published report. A fairly straightforward system is depicted in Figure 18.2. Here, systematic reviews and meta-analysis are considered the strongest and most credible of findings, while expert opinions, although still worthy of consideration, have less strength.

Clinical Significance

The clinical significance of the research finding is also an important component of evaluation. Although a statistical change can be established, consideration of the study results from the perspective of clinical practice is warranted (Mathuna et al., 2011). Research may indicate that an intervention made a difference in a patient outcome, but was the difference sizeable enough to make a practical difference (Brown, 2009)? A significant change in practice must make a substantial clinical difference to be worthy of the effort.

Applicability

A third area of research evaluation is applicability. This can be of particular concern for correctional nurses. With little clinical research focused in the correctional setting, nurses must carefully review research from other clinical settings for application to the specialty. Consideration should be given to the setting, the patients, and the resources available (Brown, 2009).

Consider the setting of the research as compared to the correctional setting. Correctional health care can be primarily categorized as ambulatory, emergency, and sub-acute. Research findings from a critical care or tertiary care setting should be

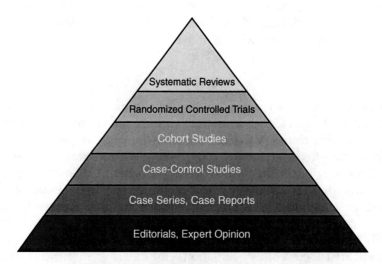

FIGURE 18.2   Evidence evaluation hierarchy.

carefully evaluated for application. However, EBPs from a pre-hospital setting may be very applicable to corrections.

Generalizability, discussed earlier, has direct bearing here. If a research study has been sufficiently randomized and the study patient population is substantially similar to the patient population of intended application, there is support for implementation (Jull, DiCenso, & Guyatt, 2005). Caution is needed if the research participants are extremely divergent of the patient population intended for application.

The final suggested area of evaluation for applicability is that of resources. Correctional settings are notoriously short on equipment and resources (ANA, 2007). Application of research findings must take into consideration availability of appropriate resources to accomplish a similar outcome. Research support, however, can also assist in obtaining necessary resources to improve patient care. Case Example 18.1 provides opportunity to develop skills in applying these evaluation principles.

CASE EXAMPLE 18.1

The nurses at Valley County Jail have noticed an increase in alcohol withdrawal emergencies in the last 3 months. They have gathered published research on the subject, primarily from emergency medical journals and book chapters. They are particularly interested in the results of a study applying a specific admission evaluation process for determining potential for withdrawal symptoms. How can the nurses determine if this research is credible and has potential for implementation in their setting?

PARTICIPATING IN RESEARCH ACTIVITIES

Strict requirements for informed consent and statutory regulation for vulnerable populations such as inmates, all but eliminated clinical research trials involving prisoners in the United States (Gostin, Vanchieri, & Pope, 2006). Accrediting bodies such as NCCHC (2008) and ACA (2010) also address ethical concerns for medical and other research involving the inmate population and constrain the involvement of inmate patients in research activities. Correctional nurses participating in any clinical research involving inmates should be particularly mindful of research principles assuring full understanding and consent of the research subjects.

Human Subjects Protection

A human subjects committee, often called an Institutional Review Board (IRB), is a research review committee with a goal of protecting human subjects involved in a research study. An IRB provides an unbiased review of proposed research to determine if all mechanisms are in place to protect the ethical rights of the human research subjects (Brown, 2009). An IRB review is an essential component of any research involving inmates or correctional health care staff.

One ethical principle of any research project is a strong informed consent process. Human subjects must make a knowledgeable choice to participate or decline participation in a research study. No pressure or coercion can be present and consent must be entirely voluntary (NCCHC, 2008).

Participants must also be informed of a variety of elements of the study, such as the purpose, how subjects are selected, and the risks associated with any treatment or lack of treatment provided by the researchers. Privacy, anonymity, and confidentially must be established and described. In addition, participants need to know how they will be protected from discomfort and harm (Brown, 2009). All of these components must be reviewed and approved by a human subjects committee or IRB before research can proceed.

Inmate Participation in Clinical Trials

Although both NCCHC (2008) and ACA (2002, 2010) severely limit human subjects research in jails and prisons, they have provisions for the involvement of inmates in clinical trials. The distinction is an important one. Involvement in clinical trials can be of great benefit to an inmate with a condition that currently has no effective treatment. For example, some cancer treatments are only available to individuals who enroll in a clinical trial. Correctional nurses may need to continue administering clinical trial medications or treatments while an individual is incarcerated.

Involvement in a clinical trial should be of benefit to the inmate and a possible treatment for a known condition. Common therapeutic clinical trial involvement includes treatments for cancer, human immunodeficiency virus (HIV), and Hepatitis C. The Code of Federal Regulation Section 45 CFR 46 establishes the specific situations in which research can be carried out on prisoners (National Institutes of Health, 2005). Special provisions are made for medical research that can reasonably be of benefit to the prisoner participant.

Correctional nurses asked to administer clinical trial treatments to inmates should confirm validity of the trial information with the inmate's medical provider. In addition to confirming the clinical trial with the inmate's medical provider, a discussion with the inmate should confirm informed consent and understanding of the treatment protocol. The individual should also understand that withdrawal from the trial can take place at any time. The site medical director should approve continuation of the clinical trial protocol. With all these safeguards in place, correctional nurses can participate in the continuation of therapeutic treatment research with inmate-patients. Case Example 18.2 provides opportunity to develop skill in applying these principles.

CASE EXAMPLE 18.2

Inmate West has arrived at the infirmary of Mountain Regional Correctional Center after a parole violation. He is under medical care for colon cancer and on a biologic treatment as part of a clinical trial. Infirmary nurses have been directed to continue administering the clinical trial treatment while he is their patient. What elements of the trial must be confirmed by the nursing staff prior to proceeding with treatment administration?

CORRECTIONAL NURSING RESEARCH AGENDA

Early research in correctional nursing has focused on professional practice issues in the specialty, including initial evaluation of specific characteristics of the specialty from the nurse's perspective. Research thus far has explored the unique role and stigmatization of the correctional nurse (Flanagan & Flanagan, 2001; Hardesty,

Champion, & Champion, 2007); the emotional labors involved in correctional nursing (Walsh, 2009); the experience of caring for inmates (Maeve & Vaughn, 2009; Weiskopf, 2005); and, more recently, fears involved in a nurse–patient relationship (Jacob & Holmes, 2011). In addition, the impact of a custody environment on professional nursing has been extensively studied (Maroney, 2005; Shelton, 2009; Willmott, 1997). A body of research is developing around clinical competency for correctional nursing (Shelton, Weiskopf, & Nicholson, 2010). Results of these efforts can inform the orientation and continuing education programs for nurses new to the specialty.

As this specialty practice continues to develop, a nursing research agenda would provide focus for advancing nursing knowledge. In particular, understanding the meaning of caring in the context of the nurse–patient relationship is important. A model for caring in correctional nursing would greatly advance the specialty and assist nurses in maintaining a professional practice in the midst of security challenges. Moral distress as it applies to the particular issues of correctional nursing deserves more attention, as well.

Clinical issues specific to this practice setting also warrant investigation. For example, correctional nurses need more information about appropriate application of community standards for pain management, patient teaching, end-of-life care, and substance withdrawal. As nurse researchers continue to develop the specialty practice of correctional nursing, the body of knowledge will provide a foundation for professional nursing excellence.

From the Experts . . .

"Correctional nursing is responsible and accountable for pursuing excellence in the advancement of the nursing profession through lifelong learning, research, and continuous quality improvement. The correctional environment poses unique challenges to integrating nursing scholarship into practice. Yet, it is imperative that well-designed studies of correctional nursing roles and scope of practice add to the growing body of national and international data. Creating new knowledge can support the continued transformation of the practice environment."

Constance Weiskopf, PhD, APRN, PMHCNS-BC, CCHP
Farmington, CT

SUMMARY

Conducting and using research in practice can seem daunting to correctional nurses. Lack of resources is just one of many barriers to research utilization. However, correctional nurses can use research principles in many ways. Examples of application included EBP efforts, best-practice evaluation, and quality improvement projects. Correctional nursing practice can be refined and defined through a nursing research agenda. Clinical issues specific to the specialty practice can be investigated to expand the knowledge base and improve patient outcomes.

DISCUSSION QUESTIONS

1. Review several general nursing journals and brainstorm application of knowledge to your correctional practice.
2. Discuss barriers to application of research in your practice setting.
3. Analyze a recent CQI study and identify each of the basic research principles in the study. What is missing? How can the next study be improved to include all the principles?
4. Evaluate your nursing practice over the last week. How much of it was evidence based? How can you improve this finding?
5. Name two skills you would need to develop to increase research utilization in your practice. What resources could you use right now to develop them?
6. Nurses at your facility are wondering if they are using the best practices to manage patients with seizures. They want to find evidence for a patient safety protocol. Develop a PICOT question to begin the evidence search.

REFERENCES

American Association of Colleges of Nursing (AACN). (2006). *Position statement on nursing research.* Retrieved from http://www.aacn.nche.edu/publications/pdf/NsgResearch.pdf

American Correctional Association. (2002). *Performance-based standards for correctional health care in adult correctional institutions.* Alexandria, VA: Author.

American Correctional Association. (2010). *2010 Standards supplement.* Alexandria, VA: Author.

American Nurses Association (ANA). (2001). *Code of ethics for nurses with interpretive statements.* Silver Spring, MD: Author. Retrieved from http://nursingworld.org/MainMenuCategories/EthicsStandards/CodeofEthicsforNurses/Code-of-Ethics.aspx

American Nurses Association (ANA). (2007). *Corrections nursing: Scope & standards of practice.* Silver Spring, MD: Author.

Benner, P. E., & Leonard, V. W. (2011) *Patient concerns, choices, and clinical judgment in evidence-based practice.* In B. M. Melnyk, & E. Fineout-Overholt (Eds.), *Evidence-based practice in nursing & healthcare: A guide to best practice* (2nd ed.). Philadelphia: Lippincott Williams & Wilkins.

Brown, S. J. (2009). *Evidence-based nursing: The research-practice connection.* Boston, MA: Jones & Bartlet.

Burckhardt, J. (2008). *Forward: Notes on nursing: What it is and what it is not.* New York: Kaplan Publishing.

Burns, N., & Grove, S. K. (2009). *The practice of nursing research: Conduct, critique and utilization* (6th ed.). St. Louis, MO: Saunders.

DiCenso, A., Ciliska, D., & Guyatt, G. (2005). Introduction to evidence-based nursing. In A. DiCenso, D. Ciliska, & G. Guyatt (Eds.), *Evidence-based nursing: A guide to clinical practice.* St. Louis, MO: Elsevier Mosby.

Fawcett, J., & Garity, J. (2009). *Evaluating research for evidence-based nursing practice.* Philadelphia: F. A. Davis.

Fineout-Overholt, E., & Stillwell, S. B. (2011). Asking compelling, clinical questions. In B. M. Melnyk, & E. Fineout-Overholt (Eds.), *Evidence-based practice in nursing & healthcare: A guide to best practice* (2nd ed.), Philadelphia: Lippincott Williams & Wilkins.

Flanagan, N. A., & Flanagan, T. J. (2001). Correctional nurses' perceptions of their role, training requirements, and prisoner health care needs. *Journal of Correctional Health Care, 8*(1), 67–85.

Gostin, L. O., Vanchieri, C., & Pope, A. (Eds.). (2006). *Ethical considerations for research involving prisoners.* Washington, DC: National Academies Press. Retrieved from http://www.ncbi.nlm.nih.gov/books/NBK19882/pdf/TOC.pdf

Hardesty, K., Champion, D., & Champion, J. (2007). Jail nurses: Perceptions, stigmatization, and working styles in correctional health care. *Journal of Correctional Health Care, 13*(3), 196–205.

Jacob, J. D., & Holmes, D. (2011). Working under threat: Fear and nurse–patient interactions in a forensic psychiatric setting. *Journal of Forensic Nursing, 7,* 68–77.

Jull, A., DiCenso, A., & Guyatt, G. (2005). Clinical manifestations of disease. In A. DiCenso, D. Ciliska, & G. Guyatt (Eds.), *Evidence-based nursing: A guide to clinical practice.* St. Louis, MO: Elsevier Mosby.

Mathuna, D. P., Finehout-Overholt, E., & Johnston, L. (2011). Critically appraising quantitative evidence for clinical decision making. In B. M. Melnyk, & E. Fineout-Overholt (Eds.), *Evidence-based practice in nursing & healthcare: A guide to best practice* (2nd ed.). Philadelphia: Lippincott Williams & Wilkins.

Maeve, M. K., & Vaughn, (2009). Nursing with prisoners: The practice of caring, forensic nursing or penal harm nursing?. *Advanced Nursing Science, 24*(2), 47–64.

Maroney, M. K. (2005). Caring and custody: Two faces of the same reality. *Journal of Correctional Health Care, 11*(1), 157–169.

Melnyk, B. M., & Fineout-Overholt, E. (2011). Making the case for evidence-based practice and cultivating a spirit of inquiry. In B. M. Melnyk, & E. Fineout-Overholt (Eds.), *Evidence-based practice in nursing & healthcare: A guide to best practice* (2nd ed.), Philadelphia: Lippincott Williams & Wilkins.

National Commission on Correctional Health Care (NCCHC). (2008). *Standards for health services in prisons.* Chicago, IL: Author.

National Institutes of Health. (2005). Code of Federal Regulations. §46.306 Permitted research involving prisoners. Retrieved from http://ohsr.od.nih.gov/guidelines/45cfr46.html#subpartc

Powers, B. A. (2011). Critically appraising qualitative evidence for clinical decision making. In B. M. Melnyk, & E. Fineout-Overholt (Eds.), *Evidence-based practice in nursing & healthcare: A guide to best practice* (2nd ed.). Philadelphia: Lippincott Williams & Wilkins.

Shelton, D. (2009). Forensic nursing in secure environments. *Journal of Forensic Nursing, 5,* 131–142.

Shelton, D., Weiskopf, C., & Nicholson, M. (2010). Correctional nursing competency development in the Connecticut Correctional Managed Health Care Program. *Journal of Correctional Health Care, 16*(3), 299–309.

Stillwell, S. B., Fineout-Overholt, E., Melnyk, B. M., & Williamson, K. M. (2010). Asking the clinical question: A key step in evidence-based practice. *American Journal of Nursing (AJN), 110*(3), 58–61.

Walsh, E. (2009). The emotional labor of nurses working in her Majesty's (HM) prison service. *Journal of Forensic Nursing, 5,* 143–152.

Weiskopf, C. S. (2005). Nurses experience of caring for inmate patients. *Journal of Advanced Nursing, 49,* 336–343.

Willmott, Y. (1997). Prison nursing: The tension between custody and care. *British Journal of Nursing, 6,* 333–336.

Zalon, M. L. (2011). Translating research into practice. In P. S. Yoder-Wise (Ed.), *Leading and managing in nursing* (5th ed.). St. Louis, MO: Elsevier Mosby.

NINETEEN

Professional Practice

Mary Muse

Correctional nurses face a unique set of circumstances in their work environment that can challenge adherence to the standards of professional practice. Changes in the health care field and the impact of disease trends in the populations incarcerated in jails, prisons and detention facilities also require correctional nurses to incorporate new knowledge and improve their practice continuously. Understanding and attending to professional nursing practice issues are keys to success in correctional nursing. Peer review, personal performance review, and competency assessment are discussed in this chapter because they are methods individual nurses use to enhance clinical performance.

The correctional nurse is expected to demonstrate the essence of nursing in their practice. This implies providing competent, knowledgeable patient care; notwithstanding the individual's reasons for incarceration, the environment, or varying viewpoints about inmates' rights to health care. The correctional nurse is expected to approach and treat the inmate-patient in a holistic manner and place the patient at the center of care. This includes anticipating and then responding both appropriately and in a timely fashion to the health needs of inmate-patients. In addition to the inmate-patient, correctional nursing includes consideration of the family and in some instances the entire correctional population. Staying grounded in nursing practice and role accountability requires perseverance and balance from the correctional nurse. It is reasonable to expect that the correctional nurse will be challenged when providing nursing care to inmates, especially when demonstrating care and compassion for this population.

From the Experts . . .

"I do not profess to know or understand why Correctional Nursing is pro-
foundly different from any other nursing specialty. I can, however, attest to Correctional Nurses' unique devotion, advocacy, and passion to provide care to an
indigent and medically under-served prison population that is more often than
not forgotten."

Karen Rea, PHN, MSN, FNP
Sacramento, CA

CORRECTIONAL NURSING PRACTICE

The American Nurses Association defines correctional nursing as "the practice of
nursing and the delivery of patient care within the unique and distinct environment
of the criminal justice system. The criminal justice system includes jails, prisons,
juvenile detention centers, substance abuse treatment facilities, and other facilities"
(2007, p. 1). Today, correctional nursing is in a very different place than it was even
10 years ago. As correctional nurses share their knowledge, others within the
nursing discipline are paying attention to the promise and opportunity of correctional health care. In addition, there have been increased opportunities for students
to have clinical experiences within correctional settings as part of their community,
public health, and mental health curriculums (Fuller, Alexander, & Hardeman,
2006). As the visibility of correctional nursing practice has increased, students and
nurses are more attracted to the specialty. Areas of nursing shortage, fiscal restraint,
and downsizing of staff in traditional health care settings as well as the complexity of
patients with chronic diseases has attracted increasing numbers of advanced practice
nurses to the specialty area.

Correctional nurses are the primary caregivers in any correctional setting and
the backbone of correctional health care. Much of correctional nursing is focused
on independent practice and autonomy (Smith, 2005). This independence and autonomy obligates the nurse to be accountable for their practice and ensure that it
conforms to the state nurse practice act. The ANA standards emphasize that correctional nurses must recognize their professional responsibility for quality nursing care
according to recognized standards (ANA, 2007). The correctional nurse is held
accountable for having the knowledge and competence to meet the health needs of
the patient population. Accountability for informed and competent professional
practice is placed with the individual nurse and is necessary for public trust and confidence (Milton, 2008).

Most correctional nurses work in an interdisciplinary team with other nurses,
physicians, and mid-level providers. A unique aspect of correctional nursing is that
the team often includes dental and mental health professionals as well. Physicians
provide important medical leadership, however, their availability varies depending
on the correctional facility and its location. Some larger and urban facilities have a
physician onsite seven days a week. Others have limited physician coverage; for
example, smaller correctional facilities may only have a physician onsite once a

week. Nurses need to be very clear about the limits of their authority under the nurse practice act and not assume responsibility for care that can only be provided by a physician or advanced practice provider.

The loss of freedom when individuals are detained within the criminal justice system means that they are unable to seek health care on their own in the community. It is this loss of freedom that creates the obligation to provide health care for persons who are incarcerated or detained. The courts have defined care that is needed as that which is required to meet "serious" medical and mental health needs (Rold, 2008). While this definition seems to limit the type and amount of health care that must be provided, the correctional nurse should be mindful that a health need that in isolation seems unimportant can collectively cause or increase harm to the patient. Nurses can play a key advocacy role in ensuring that inmates can access the care that is needed. Case Example 19.1 describes an advocacy situation correctional nurses sometimes encounter.

CASE EXAMPLE 19.1

One evening during medication administration, the nurse observes a patient having difficulty breathing. The patient tells the nurse that he is asthmatic so she requests that custody staff bring the patient to the clinic for examination. The officer replies "You don't want to start that. These guys are manipulative and they will have you running back and forth. Besides, he is faking, he does this to all new nurses." The nurse knows she should examine this patient but is intimidated by the officer's presence and comments. Although she is uncomfortable, she requests again to have the inmate brought to the clinic.

Discussion Questions:

1. What is the basis for the nurse's insistence that the patient be brought to the clinic?
2. What factors in your work environment would assist the nurse in this situation?

The Role of the Correctional Nurse

The role of the nurse is to provide holistic care for the patient. The National League for Nursing, which accredits nursing educational institutions, identifies four core values of professional nurses; these are caring, integrity, diversity, and excellence (Mission/ Goals/Core Values, n.d.). The correctional nurse often struggles to find ways to provide care consistent with the values of professional nursing while respecting the corrections culture and security rules. This struggle has implications for the nurse, because of the accountability for licensure and the professional nurse's duty to society.

The nurse's scope of practice in the correctional setting can be affected by how the nurse chooses to practice, the demands of the environment, culture, resources, and leadership. According to Muse (2011), the patient is at the core of professional nursing practice. The fact that the patient is incarcerated is only a circumstance of one's situation and should not change how nurses practice or how the nurse views the patient. In the correctional setting the nurse is frequently the first health care provider the patient encounters and the primary health professional through which the inmate has access to care.

Rena Murtha (1975) described the attitudes she found among some health care staff when she was Director of Nursing at the jail on Riker's Island in New York City. She also observed that because the inmate is not detained for the purposes of improving his health, there is an unresolved opposition of goals between providing nursing care and maintaining security. The implications for the nurse who fails to maintain professional practice in the correctional setting can be significant. First and foremost, there is an impact on patient care and patient outcomes are jeopardized. At minimum, the nurse can be subject to discipline by the employer for deficient performance. Further implications of practice below the standard may include sanctioning, suspension, or revocation of the license to practice by the board of nursing. Nurses also can be sued for malpractice or negligence in the delivery of nursing care.

Correctional nurses are guided in decisions about the scope and details of their practice by the state nurse practice act. Other documents used by correctional nurses to define their roles and responsibilities include the agency policies and procedures and clinical protocols that direct the assessment and interventions nurses may take to address patient health complaints or concerns. There should be no inconsistencies between agency policy, procedure or clinical protocols, and the state nurse practice act.

The scope and standards of practice for correctional nursing published by the American Nurses Association (ANA, 2007) further delineates the standard of practice for the specialty area. The standards set by the National Commission on Correctional Health Care (NCCHC; 2008a, 2008b, 2011) and the American Correctional Association (ACA; 2002) are widely recognized and can also be used by nurses to guide their practice.

EVOLUTION OF CORRECTIONAL NURSING PRACTICE
Literature Review

The literature describes correctional nursing as a blurring of boundaries between nursing and corrections. Challenges to professional practice, limitations in demonstrating care and compassion for patients, and difficulties working in complex settings threaten the integrity of professional nursing practice. Moore (1991) describes correctional nurses as uniquely positioned to influence inmate access to care. Dores (1994) described the influence of custody on nursing practice as a continuum of tolerance, from acknowledged to contentious. She suggested that nurses with increased levels of education and clinical experiences in public health, primary care, and psychiatric nursing were better prepared to provide health care in this setting. Similar findings and conclusions about correctional nursing have been published by Maeve (1997), Shields and de Moya (1997), Wilmont (1997), and Weiskopf (2005).

Articles published on correctional nursing since 1989 were reviewed. Emerging themes include:

- Conflict with professional practice,
- Negative attitudes among custody staff and nurses about inmate health care,
- The influence of custody staff on nursing practice,
- Feelings of conflict, stress, alienation, isolation, frustration, and powerlessness.

Nurses who work in correctional settings have been described as marginalized, labeled, and stigmatized. These studies identified limitations on practice, compromised quality of care, and a lack of caring by some nurses (Dhoneda, 1995; Kinsella & Friel, 1995; Maeve, 1997; Shields & de Moya, 1997). More recent publications still report similar themes (Flanagan, 2002, 2006; Gadow, 2003; Hardesty, Champion, & Champion, 2007; Holmes, 2005; Peternelj-Taylor, 2004, 2005; Shelton, 2009; Smith, 2005; Weiskopf, 2005).

Maeve and Vaughn (2001), while addressing the rise in incarceration rates in jails and prisons in the United States, discuss why prisons and jails are difficult to staff. They offer the following explanation; the value placed on prison health care is evidenced through the budget limitations, inequities in salaries, and limited educational preparation of nurses. Licensed practical nurses are the predominant category of nursing in these settings. The authors state that when registered nurses are present they frequently hold a 2-year degree and that those professional nurses with a bachelor's or master's degree find employment in the larger health care community. Other contributors to inappropriate staffing were the tendency of some health staff to focus on control and punishment, practicing outside of the nursing scope of practice, focus on control and punishment, issues with the death penalty, and other ethical problems.

The inherent conflicts in the mission of incarceration and delivery of health care make it difficult for correctional nurses to uphold their obligation for professional practice and remain committed to the essence of nursing care. More positively, the description of correctional nursing is moving away from the delineation of tasks to the concepts of holistic care. In Shelton's (2009) recent study, nurses were more highly educated, and a considerable number held certification in correctional health care. Nurses in the study identified health promotion, implementation of nursing principles, and the provision of care as their priority. There is more emphasis on professional practice; nursing leadership is beginning to emerge and a commitment to patient care is being expressed (Brodie, 2001; Hardesty et al., 2007). Issues of professional practice and work environments that support nursing continue to need attention. Nurses also need to promote and foster the understanding and knowledge of the role of nurses at all levels of correctional leadership along with furthering the development of collaborative relationships with custody.

Organizations Shaping Correctional Nursing

Several organizations have had a significant impact on the growth and visibility of correctional nursing. Foremost among these is the American Nurses Association (ANA), which recognized the specialty area and developed the first version of the scope and standards of practice for correctional nursing in 1985. The scope and standards document defines correctional nursing practice, articulates the standards of practice, and applies the nursing process (2007). The ANA corrections nursing scope and standards are drafted by a voluntary workgroup of nurses with varied and diverse backgrounds and experience in correctional health care. The draft is widely disseminated among nurses for public comment and revised again based upon input from practicing nurses in the field. The final document is reviewed and endorsed by the Congress on Nursing Practice. The current version of the scope and standards of practice are undergoing review and revision for publication in 2013. The ANA website, www.nursingworld.org, provides nurses the opportunity to review and comment on the proposed 2013 revision. The ANA standards are used by nurses as the basis for their practice in correctional settings. The standards provide guidance for development of policy, establishment of practice standards, nursing documentation, orientation to correctional settings, continuing education, performance review, and peer review.

Standards such as those published by the National Commission on Correctional Health Care (NCCHC) and the American Correctional Association (ACA) provide a framework for the organization and operation of health care delivery in correctional facilities. These standards address expectations for credentialing, training, and enhancement of clinical performance for all health care professionals. The standards also set expectations for compliance in the areas of governance and administration, access to care, safety, delivery of health care, health records, and medical–legal issues. These organizations accredit correctional facilities as a voluntary recognition of compliance with national standards for delivery of health care.

The National Commission on Correctional Health Care (NCCHC) is comprised of representatives of major national organizations in the fields of health, law, and corrections. The American Nurses Association is the only nursing organization represented on the NCCHC. There are usually several other nurses on the Board representing interdisciplinary organizations. In addition to the standards for delivery of health care in correctional facilities, the NCCHC publishes position statements and clinical guidelines, a quarterly peer-reviewed journal, a quarterly magazine, and holds two major educational conferences each year (About NCCHC, n.d.).

From the Experts ...

"Membership in professional organizations such as the American Correctional Health Services Association, the American Correctional Association, and the Academy of Health Care Professionals has afforded me the opportunity to network with peers, to keep current with nursing practice issues specific to corrections, and to have a better understanding of the complexities of Correctional Nursing.

Becoming active in these professional organizations has allowed me to have a voice in important issues that affect correctional nurses, to collaborate with Correctional Nursing leaders and, ultimately, to influence the future of Correctional Nursing as a Specialty. I encourage all correctional nurses to join, and become active in, their professional organizations."

Lori E. Roscoe, PhD, MPA, BSN, BSEd, CCHP-RN
Monticello, GA

The American Correctional Association (ACA) is a membership organization open to individuals interested in improving the criminal justice system and includes a special membership category for health care professionals (ACA Healthcare Professional Interest Section, n.d.). The organization includes geographic chapters, affiliate organizations comprised of professional associations, other criminal justice organizations, and student organizations. In addition to the standards for the operation of criminal justice organizations, the ACA develops positions on public policy and advocates for criminal justice issues. It publishes a magazine, *Corrections Today,* that at least annually is solely devoted to health care issues, has started a peer-reviewed health care journal, and holds two major educational conferences each year.

The American Correctional Health Services Association (ACHSA) is a membership organization for individuals in the correctional health care field. The mission of the organization is to serve as a forum for current issues and needs confronting health care professionals (Mission and ethics statement, 2011–2012). The organization is comprised of geographic chapters, although individuals may join the national organization even if there is no state or local chapter. ACHSA publishes position statements and distributes a periodic newsletter. The organization holds one major educational conference each year and each of the chapters has at least one conference annually. ACHSA is one of the organizations represented on the NCCHC Board of Directors and it is a professional affiliate of ACA.

The Academy of Correctional Health Professionals (ACHP) is a membership organization open to any individual interested in correctional health care. The purpose of the Academy is to create a professional community for the advancement of correctional health care by providing educational and professional development (Mission & Goals, 2009). The Academy is also represented on the NCCHC Board of Directors. Membership in the Academy provides subscriptions to the *Journal of Correctional Health Care* and the magazine *CorrectCare*, published by NCCHC, as well as membership discounts on registration fees and other NCCHC products.

RESPONSIBILITIES OF PROFESSIONAL PRACTICE
Orientation

The complex needs of patients cared for in correctional systems require nurses with specialized knowledge and skill (LaMarre, 2006; Muse, 2009). This population is vulnerable, has been underserved, underrepresented, and lacks adequate health care. In many cases, inmates are disenfranchised, experience health disparities, and lack family and social support. Nurses must develop proficiency in the areas of health care that reflect the needs of the patient population.

Correctional health systems can have difficulty recruiting and retaining nurses (Muse, 2009, 2011; Shelton, 2009; Storey, 2006; Wilmont, 1997). The findings from the literature provide evidence that practice environments that do not adequately orient and support their new hires will experience frequent turnover and have difficulty retaining nurses (Ebright, 2010). In some situations the nurse is expected to jump in and begin practicing as if one has several years of experience, without sufficient orientation, or worse, without any orientation. Without sufficient orientation support retention rates can be low and nurse turn over can be high (Jones & Gates, 2007). This approach is unacceptable, unsafe, and leads to potential patient and staff safety issues.

Competence

Each licensed nurse has a responsibility to their patients, the public, and themselves to maintain proficiency and competency in one's area of practice. Whelan (2006) defines competency as the assessment of the employee's ability to perform the skills and task of one's position as defined in one's job description. The National Council of State Boards of Nursing (2005) defined competence as the application of knowledge and skills necessary for practice.

Assessing and developing necessary competence is an important aspect of continuing professional development. Some recent work has been published on the development of core competencies for correctional nurses (Cashin, Chiarella, Waters, & Potter, 2008; Shelton, Weiskopf, & Nicholson, 2010). An example of a plan to address orientation and continued competency adapted from their work is found in Table 19.1.

TABLE 19.1 Phases of Timeline, Content Focus, and Content Design for Correctional Nursing Competency Plan

PHASES	PHASE 1	PHASE 2	PHASE 3	PHASE 4	PHASE 5
Timeline	Pre-orientation	Prior to facility placement	4–6 weeks close mentoring and supervision	Mentored through the first year	Lifelong learning process
Content Focus	DOC Academy Security and safety focus	Nursing orientation What is a correctional nurse	Nursing orientation in assigned facility Probationary period	Extended nursing orientation May rotate to other units and other facilities	Professional development Demonstrate continued nursing competency with annual evaluations
Content Design	Self-assessment of skills Alignment with correctional nursing values	Key points to hit the ground running Nurse point of entry issues High use/high risk clinical skills focus	Begin the mentoring relationship—retention requires this Develop the correctional nurse envisioned for retention	Continue mentoring Have more than one expert mentor Supervisor has special responsibility for retention—frequent meetings	Shift in responsibility for proof of continued competency to nurse with support Standards-based portfolio Nursing rounds: Literature and case review groups Award CEU, certification

Source: Adapted from Shelton et al. (2010).

Lifelong Learning

The Institute of Medicine (IOM; 2001) reported that health professionals were not adequately prepared academically, or through continuing education for delivery of safe patient care. Finkelman (2006) noted the IOM's emphasis on four core competencies (Exhibit 19.1) and suggested that these are achieved by lifelong learning. Lifelong learning can be accomplished in a variety of ways; attendance at employer-required education and training, orientation for a new position, pursuing formal education, maintaining current knowledge of the literature in the specialty area, conducting literature reviews, and reviewing scholarly journals and specialty magazines. The ANA has developed a framework for professional development that focuses on continuing competencies and lifelong learning. The ANA's framework includes staff development, continuing education, and academic education (Finkelman, 2006). Maintaining a professional portfolio will assist the nurse in identifying learning needs and documenting learning.

EXHIBIT 19.1
Four Core Competencies

1. Provide patient-centered care.
2. Work in interdisciplinary teams.
3. Employ evidenced-based practice.
4. Use informatics to extend beyond the practice setting to acquire new knowledge.

Source: Finkelman (2006).

State boards of nursing encourage continuing education and some require specific numbers of educational hours for relicensure. The NCCHC standards require full-time employees to have 12 hours of continuing education annually (NCCHC 2008a, 2008b, 2011). Nurses who are certified correctional health professionals (CCHP) are required to obtain 18 hours of continuing education annually, of which 6 hours must be in correctional health care (Continuing Certification). Specialty certification in correctional nursing also requires evidence of continuing education.

ENHANCING CLINICAL PERFORMANCE

Enhancing clinical performance is part of the professional nurse's commitment to practice. Standards 8 and 9 of the Corrections Nursing: Scope and Standards of Practice set concrete expectations for correctional nurses to maintain knowledge and competency reflective of current nursing practice and to periodically evaluate one's own practice in relation to recognized standards (ANA, 2007). The registered nurse enhances one's clinical performance by participating in self-reflection, setting goals for professional development, participating in on-going education, receiving feedback from supervisors through performance appraisals, reviewing the literature for best practices, and participating in peer review and quality improvement opportunities.

Peer Review

Peer review is a useful tool to promote professional growth, improve quality of patient care, and to account for performance (Hagg-Heitman & George, 2011). When implementing peer review, it is important to structure the review so that expectations, parameters, and guidelines are clear. Peer review involves feedback from colleagues on nursing practice and performance of certain activities such as emergency response or sick call. The focus is on improving quality, meeting standards, and promoting best practices. The ANA defines peer review as a "collegial, systematic, and periodic process by which registered nurses are held accountable for practice and that fosters the refinement of one's knowledge, skills, and decision-making at all levels and in all areas of practice" (ANA, 2010, p. 66). Peer review may be accomplished by clinical rounds, on-site peer review and collaboration, and retrospective record review or other processes. A peer-review example is provided in Case Example 19.2.

CASE EXAMPLE 19.2

You are observing a nurse you work with regularly administer medication as part of the peer-review program. The nurse calls each inmate by name and hands pre-poured medications to the inmate without verifying who the inmate is or that it is the right medication for that patient. You know that the facility schedule only allows a 30-minute window for medication administration to take place and the nurse has to administer medication over 60 patients in that time period.

Discussion Questions:

1. What are the factors that may be challenging this nurse's practice?
2. What could you do as a peer to address the problem this nurse is having?

Professional Practice Portfolio

The professional practice portfolio is used to document professional achievements of the nurse and to assist the nurse in assessing and promoting their learning. It may be used in performance reviews, in professional development, and in career planning.

Oermann (2002) defines a professional portfolio as a collection of carefully selected materials that document the nurse's competencies and illustrates the expertise of the nurse. The portfolio is a compilation of the nurse's career development; it contains select documents that reflect accomplishments, certifications, recognitions, publications, and resume or curriculum vitae. A professional portfolio contains evidence to support the knowledge, skills, and accomplishments that are documented in the nurse's resume and/or curriculum vitae. Elements of a professional portfolio are listed in Exhibit 19.2.

As the nurse achieves identifiable and measurable goals and is developing competency, he or she also participates in self-reflection. Eckroth-Buchner (2010) states self-awareness has long been addressed as fundamental for the professional nurse with the accepted view that self-awareness will lead to greater competence. Self-reflection should be designed to build on self-respect, self-confidence, and pride in the nurses performance.

EXHIBIT 19.2
Elements of a Professional Portfolio

Resume
- Job description
- Goals and learning objectives
- Clinical practice summary and competencies
- Achievements
- Self-reflection
- Feedback

Source: William and Jordan (2007).

An example of self-reflection is journal writing. The nurse uses a journal to record clinical experiences, lessons learned, and achievements for some period of time (a day or a week) or perhaps related to a particular situation. Reflection provides the nurse with an opportunity to review experiences for the purpose of enhancing performance. The journal is also useful in preparing and participating in the formal performance appraisal.

Credentialing and Specialty Certification

According to Finkelman (2006), credentialing is a review process used by health care organizations to ensure that a health professional is appropriately trained to provide care to patients. Credentialing includes evaluation and verification of education, license, certification, and, for advanced practice providers, evidence of malpractice insurance and review of claims history.

Briggs, Brown, Kesten, and Heath (2006), cite the most common reason for supporting certification is to protect the public. In addition, certification is thought to improve the quality of patient care. The authors state that the data supporting the impact of certification on quality is limited, but reports are encouraging. In one study, the performance by certified nurses was rated higher by supervisors than the performance of noncertified nurses. Not only does certification enhance the quality of care and protect the public, but certification enhances the nurse's self-confidence and self-esteem as well. Briggs et al. (2006 p. 53) state, "Clearly certification is a win-win proposition. Nurses gain self-esteem, job satisfaction, respect, and possible financial rewards, as well as knowledge."

Both NCCHC and the ACA offer specialty certification in correctional nursing. The development of specialty certification for correctional nursing is described by Muse (2009) as a milestone. She believes that certification helps to legitimize the specialty of correctional nursing and validates that these professionals possess a unique body of knowledge and skills. It inspires other correctional nurses to seek certification and stimulates interest in correctional nursing research. Correctional nursing certification is another action that enhances and fosters professionalism in the specialty.

The NCCHC established a certification program in 1991, the Certified Correctional Health Professional (CCHP). This certification is available to all health care professionals and demonstrates knowledge of the standards established by NCCHC. Specialty certification for correctional nurses was initiated in 2009 and is the first discipline-specific certification to be offered by the NCCHC (Continuing Certification n.d.).

Nurses wishing to seek certification (CCHP-RN) are required to be licensed as a registered nurse, possess certification as a Correctional Health Professionals (CCHP), have worked in correctional nursing for at least 2 years, and have completed in the last 3 years 54 hours of continuing education in nursing with 18 specific to correctional health care. The CCHP-RN exam measures knowledge in the clinical management of patients, promotion of a safe and secure environment for health care delivery, health promotion and maintenance, and professional roles and responsibilities in correctional nursing.

The ACA offers certification in the areas of nursing as well as adult corrections, juvenile justice, security threat groups, and correctional officer. Two types of nursing certification are offered; one for nurses in line staff positions and the other for nurse managers. A Certified Correctional Nurse (CCN) has passed a multiple choice exam, has 1 year of experience in the current position as a nurse in correctional health care, and is licensed as a nurse (RN, LPN, LVN). Certification is a demonstration of knowledge and professionalism in health care in a correctional environment, correctional law, nursing practice and standards of care, supervision, interacting with offenders, and developing/maintaining expertise in the corrections field. The Certified Nurse Manager (CCN/M) is limited to registered nurses who have at least 1 year of experience supervising correctional health care personnel. Additional areas of knowledge tested on the exam include managing human resources and conflict.

THE FUTURE OF CORRECTIONAL NURSING

Globally and nationally advancing the profession of nursing will include strategic initiatives that propel nursing to its next level. The Institute of Medicine (2011) report *The future of nursing: Leading change, advancing health* is a catalyst in advancing the profession of nursing. This report calls on nurses, educators, nurse leaders, and policy makers to take collective action to reform education and to strengthen nursing's role. The report contains four key messages;

- Nurses should practice to the fullest extent of their education and training.
- Nurses should achieve higher levels of education and training through an improved education system that promotes seamless academic progression.
- Nurses should be full partners with physicians and other health care professionals in redesigning health care in the United States.
- Effective workforce planning and policy making, requiring better data collection and improved information infrastructure.

Correctional nursing is poised for change, growth, and to have a voice in the future landscape of correctional health care. Nurses must take responsibility for defining and accounting for their practice in the correctional setting. First and foremost, correctional nurses must embrace their role as professional nurses and care givers. The correctional nurse's practice must be based on knowledge, evidence from the field, and experience in practice.

SUMMARY

Developing higher level thinking and competency of nurses to meet the health needs of the population and building knowledge in areas of litigation, advocacy, health literacy, and enhancing proficiencies triaging and managing clinical care is needed. Building nurses' skills in communication, collaboration, professional and ethical judgment, caring, negotiation, assessment, and problem solving are areas that need on-going focus. Addressing the stresses that come with practice in a rigid and controlling environment must receive attention. Assisting correctional nurses with skills in systems and organizational theory and continuing to build a focus consistent with the underpinnings of professional nursing practice is advocated.

DISCUSSION QUESTIONS

1. What are the characteristics of a professional practice environment for correctional nursing?
2. What strategies can be implemented to enhance professional practice in corrections?
3. How might the correctional nurse utilize the professional practice portfolio?
4. What are your thoughts on implementing peer review?

REFERENCES

Academy of Correctional Health Professionals. (2009). *Mission and goals*. Retrieved January 16, 2012, from Correctional Health: http://www.correctionalhealth.org/about/mission.html

American Correctional Health Services Association. (2011–2012). *Mission and ethics statement*. Retrieved January 16, 2012, from The American Correctional Health Services Association: http://www.achsa.org/index.html

American Correctional Association. (n.d.). *ACA Healthcare Professional Interest Section*. Retrieved January 16, 2012, from American Correctional Association: http://www.aca.org/hpis/

American Correctional Association. (2002). *Performance based standards for correctional health care in adult correctional institutions*. Alexandria, VA: Author.

American Nurses Association (ANA). (2007). *Corrections nursing: Scope & standards of practice*. Silver Spring, MD: Author.

American Nurses Association. (2010). *Nursing: Scope and standards of practice* (2nd ed.). Silver Spring, MD: Nurses Books.

Briggs, L., Brown, H., Kesten, K., & Heath, J. (2006). Certification: A benchmark for critical care nursing excellence. *Critical Care Nurse, 26,* 47–53.

Brodie, J. S. (2001). Caring: The essence of correctional nursing. *Tennessee Nurse, 64,* 10–12.

Cashin, A., Chiarella, M., Waters, D., & Potter, E. (2008). Assessing Nursing Competency in the Correctional Environment. The creation of a self-regulation learning and development tool. *Journal for Nurses in Staff Development, 24*(6), 267–273.

Dhoneda, R. (1995). An ethnographic study of nurses in a forensic psychiatric setting: Education and training implications. *Australia and New Zealand Journal of Mental Health Nursing, 4,* 77–82.

Dores, N. S. (1994). Correctional nursing practice. *Journal of Community Health Nursing, 11*(4), 201–210.

Ebright, P. R. (2010). The complex work of RNs: Implications for healthy work environments. *The Online Journal of Issues in Nursing, 15*(1), 11.

Eckroth-Buchner, M. (2010). Self-awareness: A review and analysis of a basic nursing concept. *Advances in Nursing Science, 33*(4), 297–309.

Finkelman, A. (2006). *Life long learning: Nursing professional development. Leadership and management in nursing* (396 pp.). Upper Saddle River, NJ: Pearson Hall.

Flanagan, N. (2002). An analysis of the relationship between job satisfaction and job stress in correctional nurses. *Research in Nursing and Health, 25*(4), 282–294.

Flanagan, N. (2006). Testing the relationship between job stress and satisfaction in correctional nurses. *Nursing Research, 55*(5), 316–327.

Fuller, S. G., Alexander, J. W., & Hardeman, S. M. (2006). Sheriff's deputies and nursing students-service learning partnership. *Nurse Educator, 31*(1), 31–35.

Gadow, S. (2003). Restorative nursing: Toward a philosophy of postmodern punishment. *Nursing Philosophy, 4,* 161–167.

Hagg-Heitman, B., & George, V. (2011). Nursing peer review: Principles and practice. *American Nurse Today, 6*(9), 1–4.

Hardesty, K., Champion, D., & Champion, J. (2007). Jail Nurses: Perceptions, stigmatization, and working styles in correctional health care. *Journal of Correctional Health Care, 13*(3), 196–205.

Holmes, D. (2005). Governing the captives: Psychiatric nursing in corrections. *Perspectives in Psychiatric Care, 41*(1), 3–13.

Institute of Medicine. (2001). *Crossing the quality chasm: A new health system for the 21st century.* Washington DC: National Academy Press.

Institute of Medicine. (2011). *The future of nursing: Leading change, advancing health.* Washington, DC: The National Academy Press.

Jones, C. B., & Gates, M. (2007). The costs and benefits of nurse turnover: A business case for nurse retention. *Online Journal of Issues in Nursing, 12*(3), 7.

Kinsella, C., & Friel, C. (1995). Job satisfaction in a medium security unit a comparative study of male and female secure unit nurses. *Psychiatric Care, 2*(1), 12–16.

LaMarre, M. (2006). *Nursing role and practice in correctional facilities. Clinical practice in correctional medicine* (2nd ed., pp. 417–424). Philadelphia, PA: Mosby Elsevier.

Maeve, M. K. (1997). Nursing practice with incarcerated women: Caring within mandated (sic) alienation. *Issues in Mental Health Nursing, 18*(2), 495–510.

Maeve, M. K., & Vaughn, M. S. (2001). Nursing with prisoners: The practice of caring? *Advances in Nursing Science, 24*(2), 47–64.

Milton, C. (2008). Accountability in nursing, reflecting on ethical codes and professional standards of nursing practice from a global perspective. *Nursing Science Quarterly, 21*(4), 300–303.

Moore, J. (1991). Exploration of factors affecting the nursing shortage in a correctional health care delivery system. *American Jails, 5*(4), 10–20.

Murtha, R. (1975). It started with a director of nursing. *The American Journal of Nursing, 75*(3), 421–422.

Muse, M. (2009).Correctional nursing: The evolution of a specialty. *Correct Care, 23*(1), 3–4.

Muse, M. (2011). Correctional nursing practice: Ethical and legal issues. *Correct Care, 25*(1), 16–17.

National Commission on Correctional Health Care (NCCHC). (2008a). *Standards for health services in prisons.* Chicago, IL: Author.

National Commission on Correctional Health Care (NCCHC). (2008b). *Standards for health services in jails.* Chicago, IL: Author.

National Commission on Correctional Health Care (NCCHC). (2011). *Standards for health services in juvenile detention and confinement facilities.* Chicago, IL: Author.

National Commission on Correctional Health Care. (n.d.). *About NCCHC.* Retrieved January 16, 2012, from National Commission on Correctional Health Care: http://www.ncchc.org/about/index.html

National Commission on Correctional Health Care. (n.d.). *Continuing certification.* Retrieved December 31, 2011, from National Commission on Correctional Health Care: http://www.ncchc.org/CCHP/continuingcert.html

National Council of State Boards of Nursing. (2005). *Meeting the ongoing challenge of continued competence.* Retrieved January 13, 2012, from www.ncsbn.org/pdfs/Continued_Comp_Paper_TestingServices.pdf

National League for Nursing. (n.d.). *Mission/Goals/Core values.* Retrieved January 12, 2012, from National League for Nursing: http://www.nln.org/aboutnln/corevalues.htm

Oermann, M. (2002). Developing a professional portfolio in nursing. *Orthopeadic Nursing, 21*(2), 73–78.

Peternelj-Taylor, C. (Dec. 2004). An exploration of othering in forensic psychiatric and correctional nursing. *Canadian Journal of Nursing Research, 36*(4), 130–146.

Peternelj-Taylor, C. (Winter 2005). Engaging the "other". *Journal of Forensic Nursing, 1*(4), 179, 191.

Rold, W. J. (2008). Thirty years after *Estelle v. Gamble*: A legal retrospective. *Journal of Correctional Health Care, 14*(1), 11–20.

Shields, K. E., & de Moya, D. (1997). Correctional health care nurses' attitudes toward inmates. *Journal of Correctional Health Care, 4*(1), 37–59.

Shelton, D. (2009). Forensic nursing in secure environments. *Journal of Forensic Nursing, 5*, 131–142.

Shelton, D., Weiskopf, C., & Nicholson, M. (2010). Correctional nursing competency development in the Connecticut Correctional Managed Health Care Program. *Journal of Correctional Health Care, 16*(4), 38–47.

Smith, S. (2005). Stepping through the looking glass: Professional autonomy in correctional nursing. *Corrections Today, 1*–5.

Storey, L. (2006). *Nursing in a secure environment: A British and Australian perspective.* Retrieved from http://www.forensicnursmag.com/articles/371corrections.html

Weiskopf, C. (2005). Nurses' experience of caring in inmate patients. *Journal of Advanced Nursing, 49*(4), 336–343.

Whelan, L. (2006). Competency assessment of nursing staff. *Orthopaedic Nursing, 25*(5), 3571–3606.

William, M., & Jordan, K. (2007). The nursing professional portfolio: A pathway to career development. *Journal of Nurses in Staff Development, 23*(3), 125–131.

Wilmont, Y. (1997). Prison nursing: The tension between custody and care. *British Journal of Nursing, 6*, 333–336.

Index